Home Care Manual

MAKING THE TRANSITION

Home Care Manual

MAKING THE TRANSITION

Sheryl Mara Zang, RN, MS
Instructor
College of Nursing
Health Science Center
State University of New York
Brooklyn, NY

Nellie C. Bailey, RN, MS, MA, CS
Assistant Professor and
Associate Dean for Academic Programming
College of Nursing
Health Science Center
State University of New York
Brooklyn, NY

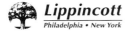

Lippincott
Philadelphia • New York

Acquisitions Editor: Susan Glover, RN, MSN
Project Editor: Gretchen Metzger
Production Manager: Helen Ewan
Production Coordinator: Patricia McCloskey
Design Coordinator: Doug Smock
Indexer: Michael Ferreira

9   8   7   6   5   4   3   2   1

Library of Congress Cataloging in Publication Data
Home care manual : making the transition / [edited by] Sheryl Mara
   Zang, Nellie C. Bailey.
      p.   cm.
      Includes bibliographical references and index.
      ISBN 0–397–55401–X (pbk. : alk. paper)
      1. Home care services—Handbooks, manuals, etc.   I. Zang, Sheryl
   Mara.   II. Bailey, Nellie C.
      [DNLM: 1. Home Care Services.   WY 115 H7638 1997]
   RT120.H65H656 1997
   362.1′4—dc20
   DNLM/DLC
   for Library of Congress   96–26199
                                                                CIP

Care has been taken to confirm the accuracy of the information presented and to describe generally accepted practices. However, the authors, editors, and publisher are not responsible for errors or omissions or for any consequences from application of the information in this book and make no warranty, express or implied, with respect to the contents of the publication.

The authors, editors and publisher have exerted every effort to ensure that drug selection and dosage set forth in this text are in accordance with current recommendations and practice at the time of publication. However, in view of ongoing research, changes in government regulations, and the constant flow of information relating to drug therapy and drug reactions, the reader is urged to check the package insert for each drug for any change in indications and dosage and for added warnings and precautions. This is particularly important when the recommended agent is a new or infrequently employed drug.

Some drugs and medical devices presented in this publication have Food and Drug Administration (FDA) clearance for limited use in restricted research settings. It is the responsibility of the health care provider to ascertain the FDA status of each drug or device planned for use in their clinical practice.

This book is dedicated to my father Philip Cohen, the inspiration in my life. To my wonderful husband Steven, to Ivy and Andrew, thank you for being with me every step of the way.

—Sheryl

I dedicate this book to all my clients. They gave me the opportunity, as a home health nurse, to provide care and gain knowledge and experience simultaneously. Thank you so much.

—Nellie

Contributors

Terese Acampora, BSN, MA
Director of Patient Services
Metropolitan Jewish Geriatric Center
Brooklyn, NY

Sandra Ceslowitz, RN, EdD
Associate Professor
SUNY Health Science Center at Brooklyn
Brooklyn, NY

Phyllis Cohen, MSW
Manager of Social Services
Visiting Nurse Association of Brooklyn
Brooklyn, NY

Maritza Cunningham, RN, BSN
Wound Ostomy Continence Clinical Nurse Specialist
Visiting Nurse Service of New York
Brooklyn, NY

Eileen M. Hanley, RN, BSN, MBA
Administrator, Hospice Care
Visiting Nurse Service of New York
New York, NY

Diane S. Harper, RN, MSN, CANP
Instructor
Molloy College
Rockville Center, NY

Lawrence Jacobsberg, MD, PhD
Psychiatrist, AIDS Program
Visiting Nurse Service of New York
New York, NY

Anne Dolores Kelly, RN, MSN
Patient Service Manager
Visiting Nurse Service of New York
Brooklyn, NY

Silvia M. Koerner, RN, MSN
Director of Quality Management Services
Visiting Nurse Service of New York
New York, NY

Emma Kontzamanis, RN, BSN, MA
Director of Professional Services
Metropolitan Jewish Geriatric Center
Home Care Division
Brooklyn, NY

Leila Laitman, MD
Psychiatrist, Geriatric Program
Visiting Nurse Service of New York
New York, NY

Patricia Lang, RN
Account Manager
Byram Healthcare Centers
Greenwich, CT

David Lindy, MD
Chief Psychiatrist
Visiting Nurse Service of New York
New York, NY

Rose Madden-Bear, BSN, MSN
Administrator for Quality Management, Corporate
Metropolitan Jewish Health Systems
Brooklyn, NY

Kathleen P. Murtagh, RN, MSN
Assistant Administrator
Metropolitan Jewish Geriatric Center
Home Care Division

Patrice Kenneally Nicholas, RN, DNSc, ANP
Associate Professor
Chairperson, Advanced Practice
Massachusetts General Hospital Institute of Health Professions
Boston, MA

Phyllis B. Parness, RN, MSN
Vice President for Clinical Services
Revival Home Health Care, Inc.
Brooklyn, NY

Arlene Pericak, RN, FNP-C, MSN
Instructor
Nursing FNP Program
The Sage College
Troy, NY

Neil Pessin, PhD
Clinical Director
Community Mental Health Services
Visiting Nurse Service of New York
New York, NY

Rosalie Rothenberg, RN, EdD
Acting Dean
SUNY Health Science Center at Brooklyn
College of Nursing
Brooklyn, NY

Joan Schmidt, RN, MS/MPH
Clinical Instructor
AIDS Services
Visiting Nurse Service of New York
New York, NY

Laila N. Sedhom, PhD
Professor/Acting Associate Dean for Graduate Nursing
SUNY Health Science Center at Brooklyn
College of Nursing
Brooklyn, NY

Karen Sherman, RN C, MPA
Director, Quality Assurance
Visiting Nurse Association of Brooklyn
Brooklyn, NY

Sally A. Sobolewski, RN, MSN
Assistant Director of Education
Visiting Nurse Service of New York
New York, NY

Gale O. Surrency, RN C, MA
Director of Patient Services
Visiting Nurse Association of Brooklyn
Brooklyn, NY

Marilyn Tillim, RN, BSN
Geriatric Care Consultant
Visiting Nurse Service of New York
Brooklyn, NY

Meryl Weinberg, RN, MA
Chief Operating Officer
Revival Home Health Care, Inc.
Brooklyn, NY

Preface

This manual is based on a very successful course, "Transition Into Home Care," that was created at the Health Science Center at Brooklyn, College of Nursing by the two authors. The authors saw the need for a course that would prepare nurses for the transition into the field of home care. The need was great, as restructuring and downsizing of hospitals and other places of employment gives nurses a new chance to look at home care as an exciting nursing challenge. There was also a great need for nurses already practicing because they have many concerns and issues that emerge as they are exposed to new experiences providing care to clients in the home.

There was one question that always emerged when we taught the course: "Why don't you put all this valuable hands-on experience into a book?" We recognized that there was a strong need for a book that would provide in-depth comprehensive information on all aspects of home care.

We have taken the entire course, divided it into chapters, and had some of the best and brightest specialists in the field write the chapters. Their chapters portray the highest professional standards in home care nursing. The contents of the manual include all aspects of home care, from the initiation of the referral, to what the nurse needs to be familiar with before the visits are made, to the actual visits and all the steps involved in discharging the client. Steps for physical assessment of the home care client and the latest skin and wound care information are included.

With this manual, the nurse will become familiar with all aspects of the Health Care Financing Administration (HCFA) 485, the initial admission, the revisit, and the sixty day/discharge summary forms. Requirements for each aspect of documentation will be discussed in terms of quality assurance, professional accountability, and reimbursement procedures.

Different home care specialties are introduced in this book as well as the clinical challenges that we face. Each chapter in the manual can stand alone as a resource, but the authors envision that the manual be read from chapter one through chapter twenty-four as it tells the story of home care.

This manual will help with documentation, goal planning, teaching and learning, and formulating care plans for paraprofessionals. We hope this book becomes a vital part of your nursing bag. Remember, you are no longer alone in the field, we are all along to help you.

Acknowledgements

The opportunity to bring so many specialists together in one home care book has been an invaluable experience for everyone involved. The contributing authors are the reason why the standards in home care remain high. We thank each and every author and we certainly learned from each contribution written.

We want to thank Dr. Rosalie Rothenberg, Acting Dean of the College of Nursing, Health Science Center at Brooklyn, for her valuable guidance, encouragement, and her willingness to share her knowledge and resources. We thank all our home care clients who have opened up their homes and hearts to us and who have enriched our lives with their experiences. We thank all the home care nurses out in the field for sharing and caring.

A special thanks and appreciation to the Visiting Nurse Association of Brooklyn and Metropolitan Jewish Geriatric Center Home Health Care Systems. Many thanks to Professor Yvonne Gray for always being encouraging and supportive. Special thanks to Elizabeth Snell, who was always ready to teach the inside of home care.

Acknowledgments

Contents

Home Care Manual

MAKING THE TRANSITION

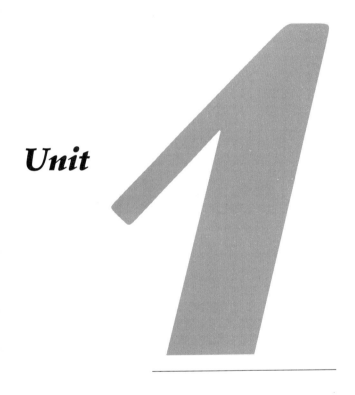

Unit

PREPARING FOR HOME CARE

1

Types of Referrals and Purpose of Home Care

Terese Acampora, BSN, MA

The Role of the Home Care
   Planner
The In-Hospital
   Assessment

The Community Referral
Pre–Hospital Discharge
Home Health Care Providers

The length of in-hospital stays has decreased dramatically in this era of escalating health care costs, extensive budget cuts, managed care, rapid advances in technology, and advances in modes of service delivery. As either a direct cause or a direct effect of these variables, the home health care industry became the vehicle by which costs were to be kept down and length of stay decreased. As a result, the home care industry itself has expanded so that it has become a complex maze that must be negotiated with great care if one is to effect the best outcome for each individual.

    This chapter focuses on the types of referrals that can be made when seeking to help a client make the transition from hospital to home. It focuses on the role of the home care planner, the process of the in-hospital assessment, the community referral, and continuity of care issues. The structures of the certified home health agency, long-term home health care program, and licensed agency also are discussed.

THE ROLE OF THE HOME CARE PLANNER

In response to escalating health care costs and as a result of the need to develop a more effective health system, hospitals are discharging clients sooner than they may be ready. These pressures dramatically emphasize the pivotal role the home care planner plays in coordinating the care that the client will receive on discharge to the home. The home care planner is the case finder in the hospital and is the liaison between the hospital and the home care agency.

The home care planner must have the ability to anticipate and resolve complex client care needs. This nurse not only must be highly trained in the area of clinical nursing practice, but also must be well versed in the economics of health care, the regulations that guide practice, and the community resources and technology available.

The home care planner's responsibility is to ensure that all of the client's needs can be met safely and cost-effectively at home. This role may involve collaboration with other health professionals at discharge planning meetings to ensure a successful transition to the home. The home care planning nurse provides information about community resources that will aid the physician and client in making the appropriate discharge plan. The nurse also must use clinical skills to assess the client's physical impairments, psychological status, ability to perform simple activities of daily living (ADL), and the skilled care procedures.

Often, the home care planner's job description includes the presentation of educational seminars to health professionals in the hospital. This is done to increase the health care professionals' knowledge of home health care programs, regulations, and new services available. The successful home care planner has the ability to combine all of these skills to ensure that clients receive the highest quality of care in the most effective, appropriate setting.

THE IN-HOSPITAL ASSESSMENT

The in-hospital assessment is an important step in moving the client along the continuum from hospital to home and ultimately to an optimal level of independence. The success of the planning process depends on coordination between hospital and home health providers. It is necessary to exchange as much information as possible during the assessment phase to avoid delays in discharge and to ensure continuity of care.

Once a client is referred to the home care agency, the home care planner must assess the client's medical, social, nursing, and rehabilitative needs to determine if the client is eligible for services. Eligibility criteria are defined by both the type of program and the insurance coverage. If the client is found to be eligible for the program referred, the home care planner should begin the assessment and should incorporate the following to achieve continuity of care and positive patient outcomes:

- *Review of the Hospital Record:* A review of the hospital record allows the nurse to identify the primary and secondary diagnoses, the client's medical history, pertinent laboratory values, medication regimen, education initiated, equipment needs, and treatment modalities. By reviewing the medical record, the nurse can assess the needs of the client and begin to develop the plan of care.

- *Patient/Family Interview:* This is the time to discuss the social and environmental aspects of the client's care at home. During the interview, the nurse is able to evaluate the adequacy of the client's support systems, the family dynamics, their understanding of the illness, and their ability to learn and perform any required care or treatment. The nurse must identify any potential problems that could develop at home that may put the client at risk. The home care planner should also address the physical nature of the home. This means that the nurse must determine how the client accesses the home; for example, are there stairs to the bedroom or bath? Is there adequate ventilation, heat, and food? The planner also assesses the need for assistive devices and durable medical equipment, such as hospital bed, wheelchair, commode, or cane.

The nurse must determine that the client will be safe at home and is willing to comply with the plan of care.

At this meeting, the home care planner must evaluate the plan of care in light of the client's financial resources. The discussion must address the type of insurance coverage and supplemental policies. In a number of cases, the insurance coverage may not be sufficient to meet all of the client's needs. Community resources or a referral to a social worker may be indicated. Perhaps the client may meet charity guidelines for free care. This is decided on an individual client basis according to agency policy. In some instances, the client may be able to pay for part of the care if it is above the coverage limits. The home care planner must obtain the client's or significant other's agreement for admittance to the program. In addition, federal law mandates that the client be informed of the right to self-determination. This is discussed in detail in Chapter 5.

Patient self-determination information should be provided at the time of first contact with the client. However, some home care agencies provide this to the client in the home in conjunction with the initial visit. All pertinent release forms, Bill of Rights, and payment materials should be signed at this time.

An important part of the interview centers around the discussion of the purpose of the program. The client must be allowed to verbalize expectations about his or her transition home and goals while on the program. The planner also must discuss the nature of the program and the need for client participation in the plan of care, and the client must agree that the program can effectively meet his or her needs.

- *Physical Assessment:* A physical assessment is a key step in the assessment process. This physical assessment establishes the baseline data that, in conjunction with the review of the hospital record and client interview, maintain continuity of care. If feasible, the nurse should observe the client or significant other demonstrate skills that will be required at home. The physical examination should be a thorough head-to-toe assessment incorporating each body system. This will focus the home care goals and make it individualized based on the specific care needs.

- *Case Conference:* After the home care planner completes the assessment, it is necessary to reconvene with the physician, discharge planner, or social worker to develop the plan of care. Continuity of care is dependent on communication between all of the parties. This is the time to identify specific goals for the client's care at home and obtain the signed physician orders (the Health Care Financing Administration [HCFA] 485) for treatment. The discharge date is agreed on, and follow-up medical appointments and transportation are arranged. Once the assessment is complete, all of the data is relayed to the home care agency. Because of the home care planner's extensive assessment, the services that will be provided should meet the client's needs and make the home care management effective. Obviously, this is the ideal situation and may not always be the case.

Sometimes the client is discharged before being seen by the home care planner, and the process may not be completed as described. Changes in the plan of care may occur once the client is home.

If the hospitalized client has not been evaluated by a home care planner, there may be certain situations when a client needs to be assessed before the agency accepts the referral. This may be indicated if the client requires many home health aide (HHA) hours or if the client's condition is medically very complex. This process is called the in-hospital assessment.

The in-hospital assessment and supporting documentation are key steps in determining whether a client is eligible to receive the services in home. The information gathered can assist in identifying potential problem areas of need that must be addressed in the development of the plan of care.

Each client's needs and the support systems that are in place vary. The level of care that is required and that the agency can provide must be looked at on a case-by-case basis. Often, the information gathered can support the need for higher HHA hours, indicate the need for therapy, identify areas that require client teaching, and focus discussion with the client, family, physician, and discharge planner.

Most home health care agencies use very specific tools to obtain data that aid in the development of the plan of care. The information obtained focuses on physical impairments, mental status, mobility, skilled nursing needs, ADL, and support systems.

The assessment of the client's physical status requires a *yes* or *no* response to questions regarding impairments of sight, hearing, speech, cardiac and respiratory function, bladder and bowel control, upper or lower extremity impairment, and ambulation difficulties. Alterations in mental status are evaluated by a *yes* or *no* response to questions about the client's alertness, judgment, ability to learn, ability to direct a worker, ability to manage affairs, impaired recent memory, problems with agitation, depression, anxiety, or episodes of wandering if left unsupervised.

If evidence exists that the client is verbally abusive or physically assaultive, has expressed suicidal ideations, or is a danger to themselves or others, a very in-depth description of the behavior must be provided, including the source of the information. A psychiatric evaluation may be needed before hospital discharge.

The assessment of mobility evaluates the client's ability to ambulate inside and outside the home, get up from a seated position, get up from the bed, transfer to the commode, or transfer to a wheelchair. Each of these behaviors is then evaluated to determine if the client can perform them independently, with the assistance of a mechanical aide, with the assistance of one person, or if the activity cannot be performed.

The evaluation for skilled nursing focuses on the following needs: decubitus care, sterile dressings, range of motion, therapeutic exercise, enemas, ostomy care, oxygen administration, inhalation therapy, catheter insertion or irrigation, intravenous therapy, injections, tube feedings, suctioning, or monitoring of vital signs. If the need for any of these is indicated, the specific frequency and who will provide or learn the treatment should be indicated.

The client's ability to perform ADL should be evaluated in the tool so that the client's needs on discharge can be clearly identified. Tasks that routinely require completion include: making or changing beds, dusting and vacuuming, light cleaning, dishwashing, shopping, laundry, meal preparation and feeding, bathing (specifically bed bath, chair bath, shower, or tub bath), grooming, and toileting.

The mode of toileting should be indicated; for instance, the client may use a toilet, commode, or bedpan. The client also may have an ostomy or Foley catheter.

Each of these items is categorized according to the level of assistance required for the client to complete the task. The client may not need assistance with a task such as feeding; however, the same client may require partial or total assistance in another area. In that case, the assessor should indicate who provides the assistance. The need for assistance with personal care and ADLs often makes the client eligible for HHA assistance.

Pertinent information about the client's support system should be solicited and documented on the tool. In the ideal situation, each client has adequate support and a backup system in place when necessary. However, this is not always the case. A careful evaluation must be completed to ensure that assistance can be accessed or can be arranged before hospital discharge. If available, the information about the significant other's relationship with the client and his or her telephone number should be obtained.

The nurse should also complete a section on the client's medication regimen and evaluate the client's ability to self medicate. The nurse should identify whether the client is independent, requires reminding to take the medication, or cannot self medicate. The nurse also should evaluate if the client can be taught to administer the medication. For instance, if the client is now on insulin daily, the planner must assess whether the client has the necessary manual dexterity and visual acuity and is willing to learn the care. If the client's ability is questionable, support systems or other backup must be arranged to ensure that the client receives the medication.

THE COMMUNITY REFERRAL

Many of the clients referred for a home care program are referred directly from a variety of sources within the community. The referrals may come directly from the physician (after an office visit), from the client or caregiver, or from agencies such as nursing homes, senior or community centers, local social services offices, and churches or synagogues.

The process of obtaining the referral is similar to that of the in-hospital referral in that the data gathered is geared toward identifying all of the client's care needs. Appropriate and necessary services can be rendered and positive client outcomes achieved if the needs are all addressed.

The referral process is completed by telephone and includes the following:

1. Pertinent demographic and insurance information is obtained from the source of the referral.
2. The diagnosis and the client's medical history are obtained through discussion with the physician. The physician must provide verbal orders for medication, diet, activities, and treatment.
3. The physician and nurse discuss the goals of the program and outcomes to be achieved. The physician must agree that the needs of the client can be met safely at home. The written confirmation of physician's verbal orders is sent out by mail.
4. Contact with the client and family is initiated to describe the home care program and the services to be rendered and to obtain a verbal agreement for services. Financial information and coverage also should be verified.

5. Clients are admitted to the program after a home assessment visit. At this time, the client admission agreement is signed, Patient Self-Determination Act (PSDA) information is provided, and the Patient's Bill of Rights is reviewed.

Whether the referral is from the hospital or made while the client is in the community, the decision to admit the client to the home care program is made on a case-by-case basis in collaboration with the nurse, physician, discharge planner, and other members of the health team. In any situation in which a case is deemed inappropriate for home health care, the client must be assisted with arrangements for services by an alternate provider. For instance, a client who resides in a home without running water, heat, or lighting may need to be sent to the hospital or may need emergency housing.

PRE–HOSPITAL DISCHARGE

The Home Evaluation

In some instances, the agency may require that, on discharge from the hospital, an in-home evaluation be completed before accepting the client into the home care program. For instance, a mother who has had no prenatal care whose child has periods of apnea may not be sent into the home environment until a home assessment can be done.

Often, agencies use a standardized form to obtain the necessary information about the home environment. The assessment tool provides information about the type of structure in which the client resides. The nurse completing the form must indicate if this is a private home or a multiple-unit dwelling. Information should be elicited about how the residence is accessed. For instance, are there buzzers? Is a key necessary? Is there an open entry? Does the client have to climb stairs, or is this an elevator building? If stairs must be negotiated, the number of stairs should be documented.

This is important information if the client is an amputee or has cardiac disease. The assessor should note the area surrounding the building or residence. Questions such as: Is the area well lit? Is it easily accessible? Are there unsavory individuals loitering around the location? If the safety of personnel is in question, escort services may need to be arranged.

Once inside the home, the internal environment should be assessed. The number of rooms in the home should be noted. The sleeping arrangements need to be evaluated. If the client needs a 24-hour live-in aide, sleeping space must be available for the aide. The nurse also must make certain that the client has electricity, running water, adequate heat and ventilation, a working stove and refrigerator, food in the home, and adequate plumbing. The home also is evaluated for adequate cooking utensils, linens, and furnishings. A working telephone is a plus, but frequently, clients do not have a phone. In that case, the nurse must determine how the client will be contacted and how the client can contact someone in an emergency.

The pets in the home should be documented. Environmental conditions such as clutter, bug or rodent infestation, or peeling paint must be documented. Faulty electricity or flooring or crumbling walls are also environmental hazards that may delay the client's discharge home. Clients who are ventilator dependent should not be discharged home until an in-home assessment is completed. The evaluation must demonstrate that the electrical output required can be supported by the wiring in the home. Floors also need to be able to support the weight of the machinery.

Once the home assessment is complete, the agency can use the information to determine if the environment is a healthful and safe one in which to provide care for the client. Family or support systems may need to be called in to clean up, fix up, or provide adequate living conditions for the client. The client, physician, and home care staff can use the information gathered on the tool to assist in the development of the plan of care.

The Patient Review Instrument Referral

Some clients may require nursing home placement. To be considered for a nursing home, clients must be evaluated, using a two-part standardized tool, the Patient Review Instrument (PRI) and Screen. The PRI assesses the client's medical conditions and the capability to perform the basic ADLs, such as eating, transferring, toileting, and mobility.

The client's behavioral patterns also are assessed. The nurse determines if the client displays verbal disruptions, physical aggression, has hallucinations, or displays infantile or socially inappropriate behaviors. The level of severity of each of the ADL capabilities and behavioral patterns is determined based on specifically defined criteria in the tool.

The second part of the assessment, the "Screen," serves two purposes. The first is to assess the client for potential mental illness, mental retardation, or de-

velopmental disabilities. The second purpose is to
evaluate the client's potential to be cared for in a community setting. The nurse evaluates whether the
client has an appropriate home in the community,
whether an appropriate community living space can
be arranged, or whether the client is eligible for care
in an adult care facility. Based on the information, a
determination is made regarding the client's eligibility
for nursing home placement. The completed forms
are submitted to nursing homes selected by the client
or family. The PRI and Screen is valid for 90 days.
Clients are reevaluated at any time in the 90-day period if their status changes.

HOME HEALTH CARE PROVIDERS

Several provider options are available when a client is
referred for home care. The goal of each of these programs is the retention of individuals in their own
homes. No one method of care is the best. The
method must be based on community resources, the
ability to develop resources through linkages and networking, and the needs of the client.

There are three major vehicles by which home
health care services are rendered: The certified home
health agency (CHHA), the long-term home health
care program (LTHHCP), and the licensed agency.

The Certified Home Health Agency

The CHHA's premise is to provide acutely ill individuals with the opportunity to receive necessary skilled
care within their own residences. The CHHA meets
the needs of individuals by providing a myriad of ser-

vices, including skilled nursing services, physical, occupational and speech therapies, medical social services, HHAs, nutritional counseling, transportation, equipment, and respiratory therapy.

In addition, the CHHA may have specialty programs such as mental health services, pediatric services, maternal and child programs, and acquired immune deficiency syndrome (AIDS) programs; high-tech services such as intravenous therapy, home chemotherapy, and pain management also may be available. The CHHA is also known as the short-term program, because services are usually of brief duration.

Eligibility for the CHHA program is evaluated individually regardless of the source of payment. Admission criteria include:

In most instances, the client is confined to the home.

The services required are "skilled" in nature. That is, they are inherently complex and require the skills of a nurse or therapist.

The services are provided under a physician's care, who specifies what is to be provided and how often services are to be rendered.

The client requires reasonable and necessary care on an intermittent basis. The client also receives daily visits if indicated.

The physician reviews and approves the plan of care every 60 days and when changes occur. Clients must have medical follow-up at least once every 60 days.

The client living alone can self-direct the care and is able to summon help in an emergency.

The client's home environment is safe and supportive. There should be adequate food, clothing, and shelter.

There is an available, willing, and capable person to participate in the plan of care as necessary.

The safety of agency personnel can be maintained while providing services.

There is a realistic assumption that there will be ongoing improvement in the client's condition toward achieving goals.

The Long-Term Home Health Care Program

The LTHHCP, or "nursing home without walls," was established to meet the needs of chronically ill individuals at home. The LTHHCP is a program that provides health and social services to Medicaid recipients who are certifiably in need of nursing home care, but who wish to receive long-term care services in their homes. The client's need for services must not exceed 75% of the average cost of long-term institutional care within the local region. This ensures that the program is cost-effective.

The LTHHCP provides skilled nursing at a minimum of every 2 weeks, physical, occupational, and speech therapies, medical social services, nutritional support, and personal care services. If eligible, the client may receive nontraditional or *waiver* services, including social day care, personal emergency response system, transportation, housing improvements, and respite care.

Clients are eligible for the LTHHCP if they meet the following criteria:

The client can be served in his or her own home.
The home environment is safe and supportive.

The client has a significant other who is willing to co-operate with and participate in the plan of care.

The client living alone can self-direct his or her care and summon help in an emergency.

The client is chronically ill and needs continuing medical supervision to remain at home.

The client has a physician who will review and sign the plan of care and who will assess the client once every 60 days.

The client's health condition is such that health care services are required on an intermittent basis.

Clients are reassessed every 120 days by the agency to determine if they still meet all of the eligibility criteria for the LTHHCP.

Clients who are on the CHHA program may be eligible for services through the LTHHCP. Once identified as a potential long-term candidate, a referral packet complete with all of the pertinent information related to the medical and social status and need for service is submitted. In addition, contact is made with the significant other to determine if he or she is willing to participate in the plan of care. The client is screened by a nurse from the LTHHCP and a representative of the local social services district. If deemed appropriate for the program, the physician is contacted, and the plan of care is developed. Once the orders are signed and returned, the client then is discharged from CHHA and admitted to the LTHHCP.

Regardless of which of these programs provides care, ongoing services are dependent on the significance of the client's health problems and the appropriateness of the service needs. Each client must be evaluated on an ongoing basis to determine if he or she remains in need of skilled care. Routine contact and coordination between the client, physician, and members of the home care team is necessary to evaluate the effectiveness in the plan of care. This coordination also allows for modification in the plans and goals and aids in determining if goals have been met or if the client condition has reached a plateau.

The Licensed Agency

The licensed home care agency offers a variety of services, many of which mirror those of the CHHA. Criteria for admission, the provision of skilled services, and the referral processes are essentially the same. However, there are distinct differences as well. The licensed agency is not a Medicare-certified agency.

If clients who have Medicare or insurance that requires that services be rendered through a CHHA choose to use these agencies, the clients need to understand that they will not be reimbursed for the services. In addition, the client is not held to the "homebound" requirements.

The licensed agency may have a professional services component that will provide the skilled services of the CHHA. The agency also may duplicate many of the CHHA's specialty programs. The largest portion of the care rendered comes from personal care services. The licensed agency provides paraprofessional services, including housekeeping, homemaker, personal care worker (PCW), and HHA level of care. These agencies may also be authorized as training sites to certify individuals as PCWs and HHAs.

The services of the licensed agency either can be provided directly to the client through private insurance or private pay arrangements, or they may be subcontracted through the CHHA or LTHHCP. For instance, many CHHAs do not have HHAs on staff and contract for their services through the licensed agency. In this arrangement, the provider agency and licensed agency work very closely to ensure that the client's personal care needs are met. Close supervision of the HHA in the home is an integral part of the program.

2

Entry Into the Home Care System and the 485

Phyllis B. Parness, RN, MSN,
and Meryl Weinberg, RN, MA

Criteria for Admission to
   Home Care
Working with the HCFA 485

CRITERIA FOR ADMISSION TO HOME CARE

It is imperative that home health agencies admit only those clients whose health needs can be safely met at home. The determination should be made by a qualified professional nurse after an assessment, which includes consideration of the health needs of the client, adequacy of the home environment, participation of informal supports, and availability of agency staff and services.

Several qualifying criteria determine whether the client is appropriate for home care services in a certified home health agency. Admission criteria are unique to the individual agencies, and each agency's policy manual defines agency-specific criteria. The following criteria are commonly employed:

Homebound

The client requiring the services must be home-bound. That is, he or she must essentially be confined to his or her place of residence. Any absences from the home should be of short duration, infrequent, and related to medical needs. When describing home-bound status, it is useful to include objective facts that demonstrate homebound status, for example, "the client is confined to bed" or "the client is severely short of breath, which restricts his/her mobility."

Need for Skilled Service

The nurse must determine whether the client needs the type of service that meets the qualifications. The client's need should be based on the diagnosis and on his or her condition. The client must have a need for at least one skilled service that is provided by the home care agency.

The skilled services usually available are skilled nursing care, physical therapy, occupational therapy, and speech therapy. In conjunction with the skilled services, the client also may receive home health aide services and, when necessary, social work services. Skilled professional services require training and expertise of the respective profession to be delivered safely and effectively. Examples of skilled nursing include:

- Observation and assessment
- Client teaching
- Medication administration
- New ostomy care
- Rehabilitation nursing
- Venipuncture
- Psychiatric evaluation and therapy

Skilled physical therapy can include:

- Assessment
- Therapeutic exercises
- Gait training
- Range of motion (ROM)
- Hot packs
- Paraffin baths
- Whirlpool baths for clients with complicated conditions

Skilled speech therapy (ST) includes:

- Assessment
- Speech and voice production
- Improvement of communicative activities of daily living (ADL)
- Aphasia assistance
- Treatment of dysphasia

Plan of Treatment

The client must be under the care of a physician who is willing to provide orders for treatment. The nurse and the physician, in collaboration with the client, develop a plan of care that is relevant to the client's primary diagnosis and prioritized health care needs. The plan of care includes all diagnoses, services, and equipment needed by the client. It also includes medications and treatments, activities permitted by the client, frequency of visits, safety measures to protect the client against injury, specific and measurable goals of care, rehabilitation potential, and discharge planning.

The client or family must be willing to participate in the plan of care. For example, if the client requires daily wound care and is unable to do this, a family member should be involved in the teaching. If the family member is unwilling or unable to provide care, the nurse must make daily visits until an alternate plan is developed or the wound is healed.

The main goal of home care is to provide the necessary skills and education to the client or family that will maximize independence in self-care. The client's response to the plan of care should be evaluated by the nurse and modified as needed during the client's course of care.

Reasonable and Necessary

The care the client requires must be of a sound nature and must be essential in promoting the health of the client. Clients are accepted for home care based on a rational expectation that the needs of the client can be met by the agency in the place where the client resides.

When the nurse makes the first visit to open the case, it is his or her responsibility to determine whether the client can be cared for safely and adequately by the home care staff in the home environment. Before the client's admission to home care, the home care planner works with the client and family to ensure that an emergency plan for care is in place during the time when the agency is not providing service.

The plan may be as simple as a call to 911 if the client is experiencing distress. At times the plan may require backup support from the family members who agree to be in the home when the agency staff are not with the client.

WORKING WITH THE HCFA 485

The HCFA 485 is a tool designed by the Health Care Financing Administration (HCFA) to be used as a generic plan of treatment (POT) for the client. The HCFA 487, Addendum to the Plan of Treatment, is used to provide additional information as necessary. The POT must be signed at least every 62 days by the physician. This is considered the certification period by Medicare. Once the determination is made that the client requires certain services, it then must be determined what the allowable level of service is. Each 485 should contain all of the Medicare-covered and noncovered services needed by the client. The HCFA 485 must be reviewed at least every 62 days. If the client needs more than 62 days of service, a new POT is required. This is known as the recertification period.

It is extremely important to fill out the 485 correctly. Proper delivery of service and reimbursement are dependent on the accurate completion of this document. The plan of treatment should always be individualized to meet the specific needs of the client while considering the unique circumstances of the client's surroundings.

The medical diagnosis of the client is not enough to determine the plan of treatment. The care provided and documentation are thoroughly reviewed by Medicare reviewers. If the nurse's documentation clearly reflects that the Medicare criteria are met, there will be no question of whether reimbursement is indicated.

Correct Completion of the 485

The HCFA 485 (Display 2-1) contains 27 numbered fields that must be completely filled in before submitting it to the physician for review and signature. Please note: The 485 may be used as the plan of treatment for other insurers if the agency absorbs the cost of reproducing. The HCFA 485 is the document that demonstrates evidence of collaboration between the nurse and physician regarding planning care. Guidelines for completing the 485 are outlined below:

Field #1: Client's Health Insurance Claim (HIC) Number

Enter the complete payor number, which may be found on the client's Medicare insurance card.

Field #2: Start of Care (SOC) Date

The start of care date is the date the initial visit was made to the client's home. Enter six digits for the date, for example, 010199. This date remains the same for all subsequent recertifications until the client is discharged from service.

Field #3: Certification Period

This date indicates the entire period that is covered by the physician's POT. Enter the six-digit date (month, day, year). If this is the initial certification period, the FROM date must match the SOC date. The TO date must not exceed a 2-month period and can be up to 62 days, depending on the months being certified. If there are subsequent recertifications, the TO date equals the prior FROM date (eg, initial certification period 030199 through 050199, recertification period 050199 through 070199). Please note: Initial certification period includes visits made from 030199 through 043099, not visits made on 050199; recertification includes visits made from 050199 through 063099, not visits made on 070199. 50199 and 070199 are the beginning of the new certification and recertification periods.

Field #4: Medical Record Number

This is an optional field that may be used by the agency to assign a unique client number to identify the client.

Field #5: Provider Number

The agency is assigned a six-digit number by Medicare. This number is entered in this field. If an error is made in this locator, the agency will not receive payment for the visits.

Field #6: Client's Name and Address

Enter the client's last name, first name, and middle initial as it appears on the client's health insurance card. The spelling must match the HCFA system for payment to be processed. This card is checked on the initial visit by the nurse who opens the case. Enter the client's address and telephone number accurately.

Department of Health and Human Services
Health Care Financing Administration

Form Approved
OMB No. 0938-0357

HOME HEALTH CERTIFICATION AND PLAN OF TREATMENT

1. Patient's HI Claim No.	2. Start Of Care Date	3. Certification Period		4. Medical Record No.	5. Provider No.
		From:	To:		

6. Patient's Name and Address

7. Provider's Name, Address and Telephone Number

8. Date of Birth:		9. Sex	M ☐	F ☐

10. Medications: Dose/Frequency/Route/(N)ew (C)hanged

11. ICD-9-CM	Principal Diagnosis	Date

12. ICD-9-CM	Surgical Procedure	Date

13. ICD-9-CM	Other Pertinent Diagnoses	Date

14. DME and Supplies

15. Safety Measure:

16. Nutritional Req.

17. Allergies:

18.A. Functional Limitations		18.B. Activities Permitted			
1 ☐ Amputation	5 ☐ Paralysis	1 ☐ Complete Bedrest	6 ☐ Partial Weight Bearing	A ☐ Wheelchair
2 ☐ Bowel/Bladder (Incontinence)	6 ☐ Endurance	2 ☐ Bedrest BRP	7 ☐ Independent at Home	B ☐ Walker
3 ☐ Contracture	7 ☐ Ambulation	3 ☐ Up As Tolerated	8 ☐ Crutches	C ☐ No Restrictions
4 ☐ Hearing	8 ☐ Speech	4 ☐ Transfer Bed/Chair	9 ☐ Cane	D ☐ Other(Specify)
	9 ☐ Legally Blind	5 ☐ Exercises Prescribed		
	A ☐ Dyspnea With Minimal Exertion			
	B ☐ Other (specify)			

Duration

19.

1 ☐ Oriented	3 ☐ Forgetful	5 ☐ Disoriented	7 ☐ Agitated
2 ☐ Comatose	4 ☐ Depressed	6 ☐ Lethargic	8 ☐ Other

Mental Status:

20. Prognosis   1 ☐ Poor   2 ☐ Guarded   3 ☐ Fair   4 ☐ Good   5 ☐ Excellent

21. Orders for Discipline and Treatments (Specify Amount/Frequency/Duration)

22. Goals/Rehabilitation Potential/Discharge Plans

23. Nurse's Signature and Date of Verbal SOC where Applicable:

25. Date HHA Received Signed POT

24. Physician's Name and Address

26. I certify/recertify that this patient is confined to his/her home and needs intermittent skilled nursing care, physical therapy and/or speech therapy or continues to need occupational therapy. The patient is under my care, and I have authorized the services on this plan of care and will periodically review the plan.

28. Anyone who misrepresents, falsifies, or conceals essential information required for payment of Federal funds may be subject to fine, imprisonment, or civil penalty under applicable Federal laws.

27. Attending Physician's Signature and Date Signed

PROVIDER

Form HCFA-485 (U-4) (02-94 Printer-Aligned)

90-0019HC (10/95)

DISPLAY 2-1. The HCFA 485.

Field #7: Provider's Name, Address, and Telephone Number

Enter the agency's name, address, and telephone number.

Field #8: Date of Birth

Enter the client's date of birth, using a six-digit number. Enter the complete year if the client was born before 1900 (eg, 09301898).

Field #9: Client's Sex

Check the applicable box.

Field #10: Medications: Dose/Frequency/Route

Enter all medications ordered by the physician, including dose, frequency, and route. The nurse also must indicate whether the medication is new within the past 30 days or changed within the past 60 days. This is done by entering an N (for *new*) or a C (for *changed*). All over-the-counter medications must be listed here. If the client has oxygen, it must be listed in this field. If there are no medications ordered, this is indicated by N/A. The HCFA 487 can be used if additional space is required for this (Display 2-2). Medications are to be evaluated in the client's home. Indicate so in this field.

Field #11: ICD-9-CM Code, Principal Diagnosis, and Onset/Exacerbation Date

HCFA requires that the client's primary diagnosis be indicated with the corresponding ICD-9-DM code. A special book is used to determine the appropriate code to be used. Using the source book, enter the code that identifies the principal diagnosis and enter the diagnosis. It is important to select the principal diagnosis based on the most acute condition of the client for which the client receives home care service. The diagnosis must be as specific as possible. A clear picture must be created of why a client requires skilled services. Certain treatments are diagnosis specific for reimbursement, such as calcitonin (osteoporosis) and vitamin B_{12} (pernicious anemia) injections. A procedure is never a primary diagnosis. It is important to remember that when certain conditions are treated in the hospital, they are no longer appropriate primary diagnoses. For example, a client who undergoes a cholecystectomy for cholecystitis would not have a primary diagnosis on the 485 of cholecystitis. The abdominal wound or other most prevalent need for home care would be an appropriate primary diagnosis.

Field #12: ICD-9-CM Code, Surgical Procedure, and Date

Enter all ICD-9-CM codes and procedures that are relevant to the client's primary condition. Procedures not relevant to the care being provided should not be entered.

Field #13: ICD-9-CM Codes, Other Pertinent Diagnoses, and Onset/ Exacerbation Date

Enter all secondary diagnoses in order of priority that are relevant to the care being provided. If the client needs recertification, all diagnoses should be evalu-

Department of Health and Human Services
Health Care Financing Administration

Form Approved
OMB No. 0938-0357

ADDENDUM TO: ☐ PLAN OF TREATMENT ☐ MEDICAL UPDATE

1. Patient's HI Claim No.	2. SOC Date	3. Certification Period		4. Medical Record No.	5. Provider No.
		From:	To:		

6. Patient's Name

7. Provider Name

8. Item
No.

9. Signature of Physician

10. Date

11. Optional Name/Signature of Nurse/Therapist

12. Date

Form HCFA-487 (CA) (4-87)

90-0021   (8/88)

DISPLAY 2-2. The HCFA 487.

ated to determine if they are still relevant to the client's needs.

Fields 11, 12, and 13 must have the date of onset or exacerbation. If the date is unknown, 000000 may be entered.

Field #14: Durable Medical Equipment (DME) and Supplies

Enter all supplies and equipment to be billed. If none are to be billed, enter *N/A*.

Field #15: Safety Measures

Enter all measures identified by the physician or agency that are necessary to keep the client safe. For example, clients with difficulty in mobility should keep walk areas clear of clutter and leave adequate room for maneuvering assistive devices. If none are necessary, enter *N/A*.

Field #16: Nutritional Requirements

Enter the prescribed diet, fluid requirements or restrictions, nutritional supplements, and enteral feedings.

Field #17: Allergies

Enter medication allergies and all other allergies reported by the client. If none, enter *NKA,* no known allergies.

Field #18A: Functional Limitations

Field 18A helps to support the client's homebound status. Be specific when describing the functional limitations of the client. Because being homebound is a requirement, the contents of this field are critical for a claim reviewer's determination regarding payment. Check all of the items that describe the current limitations of the client.

Field #18B: Activities Permitted

Check the activities as defined in the POT. If *Other* is checked, it must be specifically described.

Field #19: Mental Status

Check the boxes that most closely describe the client's current status. Mental status can contribute to the development of a case for homebound status.

Field #20: Prognosis

Check the box that most closely defines the prognosis of the client. The prognosis should relate to the type of plan created. It can support the need for teaching or treatment.

Field #21: Orders for Disciplines and Treatments

The frequency and duration of services must be documented in this section for each discipline ordered. The home health aide must have the duration of the visit delineated in hours. Interim orders can always be developed with the physician if the initial estimate does not ultimately meet the client's needs. The client's needs and the priorities of care usually determine the frequency. At times, the physician will order a specific frequency and duration. For example, the client has a sacral decubitus requiring daily nursing visits for 21 days. Most often, however, it will be up to the nurse making the initial visit, in collaboration with the physician, to determine the most suitable frequency and duration of visits needed by the client. The client who requires Foley catheter changes because of urinary retention will probably need a nursing visit once monthly for observation and assessment of urinary status, signs of urinary tract infection, and the actual Foley catheter change. It is important to identify the supplies needed for the catheter change, for example, a 16 French Foley catheter with a 5-cc balloon. The directions, frequency, and duration would then read, *Skilled Nursing (SN) needed to insert a #16 French Foley catheter 1mo2 (once a month for 2 months) and 3 PRN visits for problems with catheter function.* Another typical home care client would be a 55-year-old man post–myocardial infarction. Initially, this client should be visited more frequently, then visits should be tapered as his condition improves. For example, his visits could be three to five times a week for 2 weeks, then two to three times a week for 2 weeks. Teaching and discharge planning could be completed in the last 2 weeks with a weekly visit frequency, providing no complications arise.

When a new insulin-dependent diabetic comes home from a hospitalization, initial self-administration teaching has usually begun in the hospital. The nurse could plan to visit daily for 7 days to ensure that the client uses proper technique, rotates the injection site, draws insulin up correctly, and has adequate confidence to perform this task independently. The subsequent visit frequency will depend on other health problems and teaching that is required. The client's rate of learning will impact the frequency and duration as well.

When documenting the need for skilled care, the terms *assessment, observation, teaching, performing skilled procedures,* and *evaluation* are key elements. These terms should be used when completing this section of the 485. Avoid using nonspecific terms such as *monitor clinical status,* and words that do not denote a skilled need such as *reinforce* or *encourage.*

Field #22: Goals/Rehabilitation Potential/Discharge Plans

Enter a description of the achievable goals for the client, the client's ability to meet the goals, and estimate the time it will take to achieve the goals. Indicate what the plans are for the client after discharge. Goals must be client specific, realistic, and measurable. They also must be linked to the skilled services being provided. Examples of goals that are specific, realistic, and measurable follow:

- Client will be compliant with diet and medications within 2 weeks
- Client will prepare and self-inject insulin within 1 week
- Client will ambulate independently with a cane in 4 weeks.
- Client/caregiver will perform colostomy care in 3 days.

This field is often used to document the finite and predictable end date for daily care. Medicare does not pay for daily visits with no end date in sight. If a client requires wound care for a deep wound that cannot heal, Medicare is not the appropriate payor. However, Medicare will pay if the physician and nurse believe after 8 weeks of daily care the wound will heal sufficiently to taper visits to three times a week. The date 8 weeks after the SOC date should be identified in this locator.

Field #23: Nurse's Signature and Date of Verbal Start of Care

The signature and date in this field indicate that the nurse has spoken to the physician, has verified orders for the client, and has approval to make the visit.

Field #24: Physician's Name and Address

Enter the full name, address, and phone number of the physician who will sign the plan of treatment and certify visits or services. This physician should be the physician responsible for the client's care in the first certification period.

Field #25: Date Home Health Agency Received Signed POT

Enter the date that the agency receives the POT from the physician. If the physician has dated field #27, then the date may be omitted here. Typically, agencies date stamp all documents for the client's record when they are received.

Field #26: Physician Certification

Check whether this is the initial certification or recertification.

Field #27: Attending Physician's Signature and Date Signed

If more than one physician is involved in the client's care, the plan should be signed by the primary physician on the case.

The physician must sign the POT. Rubber signature stamps are not acceptable in place of the actual signature. If the physician does not date this field, then the agency must complete Field #25.

Completion of the 485 at the start of care is the health care team's best estimate of the client's current condition and anticipated course of care in the next 62 days. Experience is a significant factor in developing this skill. The new nurse can find assistance and supervisory input. It is always important to remember that each client's condition, ability to comprehend instructions, and task performance will vary. It is for this reason that each plan of treatment is a unique document that portrays a clear picture to any reviewer determining reimbursement.

3

Home Care Reimbursement: A Team Effort

Phyllis B. Parness, RN, MSN,
and Meryl Weinberg, RN, MA

Who Pays for Service and
    What Do Payors Cover?
Eligibility Criteria for
    Home Care

How Is the Appropriate
    Payor Selected?

Home care reimbursement in a certified home health care agency is a process that differs from other medical reimbursement. The nurse and billing staff must work in collaboration to obtain and process required information and documentation for payment of services to occur.

The home care nurse must be completely familiar with the conditions and regulations of each payor to make an appropriate determination regarding who will pay the bill. This is a unique role for the registered professional nurse. Few nursing positions require the nurse to be responsible for providing patient care while participating in the reimbursement process. In the home care setting, a clinician assesses, plans, implements, and evaluates care provided. The nurse must take the process one step further into the realm of reimbursement. The decisions made in the nursing process integrate this additional responsibility. The role of the professional nurse is expanded in scope and challenges traditional nursing practice.

The home care agency must set up systems that incorporate prospective, concurrent, and retrospective analysis of billing determinations to assist the nurse in decision making and ensure appropriate identification of payor source.

WHO PAYS FOR SERVICE AND WHAT DO PAYORS COVER?

What is a payor? A payor is an entity responsible for paying the bill. In the case of home care, the most frequently used payors are:

Medicare
Medicaid
Commercial insurers, including managed care companies
No-fault
Worker's compensation
Private pay
Free care dollars

Covered services are services delivered by the home care agency that the insurance plan agrees to pay either totally or partially. Coverage for each payor type is determined by the payor. It is understood that services provided outside the realm of covered services will not be reimbursed by that payor. It is the responsibility of the nurse to ensure that any services needed or requested are covered. When coverage is not available, clients must be informed in advance of their responsibility for payment.

Medicare

Medicare, also known as Title XVII of the Social Security Act, is a federally funded program for the elderly and disabled population. Medicare is a two-part program commonly known as Part A and Part B. Medicare Part A covers homecare for homebound clients, and Medicare Part B covers clients who may or may not be homebound. Medicare Part B is an optional program that can be purchased by the client.

The Medicare program for home care was developed to focus on short-term intermittent care. There are long-term clinical conditions that, under certain circumstances, may be reimbursable by Medicare (eg, insulin-dependent diabetes mellitus).

Because Medicare is a federally funded program, coverage criteria should be similar from state to state. The Health Insurance Manual #11 (HIM-11) is the source document used in the home care industry to answer questions about coverage and billing. This manual can be obtained for a fee from the United States Government Printing Office. It should be readily available for use at every home care agency.

There is a great deal of misinterpretation of Medicare guidelines through word-of-mouth education. It is important that the nurse provide the client with written documentation regarding Medicare criteria.

Medicare has traditionally been known as a conservative payor. It is for this reason that it has served as a guide that many other insurers use to determine coverage. Medicare covers skilled nursing, physical therapy (PT), occupational therapy (OT), speech therapy (ST), medical social service, home health aide (HHA), medical supplies, and durable medical equipment.

When determining if services are skilled nursing services, the following must be considered:

Complexity of the task
Condition of the patient
Acceptable standards of medical and nursing practice

Skilled nursing services are services that require the training and experience of a professional nurse to be safe and effective, for example, a client with an open draining wound, needing irrigation, packing, and dressing daily. The nurse would be needed to provide wound care until the wound is healed or a family member is taught to do the wound care. For a therapy service (PT, OT, ST) to be considered skilled, it must be complex enough that it can be performed safely or effectively by or under the supervision of a skilled therapist.

To be reimbursed for therapy, there must be an expectation that the client's condition will improve significantly in a reasonable period or the service is needed to establish a safe and effective home maintenance program. An example would be a client who had a total hip replacement and is ambulatory but cannot safely climb stairs. The physical therapist is needed to teach the client to safely climb and descend the stairs.

An HHA is a reimbursable service when the client exhibits a need for skilled services and is unable to meet his or her personal care needs without assistance. Personal care tasks can include, but are not limited to, bathing and skin care, transfer activities, assistance with exercise, range of motion, assistance with meals, medications, and catheter care.

A medical social worker will be paid for by Medicare when interventions have a significant impact on reducing obstacles to the successful implementation of the client's plan of care. Medicare considers social work services a dependent service. A client must qualify for Medicare based on a need for skilled nursing or therapy services.

If a skilled service is present, social work will be covered for the following types of interventions:

Psychosocial assessment
Financial/environmental assessment
Counseling
Community resources and long-range planning

Home medical equipment (HME), also known as durable medical equipment (DME), includes items that are purchased or rented for the care of an individual, for example, wheelchairs, hospital beds, and walkers.

Current Trends in Medicare

Medicare expenditures have grown considerably in the past several years ($1.6 billion in 1993 to $13 billion in 1994). As a result, the federal government is seeking ways to reduce Medicare costs. The National Association for Home Care (NAHC) is working with the Health Care Financing Administration (HCFA) to develop a prospective payment system of reimbursement for home health services. Cost containment is the objective. A total dollar cap would be established for each beneficiary for home care services, which home care agencies would use to provide service. This cap may severely limit the ability of the home care agency to be reimbursed for adequate and appropriate services to its clients. Several implementation plans have been proposed by members of Congress and by the President. These proposals differ considerably in scope. The hope of the providers of home care services is that the system of reimbursement selected maintains quality care and ensures easy access to services.

Medicaid

Medicaid, also know as Title XIX of the Social Security Act, is a joint federal–state program administered by local governments. It has been set up to provide the low-income sectors with health care services, including home care. It assists families with dependent children, the aged, blind, and disabled. Applicants for Medicaid must be residents of the area and must demonstrate financial need based on income and assets.

Guidelines for Medicaid eligibility vary from state to state. In most states, clients have the option of electing participation in the *spend-down* program. This program allows clients who are ineligible for Medicaid based on income to spend the differential on their health care expenses to establish eligibility. After the spend-down is met, all Medicaid-incurred services would be paid by the Medicaid program.

The criteria for Medicaid eligibility change periodically. Hospitals and home care agencies may assist clients in submitting Medicaid applications. Clients and their families can work directly with their local Medicaid office to submit needed documents as well.

Medicaid coverage includes community services, home care, personal care, and institutional care:

Community Services

Community services are the services of physicians, dentists, nurses, optometrists, and other professional personnel. Community services also include outpatient/clinic services, supplies, eyeglasses, prosthetic appliances, physical therapy, laboratory and radiology services, transportation for medical care, and prescription drugs.

Home Care

Home care services include nursing, PT, OT, ST, HHA, and personal care services.

Personal Care Services

Personal care attendants are persons who provide care under the Medicaid personal care benefit. They must meet the competency requirements established by the state in which they are operating.

Institutional Care

Institutional care covers care provided in hospitals, nursing homes, and other medical facilities. Long-term home health care services are also provided in some states (eg, New York State) through the Lombardi Program (Nursing Home Without Walls). Clients are also entitled to community services such as laboratory and radiology services, transportation, and prescription drugs.

Current Trends in Medicaid

When the Medicaid program was established in 1965, the program served to fund the growth of the home care industry. Recently, states have been forced to examine Medicaid expenditures with a focus on savings. It is becoming increasingly difficult, from a financial perspective, to maintain long-term and chronically ill clients at home. There is a definitive movement to reduce expenditures for Medicaid clients, particularly in the area of personal care services. If this occurs, the only option available to many clients may be institutional placement.

Commercial Insurers

Commercial insurers are insurance companies that provide health care coverage through a contract. Contracts may be purchased by individuals or employers as a benefit to employees. At times, there are co-payments and deductibles that the client will be responsible for. The following are some examples of commercial insurers:

B/C
B/S
Oxford
Aetna
GHI
H.I.P.
Magna Care

Currently, this industry is experiencing rapid growth and change. Because new plans and programs are continuously being developed, the nurse must keep current by reading related material.

Managed Care

Case management has evolved as a mechanism to control clinical services and fiscal liability of commercial insurers. An individual or individuals serve as a conduit to monitor and control services provided. It is the case manager's responsibility to ensure that the client receives adequate and appropriate home health services at a reasonable cost. When a managed care case is referred to a home health agency, the nurse is responsible for communication with the insurance company's case manager to obtain authorization for service. Each insurer determines frequency of contact with the home care agency for ongoing approval of service and frequency of visits.

The nurse plays a pivotal role in communicating with case managers of managed care companies and must obtain preauthorization, which includes a discussion of the client's insurance information, diagnosis, and initial service needs. At this time, the nurse and other disciplines usually are given approval for the initial visits. After the nurse performs the initial assessment visit, she communicates her findings to the case manager. Information can be transmitted by phone, fax, or by email.

Managed care companies appreciate efforts to report concise factual information. It is the responsibility of each nurse to present objective clinical information by which the case manager can authorize continued services. Data pertaining to the clinical assessment, interventions, and outcomes constitute the essence of the report.

For these reasons, it is a good idea to format the presentation in a standardized manner. Display 3-1 is representative of how to organize the data.

Instructions for Completion of Case Management Report

1. Name and title of caregiver completing report
2. Date of report
3. Insurance company case manager receiving report
4. Name of payor
5. Case manager telephone number with extension
6. Case manager fax number
7. Client name
8. Agency-assigned medical record number
9. Type of report being presented
10. Timeframe for visits being reported
11. State number of visits made in timeframe in item 10
12. Check discipline that is being reported
13. List all diagnoses
14. Report highest and lowest figures for period identified
15. List any relevant home or relationship information, for example, presence of support system in home, safety or accessibility of home, bathroom, and so forth
16. Include: systems assessment, functional ability, ability to perform activities of daily living, ambulation, knowledge/compliance with medications, diet, and treatment regimen. List all abnormal findings, wound status, if appropriate (eg, loca-

tion, color, size, description of drainage, type of dressing), ability to perform self-care. Include all nursing care and education provided to patient during the period of the report

17. List response to clinical intervention and client's receptivity to and retention of teaching
18. List all unresolved goals and plans to attain same
19. Next scheduled appointment with physician
20. Projected discharge date from home health services
21. Equipment or supplies ordered during report period and anticipated needs for next timeframe
22. List requested visit frequency
23. List approved visits for next service period
24. Upcoming service period being approved
25. Number assigned by case manager
26. Due date for next clinical update
27. For discharges only: Complete total number of visits for each discipline providing service

Communication is the key to successful managed care relationships. These contracts are vital to secure the future of the home care agency. A nurse who cultivates these relationships is a valued employee.

HMOs

Commercial insurance can also be provided through a health maintenance organization (HMO). Each commercial insurer specifies the scope and quantity of services that are covered. It is advisable for the nurse to become familiar with the benefits available to each client when providing service.

HMOs are prepaid health care plans through which enrollees receive all clinical services. A home

DISPLAY 3-1. Case Management Report

1. Reporting professional's name and title: _____

2. Date: _____ 3. Case Manager _____ 4. Insurance Co. _____

5. Phone # _____ ext. _____ 6. Fax # _____

7. Client name _____ 8. Med. Rec. # _____

9. Type of report ○ Initial   ○ Update   ○ Discharge

10. Service period for report film _____ to _____ 11. # Of visits _____

12. Discipline ○ RN ○ PT ○ OT ○ ST ○ MSS ○ HHA ○ Nutrition ○ Other

13. All diagnoses

14. VS Range B.P. _____ T _____ P _____ R _____ WT _____

15. Social/environmental assessment _____

16. Clinical assessment/interventions _____

17. Outcomes of treatment/teaching _____

18. Goals/plans for continued service _____

19. Next MD appt. _____   20. Anticipated D/C date _____

21. Equipment/supplies _____

Confirmation for Continued Service   **For D/C Only**

22. Visit Frequency _____   27. Total VN visits _____

23. Service approved _____ visits   Total PT visits _____

24. Auth. Dates _____   Total OT visits _____

25. Auth. Number _____   Total ST visits _____

26. Follow-up date _____   Total HHA visits _____

                                                 Total MSS visits _____

© With permission. Revival Home Health Care

health agency must have a contractual relationship with the HMO to provide reimbursable care to the participating members.

Between 1989 and 1994, health care costs for beneficiaries enrolled in HMOs dropped to 40% less than during the years before their joining a managed care program.

In New York State, 37 health care plans were chosen to participate in the DOH Medicaid Managed Care program. Enrolling recipients in these programs is projected to decrease Medicaid expenditures by 13%. Cost savings will be achieved through the government program paying an annual fee for services to the insurance company. It is the goal of the insurance company case manager to control volume and thereby costs.

No-Fault Insurance

No-fault insurance is otherwise known as personal injury protection (PIP). It pays for expenses incurred by persons in a motor vehicle accident. Persons who have and drive motor vehicles are required by law to purchase basic no-fault insurance. The nurse who makes the assessment visit in the home must determine whether the client's health problem is a result of a motor vehicle accident. In this case, no-fault would be the primary insurer. When no-fault insurance is exhausted, the home care agency may select another available payor for reimbursement. No-fault coverage varies based on each individual policy. Basic no-fault covers up to $50,000 of necessary doctor bills, hospital bills, and other health benefits, including home care.

Worker's Compensation

Worker's compensation policies are prescribed by law and vary from state to state. The legislation's intent is to provide for the payment of benefits for occupational injuries or diseases incurred by covered employed while at work. The compensation board screens claims for legitimacy and case management of employees as a mechanism to prevent overutilization of services. Benefits provided by worker's compensation policies vary from state to state as defined by state law. Nurses must work collaboratively with case managers to ensure that services provided will be covered.

Private Pay

Clients who are not covered by any insurance plan may pay for the services of a home health agency. Although agency charges are standardized, most agencies have a sliding fee scale to account for differences in clients' ability to pay. All services an agency provides may be paid for privately.

Free Care

Most agencies are required by government regulations to provide services at no charge to clients who meet specific agency-defined criteria. The nurse must be familiar with the policies and procedures of his or her agency. A fee assessment may be performed by a nurse to determine eligibility for free care. Any service that a certified home health agency is authorized to provide can be paid for through free care dollars.

ELIGIBILITY CRITERIA FOR HOME CARE

Table 3-1 delineates eligibility requirements for home care reimbursement.

HOW IS THE APPROPRIATE PAYOR SELECTED?

When the client is referred for service, all insurance information should be obtained by the intake nurse. The initial visit gives the nurse providing care the opportunity to verify the information obtained at intake. In the home, the nurse examines the source insurance documents to eliminate clerical errors that may have occurred during the intake process. The nurse should obtain information about all potential payors, including, but not limited to:

No-fault insurance
Supplemental policies
Employment status of spouse
Purchase of Medicare Part B

Although there are always exceptions, the rule of thumb for selection of primary payor should be made in the following order:

1. Worker's compensation or no-fault
2. Commercial insurance
3. Medicare
4. Medicaid
5. Private pay
6. Free care

Table 3-1
Eligibility Requirements for Home Care Reimbursement

Payor	Home-bound*	Skilled Need[†]	Under MD Plan of Treatment[‡]	Coverage Limits[§]	Part-Time/Intermittent[ǁ]	Reasonable and Necessary[¶]
Medicare	Yes	Yes	Yes	Up to 35 hours per week of skilled nursing & home health aide	Yes	Yes
Medicaid	No	No	Yes	State determined	No	Yes
Commercial	Usually	Not required	Yes	Policy determined	No	Yes
Private/Free	Agency determined	Not required	Yes	Agency determined	No	Yes

continued

Table 3-1
Eligibility Requirements for Home Care Reimbursement Continued

Payor	Home-bound*	Skilled Need†	Under MD Plan of Treatment‡	Coverage Limits§	Part-Time/Intermittent‖	Reasonable and Necessary¶
No-Fault	No	No	Yes	Policy determined	No	Yes
Worker's Compensation	No	Not required	Yes	State determined	No	Yes

*Homebound: Essentially confined to place of residence and requiring a considerable and taxing effort or the assistance of another person to leave the home.

†Skilled: Services qualifying for Medicare reimbursement that can only be performed by a registered nurse, physical therapist, speech therapist, or occupational therapist.

‡Plan of Treatment: A written plan developed by professional staff in consultation with and authorized by the physician. It supports the client's total needs and serves as the basis for service delivery.

§Coverage Limits: Maximum allowed visits or hours of services.

‖Part-Time: Coverage provided by a skilled nurse or home health aide for less than 8 hours a day, any number of days per week. Intermittent: The client's need for skilled nursing services less than daily (5 to 7 days per week), for a finite and predictable period.

¶Reasonable and Necessary: Care required is of a sound nature and is essential in promoting the health of the client.

Unique situations should be discussed with a manager to assure the appropriate decision.

A final issue related to billing involves the simultaneous use of two payors. A common term for this practice is *split billing*. This is usually done when one payor covers a limited amount or range of services. An example of split billing occurs when Medicare has covered a client for the maximum of 35 hours of nursing and HHA service. However, the client requires additional custodial HHA services. The additional hours can be billed to any other appropriate secondary source.

Knowledge, creativity, and skill are required to integrate a client's clinical needs with the agency's reimbursement needs. Teamwork among agency staff plays a significant role in the success of this effort. Professional nurses are positioned to meet this challenge in the field of home health care.

4

Time Management and Setting Priorities

Sandra Ceslowitz, RN, EdD

DETERMINING VISIT FREQUENCIES

On discharge from the hospital, a 485 form from the Health Care Financing Administration (HCFA) is completed on which visit frequency is established. This is referred to as certification. The certification lasts for 60 to 62 days. The form contains an estimation of the number of visits by the various team members for a 60- to 62-day period. The visit frequency is projected to be greater during the initial weeks and less as the caregiver/client learn to manage the client's condition. This change in the number of visits is referred to as *tapering*. For example, the following schedule illustrates tapering: daily visits for 1 week, three times a week (TIW) for 3 weeks, twice a week (BIW) for 2 weeks, and once a week (OW) for 1 week.

A clinical example illustrates tapering. A client discharged from the hospital with a burn was taught self-care. This included dressing changes and observation for signs and symptoms of infection. Initially the nurse visited the client with greater frequency. As the client progressed in being able to manage self-care independently, the nurse reduced (tapered) the visits until the burn was healed.

The frequency of visits may need to be increased. An informal clue that may alert the nurse to this need would occur when the nurse observes that something new is happening to the client or caregiver. Such incidents include new treatments, new medications, new significant physical or emotional symptoms, new diagnoses, or a new caregiver. Visits need to increase in frequency when the client's condition begins to deteriorate and acute changes occur. An example of this is when an insulin-dependent diabetic client's daughter who administers the insulin goes on vacation. If another family member needs to take over this task temporarily for the daughter, the nurse would again have to increase the visit frequency to daily until the other family member was competent in this task. If the client's or caregiver's situation changes and visit frequency is increased, physician approval is needed.

Conversely, visits may be gradually decreased when the client is responding to treatment, or the client/caregiver begins to show understanding of teaching. Therefore, reading the 485 will serve as an initial guide to visit frequency. Adjustments in frequency can be made based on the nurse's assessment and physician verification.

Time management requires planning a schedule of when home visits will be made. The following outline is a guideline for knowing the acceptable number of days that may elapse between visits: weekly, 6 to 8 days; twice weekly, 3 to 4 days; three times a week, 2 to 3 days. For example, if a patient is BIW and is visited on Monday, then the next visit should be scheduled Thursday or Friday. This allows leeway if the visit cannot be made on the exact day scheduled. Because different agencies have policies about scheduling nonemergent visits on weekends when staffing may be reduced, it is important to discuss projected weekend visits with the agency. The scheduling of frequency of visits has many facets. For example, it would be unwise to plan weekly visits for every weekly patient on a Monday because there usually are new patients who were admitted over the weekend and need to be visited on Monday. Each Wednesday the nurse should plan a tentative schedule of the clients to be visited the following week. Doing this allows the nurse to project which of the days will have a lighter schedule. Time during these days can be used to write 60-day summaries or to complete other paperwork.

TIME SPENT AT VISIT AND PRIORITIZATION OF NEEDS

The actual time spent in the home needs to be documented for statistical purposes for the agency. Generally a new visit takes an hour and a revisit a half hour. Of course, these are averages. If the nurse advises the patient who is being visited for the first time to have medicines out for checking as well as insurance information ready, the time spent looking for these items will be saved.

The time spent during the visit is based on discovering and prioritizing needs. These require that the nurse be a skilled communicator. The manner in which the nurse communicates with the client/family also influences the duration of the visit. It is appropriate to tell the client the expected duration of the visit. Doing this gives clients the opportunity to organize their thoughts and make sure that their most important concerns are expressed. The nurse may suggest that clients write down any questions that emerge between visits. The nurse also must know when to ask open-ended questions and when to ask closed-ended questions. Closed-ended questions are appropriate for rapidly gaining information. An example would be: "Have you had headache, weakness, hunger, or fainting?" (signs of hypoglycemia). An open-ended question would be: "How are you managing with your diet and insulin administration?" This question may elicit greater feelings from the client, which may be time consuming. It is unfair to clients to ask an open-ended question at the conclusion of the visit and then not allow expression of feelings. This type of question is better used at the beginning of the visit.

MANAGING A CASELOAD OF CLIENTS

The nurse, when visiting several clients in one day, needs to decide in what order to arrange the visits. Certainly, the most acute clients receive greatest priority. Clients with certain illnesses need to be visited early in the morning. An example would be a client with diabetes who does not yet know how to administer insulin or use the glucometer. If a client is being visited twice daily for wound care, the first visit also needs to be made earlier in the day to allow sufficient time between the two visits.

Other criteria in deciding the order of clients to be visited are the following: Any treatment that if postponed would result in a significant increase of discomfort would need to be scheduled early in the day. If a catheter is blocked, and needs changing, this would be a priority. It is preferable to open an initial visit in the morning because the nurse is more likely to be able to contact the physician, order supplies, and follow-up on any identified problems.

Just as it is important to know who needs to be visited first, it also is important to assess whose visits can be either postponed to later in the day or later in the week. The nurse needs to have a few patients whose visits can be postponed to accommodate new admissions or emergency situations. These would include patients who have achieved a stabilized physical or emotional state and whose visits are being tapered. An example would be a person admitted with congestive heart failure who has not had recent changes in vital signs, activity tolerance, medications, or fluid retention. Even when a visit is postponed, the frequency schedule projected on the 485 needs to be followed. If the client is not at home or refuses a visit, the nurse needs to document an attempted visit, again ensuring that the visit schedule of the 485 is adhered to.

Visits may need to be timed around when a family member is home, if this is the person who is going to be taught. The nurse may need to plan a visit when the home health aide is present so assistance can be given with such procedures as Foley insertion or wound care. At times, the nurse needs to arrange to visit at the same time when a therapist is in the home. An example is to arrange to be present when the patient is taught a difficult transfer. The nurse tries to accommodate the visit to the client's usual daily schedule as much as possible. For example, the nurse would arrange a morning visit for a client who has a sacral decubitus and needs the dressing done before being transferred to a wheelchair.

Geographic location is another influential factor. Efficient use of time warrants getting an overview of where all the clients who will be visited on any one day live and planning one's route accordingly. Map reading is an important time management tool. Whether it is a map used when driving a car or a subway or bus map, having a map available will help prevent the nurse from getting lost. Getting lost not only is anxiety producing, but it also disrupts the nurse's schedule. The nurse should call the client and apprise him or her of the situation. At times the client or family member may even be able to give directions.

When the nurses start out in the morning, they call clients and give an estimated time in which the visit will occur. It is advisable to give an hour's leeway to allow for unavoidable delays. When making this phone call, it is wise to get a cross street on which the residence is located. If a client needs daily wound care, calling each day may not be needed. Nurses simply remind them of the time of the visit the next day, or they write the time on a calendar in the client's home.

STAYING ON TOP OF THE PAPERWORK AND SUBMISSION OF PAPERWORK ON A TIMELY BASIS

The volume of paperwork in home care is time consuming. Having a positive mental attitude is important. Try to think of the paperwork as part of the care rendered, not as a separate entity. Nurses need to appreciate that documentation is essential for the patients to receive needed care, for the employees to be paid (including themselves), and for the agency to stay afloat. Having some system makes the task manageable. In home care, forms on which the nurses record home visits are called Initial Forms, Revisit Reports, or Progress Notes. Some nurses find it helpful to write routine information on the Visit Report while in the home. This would include such information as vital signs, type of wound care, and doctor's appointments. Nurses vary in being able to write the complete Visit Reports in the home. Some write the visit as soon as they go to the car, if they are driving. Others use a tape recorder after each visit to save pertinent information. However, if the neighborhood is unsafe, the nurse would not want to spend extra time and concentration in writing notes outside the home. In this situation, the nurse would document as much as possible in the home and finish the charting on completion of the day's visits. Keeping a copy of the previous visit report with you will assist you in organizing your notes. Visit Reports need to be placed in the client's record within 2 or 3 days of the visit, depending on agency policy.

Whenever a physician is called and orders change from the original 485, a form needs to be mailed to the physician for verification and signature. An example would be if the patient shows side effects of a drug and the dose is changed or if additional nursing visits are needed. The original form should be mailed to the physician as soon as possible. A copy is placed in the client's record until the signed form is returned to the agency.

Besides Visit Reports, another paperwork requirement is writing discharge summaries. It is best to write them as soon as possible at the time of discharge and hand them in with the last progress note.

For every client who receives care over a 60-day period, a recertification form needs to be completed. Six weeks from the start of care date, the nurse needs to evaluate the degree to which goals are being achieved. If the nurse believes the client will be seen

---

DISPLAY 4-1. **Master List**

Data

Client's name, address, and phone number

Name and phone number of physician

Certification period

Name of home health aide and days and hours in the home

Names and phone numbers of assigned therapist/ social worker

Paperwork Requirements (write due date and completion date or write O for Outstanding)

Recertification

Discharge summary

Home health aide supervisory visit

---

beyond the eight weeks, then the recertification form is sent to the physician. Some agencies require that the 60-day summaries be submitted 10 days before they are due. (See Chapters 13 and 14.)

Writing a master list of the names of your caseload and the documentation requirement, what was done, and what is outstanding is a good organizational strategy. Keeping the most recent 485 with you also is a good idea. Display 4-1 is an example of the information contained in such a master list.

COORDINATION WITH OTHER DISCIPLINES

The nurse may act as coordinator with other health team members. The nurse needs to call the physician after the initial visit to verify the medications and plan of care, when any changes in the plan of care needs to be made, when any significant change in the client's condition occurs, and when the patient is discharged.

Home health aides require supervisory visits every 2 weeks. Many agencies reserve a space on the Visit Report for documentation of this supervision, and the home health aide may need to sign the form.

The nurse needs to be knowledgeable about the progress the patient is making with various therapies: physical therapy (PT), occupational therapy (OT), and speech therapy (ST), and how social work plans are progressing. Reading progress notes of other disciplines on a regular basis is a way of monitoring the client's progress. The client should be asked to reserve a folder in a designated space in the home. Therapists usually leave written instructions for patients, and the nurse needs to be apprised of these instructions so that there is consistency between various disciplines.

The nurse needs to know that Medicare regulations will not allow home health aide visits unless the patient concurrently is receiving visits by a registered nurse (RN) or physical therapist (PT). According to Medicare regulations, a social worker is not allowed to be the only service in the home. Therefore, the nurse needs to assess early in the certification period if he or she thinks that the patients will require the services of a social worker. In this way the social worker will be brought into the case early, while the visiting nurse or physical therapist is still in the home.

Coordination with other disciplines by phone needs to be documented in the client's record. Many agencies require that this documentation be done in red ink. The documentation should include the date and time the phone call was made, the name of the person called, and the essence of the conversation. Phone calls to clients and caregivers, except those brief ones to announce approximate visit time, also need to be documented. Nurses who have a cellular phone or a beeper with them in the field find that these aid their communication activities. These time management suggestions, if used consistently, will become integral to the routine that you establish as a visiting nurse.

5

Clients' Legal Rights and Confidentiality

Rose Madden-Bear, BSN, MSN

CLIENT RIGHTS AND RESPONSIBILITIES

Protection of client rights and confidentiality is probably the single most important concern for home health care providers. Both regulators and accrediting bodies have set standards for client rights and confidentiality; however, it is the duty of both the home health industry and home care professionals to uphold protection of these rights.

Unlike other health care settings, the visiting nurse is a guest in the client's home. The client allows the nurse, aide, or therapist to enter his or her home, and certain basic client rights are implied. However, the nurse needs to specifically communicate each of the various rights and responsibilities to the client. Client rights that are protected by law include the following:

The client has the right to complete and competent care of the highest quality. This includes treating the client courteously, fairly, and respectfully.

The client should receive a prompt response to requests for help and assistance. This is especially true in emergency situations, where an immediate response is required.

The client should be treated equally and without regard to race, creed, sex, age, ethnic origin, national origin, disability, or insurance source. The home care nurse needs to be nondiscriminatory in his or her care and treatment of the client. This can sometimes pose as a difficult situation for the nurse who may be having religious or cultural dilemmas in caring for the client. In these situations, agencies often have ethics committees to provide guidance to the nurse in resolving these conflicts between the nurse's personal values while still treating the client respectfully.

The client has the right to know about his or her problems, plan of care, and treatment. This topic will be presented in more detail during the discussion of informed consent. The nurse must make every attempt possible to involve the client in his or her plan of care. This will ensure that the client is making informed choices and decisions.

This area also includes the client's right to be notified in advance of changes in his or her plan of care, and to know the names and titles of the nurse, aide, therapist, and so forth, who are involved in the plan of care. In addition, the client has the right to refuse treatments or medications after being fully informed and having understood the consequences of his or her actions.

The client has the right to have his or her property in the home treated with respect. This requires the caregiver being careful not to break, soil, or destroy any of the client's belongings or furnishings.

The client has the right to confidential treatment of his or her own medical information. This subject is discussed later in more detail, including preventing violations of privacy. For example, the nurse must refrain from discussing clients in hallways, elevators, and public places. In addition, the client must first authorize permission to obtain or release his or her medical information by signing a release form before this information is furnished.

The client has the right to voice grievances or objections without fear of reprisal. In addition, if a client is not satisfied with the resolution to his or her complaint, the client should be provided with a recourse. Various states now offer hotline numbers so that clients can call if they are not satisfied with their home care services.

The client has the right to be informed by the nurse when he or she will be discharged. The client should be given the opportunity to discuss any reasons, concerns, and long-term plans he or she might have with the nurse before the discharge occurs.

The client has the right to formulate an advance directive. This topic is discussed at length in the Patient Self-Determination Act section of this chapter.

Clients also have responsibilities that are communicated to them by the nurse at the initial visit. These responsibilities include:

Notifying the nurse or physician when the client has a change in functional, social, or physical status

Notifying the nurse or physician when there is a problem or change that will affect the plan of care

Cooperating with the home care nurse, therapist, aide, and other caregivers to the fullest extent possible

Following the plan of care established with his or her understanding, consent, and cooperation.

CLIENT CONFIDENTIALITY

Confidentiality is a client's right that not only protects an individual from unwarranted intrusion of privacy or discussion but also governs protection of client information. Protection of confidentiality is an implied right when the nurse agrees to care for the client. In legal terms, the nurse has established a "duty to care" for the client, and this carries a professional responsibility to be completely confidential. Protection of confidentiality addresses not only privacy of discussion of clients but also protection of clinical records.

What does this mean for the nurse in the home? There are very basic steps nurses need to follow to protect confidentiality. These include:

Nurses should never leave a client's medical record unattended, such as in a car or bag.

Nurses should not document their clinical notes in public places, where others may have access to clients' medical information.

If a nurse uses a typing service to type his or her dictated notes, client identifiers should be removed. Use client initials or registration numbers to identify the client.

Always protect the clinical record from unauthorized access such as closing the clinical record or turning clinical notes face down when leaving the room or one's desk temporarily.

Discussion of client information should only occur when it is relevant to provision of care and services. Inquiries related to client information should be relevant and kept confidential. In addition, nurses must be very careful not to breach a client's confidentiality in dealing with family members.

CONFIDENTIALITY IN THE CLIENT'S HOME

In home care, family members are very often involved in the client's care. At times, a client may share information with the nurse and have chosen not to inform family members. The nurse, as a client advocate, must protect and respect that client's right to confidentiality. As a result, the nurse should not openly share private information with family members without the client's knowledge and consent. This is especially true in cases of human immunodeficiency virus (HIV) confidentiality, or discussion of lifestyle factors such as sexual preference, intravenous drug use, and so forth.

Confidentiality is an extremely important issue with respect to the home visit itself. The nurse must never discuss the client outside the home setting, and should limit discussions with family members to locations in which others are not present. This may be difficult for home care staff, who may get bombarded with questions or comments from neighbors or friends. For example, a home health aide may be doing laundry in the client's building and be presented with inquiries from neighbors. In these cases, the nurse should instruct the home health aide to inform neighbors or friends that he or she cannot share client information with them. However, the nurse or aide should do so in a sincere, nonintimidating manner, so as not to possibly alienate the client from others in the building.

The nurse must remember that client confidentiality is a basic human right. Clients' rights are outlined in a bill of rights and, consequently, nurses should familiarize themselves with these rights. Nurses need to know under what circumstances they can release confidential information. For example, the nurse needs to inform the physician regarding client status changes or situations that may be of potential harm to the client. Often situations in the home environment can put a client in potential risk, and the physician should be aware of this. Physician involvement in the care plan is very important to guide future care decisions.

In addition, the home care nurse may need to notify various state and city protection agencies if the nurse believes that the client or others may be at risk for harm. For example, confidential medical information or information shared by a client with the nurse may pose as a threat to others. Nurses should be aware of their legal responsibilities as defined in the various nurse practice acts and laws, which may vary from state to state.

THE HOME CARE RECORD AS A LEGAL RECORD

The home care clinical record is considered a legal document and can be submitted as evidence in a court of law. Clinical records as a rule should not be altered. However, if an incorrect entry, spelling, or date is written, one line should be crossed through it and initialed and dated by the individual who made the entry. One individual should never alter the entry of another; however, in some instances, entries may need to be co-signed (such as by a supervisor). Clinical records should never contain a corrective substance such as Wite-Out® to obliterate the entry. At times it may be necessary to clarify an entry with a subsequent record entry without changing the clinical record.

In the home health industry, the use of *fee for service* staff and independent contractors is common. Therefore, professional disciplines should use carbon visit notes and retain a copy of each visit. This enables the professional to protect himself or herself in the event that submitted notes are altered. Laws differ from state to state with regard to retention of clinical record documentation. In general, 6 to 7 years may be the average requirement for retaining clinical documentation. However, legal statutes of limitations (such as for minors) may require retaining your clinical notes for much longer.

Confidentiality protection of legal records takes place through a variety of interventions. Nurses should be aware of their employers' policies for protection of clinical records. Policies that should exist include statements that govern:

Access to clinical records
Entry into clinical records
Release of clinical records

For example, organizations must regulate who has access to audit and review records and those individuals (by job position) who may make record entries. This is especially true for states that have specific confidentiality laws for HIV-positive persons or clients with other particular disabilities, such as chemical dependencies. In addition, the nurse needs to remember that disclosure of confidential medical information may not take place over the telephone to unauthorized persons. Often the nurse may be contacted by telephone for information about the client. The nurse must be aware that laws governing the release of medical information on paper usually also apply to telephone contacts. The nurse needs to ensure that those persons are in fact authorized to receive that information. The nurse should request the individuals to identify themselves and who they represent (for example, a social services agency, physician's office, etc.). The nurse then must document this information in the clinical record along with the telephone discussion that took place regarding the client.

Some client information may be of such a confidential nature that the nurse would be required to obtain a release from the client or an authorization from the requested party. In most states, family members are not automatically entitled to release of medical records unless the protected person is deceased. Therefore, in these cases, when families are requesting records, a consent is required. In all cases, release of medical information should be appropriately authorized with verification of the person signing the consent.

TERMS AND USE OF INFORMED CONSENT

Informed consent is a basic human right that allows the client to be provided with adequate information about his or her illness, plan of care, and treatments. In obtaining informed consent, the nurse or physician is required to describe to the client the medical condition, what procedure or treatment is being performed, and why. In addition, the nurse needs to describe potential side effects or adverse reactions that may occur. The home care nurse also needs to describe existing alternatives to the proposed treatment to completely fulfill the requirements of informed consent.

If the nurse has reason to believe that a client does not understand the nature of a treatment for which he or she has consented, the nurse should intervene accordingly. This includes notification of the physician immediately and documentation of actions taken.

Informed consent involves both consent to treatment and refusal of treatment, based on the information that has been provided to the individual. In home care, as in other settings, the "duty to disclose" information to obtain consent usually rests with the physician. However, legal accountability does not end there. The nurse who is performing the treatments and procedures, as ordered by the physician, needs to ascertain if the client is aware of and understands the care or treatment he or she will receive.

Essentially, there are two basic elements to the process of obtaining informed consent. The first component is imparting knowledge, and the second component is determining the client's ability to make health care decisions.

The first component, imparting knowledge, requires providing the following information:

The nurse needs to describe the nature of the client's illness or medical condition and assess his or her understanding of this information.
The nurse needs to describe the proposed treatments, procedures, and so forth, including their purposes.

In addition, the nurse would also provide the following information:

The expected outcomes, such as percentages of success
The inherent risks associated with the procedure or treatment
Any existing alternatives
The expected outcomes if treatment is refused

The second element, determining the client's ability to make health care decisions, requires that the client's education and comprehension level guide the design of the consent.

Occasionally, a client may be considered "incapacitated" in the hospital and is discharged home and shows signs of improved orientation in his or her own familiar surroundings. Family members are an essential component of providing this type of client status information to the nurse. The home care nurse has a responsibility to inform the physician and should encourage family members to provide measures to further improve the client's orientation, such as photographs, familiar visitors, etc. It is important to remember that, for informed consent to be obtained, the person must be able to make responsible decisions.

In certain situations, a consent may be implied. Implied consent usually occurs in emergency treatments, such as cardiopulmonary resuscitation, and when routine noninvasive procedures are performed that pose minimal risks, remote consequences, and the client has prior knowledge. In home care, an example would be the nurse taking vital signs or performing low-risk treatments such as ambulation training.

However, it is recommended that specific home care consents be obtained for procedures and treatments that are invasive and a general home care consent be obtained for routine care. Specific consents have been used in home health care for procedures and treatments that may possess serious side effects or complications, such as peripherally inserted central catheters. In addition, specific consents are used for administration of certain medications that may potentially harm a client. Examples of consents used in home health care include:

General releases to obtain or release client information

General consents to receive care and services by the home health agency and its employees/contractors

Administration of chemotherapy

Administration of investigational drugs in the home setting

Care provided by family-employed substitutes

Advance directive consents

Insertion of various venous catheters

Home health care clients must be given the opportunity to make informed choices. Actions should be taken to ascertain whether in fact the client has actually made an informed decision, and subsequently, should be substantiated by documentation of the home care interventions.

Clinical Record Documentation for Obtaining Consents

What information was presented

Who was present, and whether the consent was witnessed

Whether the client has been given the opportunity to ask questions and understand responses

What amount of time was spent in obtaining the consent

What teaching materials were used

Any additional client discussions that took place before decision was made

That consent is given freely, voluntarily, and without
coercion

Age verified in cases of minors and emancipated minors (for example, in some states, emancipated
minors are individuals younger than age 18 years
who are married or have a child)

Each of these items written in the clinical record
will protect home health agencies and professionals
from allegations of malpractice or negligence arising
from lack of informed consent.

THE PATIENT SELF-DETERMINATION ACT

In 1990, as part of the Omnibus Budget Reconcilia-
tion Act, the federal government enacted legislation
titled the Patient Self-Determination Act (PSDA). The
PSDA requires states to pass laws stating that adult
patients shall be provided with written information
about advance directives. This law took effect on December 1, 1991. Essentially, PSDA is a federal law
that requires health care providers (such as hospitals,
nursing homes, and home health agencies) to provide
clients with information about the right to direct their
own treatment and execute an advance directive. In
addition, health care providers are also mandated to
inquire from the client whether he or she has an existing advance directive.

In the home care setting, a variety of interventions have taken place to meet this requirement.
Home care nurses are responsible to distribute this
information about available advance directives to
clients at the initial nursing visit. If the client is not

capable of understanding the information, it is given to a family member or a significant other. The home care nurse is responsible to explain the PSDA, client's rights included in the law, and the availability of advance directives in his or her state.

The nurse would explain to the client about the PSDA and then provide the following written information:

Information regarding the client's right to make decisions about his or her medical care

How to plan in advance regarding medical care decisions, and what instructions or choices should be specified

Specific information regarding the various advance directives available to the client as according to his or her state laws

The nurse then would also provide an acknowledgement form for the client or significant other to sign, as validation that the information has been received.

In the home setting, the client may be overwhelmed with the type and amount of PSDA information and therefore may request family members to be present to read and hear the information on subsequent visits. The nurse would then obtain documentation that the client received the information on the initial visit and then continue the teaching on subsequent visits.

All attempts must be made to ensure that the client understands the information given. If the client requests an advance directive, the nurse will assist the client as needed in formulating an advance directive or refer the client to a social worker for guidance and assistance. Each client is asked if he or she has an advance directive, and the response is noted in the clinical record. If an advance directive exists, a copy should be made and filed in the clinical record.

ADVANCE DIRECTIVES

The PSDA preserves a client's right to autonomy and self-determination with regard to treatment decisions, refusal of treatments, and formulation of advance directives. Advance directives are documents with written instructions relating to health/medical care decisions that will be made in the event a person becomes incapacitated. Advance directives may take different forms. Examples include, but are not limited to, living wills, proxies, and consents for issuance of do not resuscitate (DNR) orders. Individuals execute these documents while they still have capacity to make their health care decisions. These documents would then become effective when the client is incapacitated.

Advance directives provide a clear indication of a person's wishes or preferences regarding emergency measures and life-sustaining treatment. The document guides treatment decisions while respecting the individual's wishes and values.

Living Wills, Health Care Proxies, and Do Not Resuscitate Consents and Orders

Most, if not all, states have some form of advance directive legislation. There are important distinctions between advance directives. Some directives may specify actual instructions, and others may designate a surrogate decision maker. Advance directives may take the form of a living will or a client-signed DNR consent. These documents should provide "clear and convincing evidence" of the client's own wishes regarding life-sustaining treatment and cardiopulmonary resuscitation. These documents also should provide clear direction to the physician and nurse regarding health care decisions.

Living Wills

Living wills are documents that outline specific instructions about the client's wishes for various health care choices or treatments. These documents usually outline specific treatments or interventions that the client does not want to receive. For example, a living will may specify instructions regarding kidney dialysis, mechanical ventilation, antibiotic therapy, and cardiopulmonary resuscitation. Some living wills may even include specifics about organ donation wishes.

Do Not Resuscitate

A second advance directive is a consent for the issuance of a DNR order. Essentially, the client consents to a DNR order, and the physician then issues the DNR order. DNR consents and protocols in home care may differ from hospital protocols, depending on state regulations. For example, in New York State, a Non-Hospital Do Not Resuscitate Order (NHDNR) must be obtained before a DNR consent is considered valid.

Essentially, this requirement takes effect when a client has a DNR consent issued while he or she is at home. The client's physician must also sign a specific NHDNR order for the DNR order to take effect.

Hence, the nurse needs to verify that the physician's NHDNR order has been signed and dated.

DNR orders generally take effect as soon as the physician signs the order; however, this may vary from state to state. DNR orders may be in effect for a specified period as according to state law, such as from 60 to 90 days. Therefore, it is reasonably prudent to have DNR orders reissued every 62 days on renewal of the plan of treatment.

The home care nurse would explain to the client how to complete the document and answer any questions the client may have. The nurse also may want to refer the client to a social worker, because the client may need supportive counseling to reach a decision. In most client situations involving discussion and completion of advance directives, there would be family members involved if they are available.

Health Care Proxies

Advance directives may also take the form of *surrogate* or *proxy* decision making. Essentially, the law presumes that the client has the right to consent or refuse treatment until the client no longer has the capacity to do so. At this point, surrogate decision making would take place.

Health care proxies are documents that delegate to another adult the authority to make medical care decisions on behalf of the client. These proxy individuals may be called an *agent*, *surrogate*, or a *power of attorney* for health care decisions, depending on each state's laws and regulations.

The authority dictated by the proxy document to make medical decisions may include choices regarding withdrawing or withholding life-sustaining treatments as well as cardiopulmonary resuscitation. This authority only takes place when the client becomes incapable of making his or her own decisions. The home care nurse would explain the health care proxy to the client at the time of the visit. This would include answering questions such as:

How is the document completed?
Who can witness the proxy?
Who can be an agent?
What instructions should be included?

These questions are important to ensure a proper valid document. For example, in New York State, the client's nurse is prohibited from being the client's agent. States may differ in their definition of surrogates, proxies, or health care agents. Surrogate decision makers are usually family members or next of kin. However, surrogates or agents may include other individuals (such as a friend or neighbor) whom the client designates and believes would know his or her wishes after considering the facts and circumstances of the health care decision.

Surrogate or proxy decision making requires a determination of lack of capacity. This determination may vary from state to state; however, usually two physicians are required to attest to the client's incapacitation. The incapacity determination would then be filed with the consent in the clinical record. Surrogate DNR consents, health care proxies, and powers of attorney for health decisions require the nurse or physician to discuss instructions about medical care decisions with the agent or surrogate. However, a proxy also may actually dictate specific instructions on the document.

Revocation and Revision of Advance Directives

Advance directives such as proxies, living wills, and DNR consents usually can be revoked at any time, orally or in writing. This revocation needs to be documented in the clinical record. It is also recommended that an *X* be written on the document to signify revocation.

The client always retains the right to revise or revoke the advance directive. For example, a terminal client's wishes may change over a period of months, depending on issues such as religious beliefs, perception of pain, and quality of life concerns. Therefore, that client may choose to alter the advance directive based on changed wishes or values.

The nurse should notify the physician immediately in the event that there is a change in the status of a client's advance directive. This includes execution, revocation, or any modification in the text of the advance directive. Notification of the physician and the status of the advance directive then are documented by the nurse in the clinical record.

Determining the Point When Advance Directives Take Effect

Advance directives survive the length of the person's incapacity, in that they will apply as long as the person is incapable of making his or her decisions, and providing that the client has not specified any expiration instructions or limitations. It is important to remember these documents do not take effect until an incapacity determination is made. Clients always have the right to make their wishes known orally or in writing, while they still are capable of doing so.

Advance directives can cover all health care decisions, such as treatment consents, treatment refusals, or withdrawal of treatment. The document may express limits, restrictions, and instructions to guide health care practitioners about the client's wishes regarding medical care. Surrogates or health care agents also may request specific medical information to make an informed decision. Advance directives may be executed well before health care decision making is needed, or immediately, as in emergency situations.

If a client has an advance directive, the nurse should instruct clients or family members to prominently display this document in the home. For example, advance directives can be posted in visible areas such as on the refrigerator or on a bedroom wall. Doing so would facilitate access to the directive by the home care team (nurse, physician, aide, etc.) and emergency medical services (EMS), so they could honor the advance directive as specified.

Home health care is a unique industry in many ways in its implementation of advance directives. According to the PSDA, clinical record documentation must always indicate whether an individual has executed an advance directive. In addition, home care providers are required to have evidence of the directive in the clinical record. However, providers may choose to retain copies and not the original copy of the document. The purpose of this procedure is to ensure that the client/family has the original directive, in the event of hospitalization or emergency medical care.

Secondly, determining the point when an advance directive takes effect may also differ greatly between the hospital and home care setting, as was described earlier. Consequently, home care nurses need to be aware of what protocols and documents must be in place before the advance directive actually takes effect. In addition, a nursing home or a hospital DNR order may not necessarily apply in the home setting, as various state laws dictate. The home care nurse needs to be knowledgeable of his or her agency's policies and procedures and the laws applicable to his or her own state's advance directives. For example, the home care nurse would be responsible to verify that a DNR order has been signed and received from the client's physician for the DNR consent to be honored by emergency services personnel.

In summary, the home care nurse carries significant responsibilities with respect to confidentiality and clients' rights. This is especially true of the rights of clients to informed consent, to participate in their health care decisions, and to execute advance directives. The role of home care nurses is to respect these rights and to encourage client self-determination and autonomy.

However, home care nurses must also protect their clients from actual or potential threats of harm or injury as they exercise these rights. Nurses must help their clients and families understand the benefits and consequences of their health care decisions. This is an essential part of the nursing role as health educators and client advocates in a home health care setting.

6

Safety
in the Home,
Community,
and Emergency
Situations

Karen Sherman, RN C, MPA

All home care nurses must consider safety factors when they make home visits. This chapter will guide the new or experienced nurse in the safe planning of a home visit and client safety in the home.

Home visiting is significantly different from providing care in an institutional setting. In particular, hospital nurses focus more on patient safety rather than on their own personal safety. Nurses making the transition to home care must develop an awareness of personal safety issues. The nurse's safety is of prime concern before, during, and after the home visit. The home care agency should provide necessary referral information about the client to assist in visit planning and implementation of safety measures.

Safety precautions need to be taken at all times. Many home care nurses do not consider all the risks to which they are exposed while working. The home care nurse who works in a high-crime area of a large city is confronted with different priorities than someone who works in a predominately rural or suburban location. In reality, crime is everywhere, and it is an occupational hazard for home care nurses. However, preventative measures can help reduce the incidence of nurses becoming crime victims.

Home safety is also important. Home health nurses need to assess for environmental hazards that may cause injury or accidents in the home. It is part of the nurse's role to teach clients home safety, including proper use of equipment, prevention of falls, fire safety, and emergency precautions.

Staff education about field and home safety should be conducted during orientation to the agency and on an annual basis through in-service programs. Agency policies and procedures pertaining to safety must be discussed. Staff will be more receptive to safety education when they understand the rationale for procedures, take precautions to protect themselves, report unsafe situations, and share apprehensions or fears with their supervisor.

When accidents occur to either staff or clients, an incident report is usually filed at the agency so that corrective action can be taken.

ASSESSING FOR SAFETY

Previsit planning begins with verifying the client's address, cross streets, and specific entry information. For apartment buildings, it is especially important to know apartment or intercom numbers. A telephone call to the client can serve both to schedule the visit and to obtain additional travel information. Clients and families can provide helpful information regarding parking or locations for public transportation. Collaboration with other nurses who are familiar with the area is valuable, but never divulge home telephone numbers. Many clients have caller ID service from the phone company and can easily find out nurses' home phone numbers and addresses. There is potential for harassment with this unauthorized use of personal information.

All home care nurses should know how to use a map. Even nurses who are familiar with the neighborhood or area should consult a map when unknown streets are encountered. It is important to know how to get to the client's home from the office and which routes to take when traveling from one client's home to the next. For nurses working in areas served by bus or subway, carrying these additional maps is also recommended.

Some agencies have used security escort services to improve staff safety in the inner city. The primary intent is to have another person accompany the nurse into areas that are unsafe. Escorts are usually unarmed and have been trained in street safety. Client confidentiality must be maintained when escorts enter the home and wait for nurses. Escorts may be hired for full-time or on an on-call basis. Some agencies follow a similar approach using a buddy system, whereby other agency staff accompany nurses in the field.

It is important to consider not only where the nurse is going, but when. Planning of visits should take into consideration the time of day. There are communities where staff are encouraged to avoid late afternoon or evening visits because of drug or gang activity. Requesting the assistance of city or housing police is an option occasionally used.

GUIDELINES FOR PERSONAL SAFETY

Nurses should take reasonable precautions to protect themselves at all times. New home care nurses tend to be more cautious and anxious. Experienced nurses have learned the streets and may use good judgment most of the time, but occasionally take unnecessary risks (Display 6-1).

Learning how to become street smart is crucial to working in the community. One of the most important rules to remember is to always be alert and observe surroundings. Do not appear lost or uncertain about where you are going. Some nurses may be so preoccupied with client care needs or problems that they become distracted while traveling. Keep your mind on getting safely to your destination. Try to be aware of people near you and their activities. Take note of odd or unusual events.

Nurses should maintain an image of professionalism in their appearance. Adherence to the dress code could have an impact on safety in the community. Many home health agencies have discontinued the use of uniforms or lab coats. In the past, the home

DISPLAY 6-1. **Ten Personal Security Tips**

1. Carry a minimal amount of money, your driver's license, and ID.
2. Do not take purses/wallets with you on visits. Use a fanny pack to carry keys.
3. Be aware of surroundings at all times and know exactly where you are going.
4. Be alert to people or groups; notice body language and eye contact.
5. Avoid walking in dark, deserted places. Do not take shortcuts through secluded alleys or vacant lots.
6. Walk in the center of sidewalks away from buildings, parked cars, and tall hedges.
7. Look for working public telephones or use a cellular phone.
8. Do not ask a stranger for directions; call your office or ask police for help.
9. If you suspect someone is following you, enter a business establishment.
10. If a group of people look threatening, cross to the other side or walk in the street.

care nurse was readily identified by a uniform, and people respected and welcomed the nurse to the community. However, uniforms and nursing bags can draw attention to the nurse, who may be carrying needles, syringes, or other valuable medical instruments. Wearing street clothes allows the nurse to blend in with the community. To avoid robbery, especially by chain-snatchers, jewelry should be kept to a minimum. Also, comfortable shoes should be worn for routine walking or unexpected running. Overall, it is best to dress appropriately for the weather and within the guidelines established by the agency.

When home care nurses are assigned to a particular area, they need to know as much about the community as possible, including local businesses and merchants, public areas, and emergency resources. Some nurses work very well in their own community because they know the neighborhood and are familiar faces. Even nurses working in new areas quickly become familiar to local merchants and people who "hang out" in the community. It is a good idea to know the location of public buildings such as the post office, library, and schools, in case assistance is needed. The location of emergency resources such as local hospitals, police, and fire departments should be noted for future reference.

TRAVEL PRECAUTIONS AND CAR SAFETY

Many nurses rely on their own vehicles for traveling. Special safety precautions and regular car maintenance will help both new and experienced nurses use their cars safely. Proper maintenance of cars will prevent unexpected breakdowns, thereby avoiding vulnerable situations. Cars should be equipped with emergency items, including tools, flashlight, jumper cables, flares, and a spare tire. In winter weather, it is also a good idea to keep a survival kit containing food, additional clothing, and a blanket (Display 6-2).

Even with the best travel plans, getting lost is inevitable. To avoid appearing lost, first drive down the street until the building is located, then park. A build-

DISPLAY 6-2. **Ten Car Safety Tips**

1. Keep car doors locked and windows partially opened while driving.
2. Carry car keys in your hand for immediate entry.
3. Before entering your car, check the back seat and floor. When approaching your car, look under the car.
4. Do not leave valuables, including the nursing bag or client records, in the car.
5. If using your car trunk, place items in it when leaving the office, your home, or a client's home and not before entering a building.
6. Do not pick up hitchhikers.
7. Park your vehicle in well-lighted areas.
8. Carjacking tips: Drive in the center lane unless making turns. Avoid the curb lanes. Leave enough distance in front of your car to make a quick turn.
9. Use antitheft devices.
10. In winter weather, keep your gas tank more than half full.

ing or address may not be visible, and it is not a good idea to make your search obvious. Try to park as close to the address as possible. Nurses should look for safe parking areas on streets, driveways, parking lots, or garages. Park in well-lighted areas, and avoid streets that have either abandoned or vandalized cars. If you have to double-park your car, place an agency card on the windshield to identify the vehicle. Pay attention to parking rules and regulations so that your car will not be towed or ticketed. It is a costly inconvenience to return to find your car gone.

Many agencies offer driver safety courses to teach basic and defensive driving skills. This may help to reduce personal and agency insurance liability. It is also a good idea to attend lectures conducted by the police on safeguarding yourself and your car.

HOME VISIT PRECAUTIONS

Again, assess safety before entering the client's home. Nurses need to be cautious when approaching a building or private residence. It there are any doubts or fears about a certain visit, it should not be made until it is discussed with the agency. Sometimes the client may not be home, and nurses must assess the situation. For safety reasons, do not wait around unnecessarily. When there is no response to knocking, it is appropriate to leave a note under the door or in a mailbox. In most cases, a phone call to confirm a return visit may be possible (Display 6-3).

Nurses need to use extreme caution when making visits to clients who live in large public housing units. These may be high-rise buildings or smaller units situated in a complex.

When approaching buildings, observe all activity and note unusual entrances. Security at many apartment buildings is nonexistent, and front doors may be unlocked and intercoms or bells broken. In the absence of an escort, family members can be helpful by meeting the nurse at the entrance or keeping a lookout from a window.

Special precautions must be followed for the safe use of stairs and elevators. Closed stairwells and elevators generally classify a building as a safety risk no matter the location. Nurses should try to avoid stairs

---

DISPLAY 6-3. **Ten Community Safety Tips**

1. Use caution with all elevators.
2. Use open and well-lit stairs.
3. Have a family member meet you at an outside entrance as an escort.
4. Plan to make visits in the morning in areas you feel less comfortable in.
5. Never enter a building that appears unsafe.
6. Be cautious of pets and ask that animals be put away.
7. Exit the home immediately if there is a threatening situation.
8. Keep the nursing bag and other items in sight.
9. If the client is not home, leave a note under the door or in a mailbox. Do not hang around.
10. Notify the office if you are working after normal business hours.

---

that are poorly lit or enclosed in stairwells with doors. Always look before you enter an elevator. The best advice is not to get on an elevator if there is any question about the other occupants. When on the elevator, stay near the door and control panel. Be observant of other occupants who enter the elevator. Feel free to exit the elevator if you feel uncomfortable. Having a ready-made excuse, such as "I forgot something," may reduce any possible embarrassment. If you must exit the elevator, wait for another one and do not use the stairs. If an elevator has access to the basement, push the down button and allow the elevator to come up empty or occupied.

Always know the apartment number and do not search for clients by knocking on strange doors or ringing other doorbells. Always find out who the person is that answers the door. If an unfamiliar person answers the door, find out if the client is home before entering.

Nurses should exit the home immediately if there is a threatening situation, such as weapons, drug activity, or potential for physical abuse. It is always important to assess the client's safety, but if the nurse's safety is in jeopardy, then it is appropriate to leave the home. Once in a safe environment, the situation should be discussed with the appropriate office manager and the client contacted to resolve the problem.

Nurses should be careful not to attempt to break up a domestic argument, as the situation could quickly turn against them. If a nurse should encounter an intoxicated or mentally unstable person in the client's home, it is advisable to keep an eye on them at a distance. To prevent becoming trapped, be aware of all possible exits and entrances, doors, and hallways.

It is important to keep the nursing bag and other items within sight. The bag should be closed when not in use, as this will prevent access by children and pets. Do not take chances with animals, because they can be unpredictable. Always ask that pets be put in another room during the visit.

SAFETY IN THE HOME

Patient safety is a major concern for all home care providers. It is the responsibility of the home health agency and the nurse to ensure that basic home safety is evaluated and taught to clients and caregivers. Home care nurses and other field personnel must be able to assess and plan appropriate interventions related to client safety.

The goal is to establish and maintain a safe home environment. The home should be assessed for safety factors such as fall prevention, fire safety, medication use, equipment, infection control, and emergency preparedness. Home safety measures are necessary to identify and reduce accidents in the home. Unlike the hospital, the client's home may need modifications to make it a safe environment. Unfortunately, falls, medication errors, and accidents do occur, and these must be reported as incidents.

The client and family must be taught basic home safety and how to make changes in their home. Specific measures depend on the client's medical problems and related nursing diagnoses.

On the initial visit, the nurse should conduct a thorough assessment of the client's home. Each room should be assessed with the client or family to point out safety hazards. General safety measures should be discussed at this time, and on subsequent visits, the nurse should reevaluate the home to monitor improvements.

Accidents caused by falls can occur in any part of the home, but particularly in the bathroom and bedroom, where assistive devices are frequently used. Most falls can be prevented by teaching clients proper transfer and ambulation techniques.

The elderly are more prone to falls because of poor eyesight, use of medications, and problems with ambulating. Safety teaching should be directed toward keeping pathways clear, using throw rugs with nonslip backing, and proper lighting. Clients also should be instructed to wear shoes with rubber soles and to keep side rails up on hospital beds.

Fire safety and burn prevention must be explained to the client, family, and caregivers. All homes should be equipped with smoke detectors and have fire evacuation plans. The plan should take into consideration anyone in the home who is handicapped or has special needs. Electrical safety and smoking precautions should be included with fire safety. Clients who use oxygen must be taught specific precautions. Fire hazards, if present, must be identified and discussed with the client to prevent serious injury.

The client should be instructed about the correct use of any medical equipment and how to report problems. An instruction manual and telephone number of the home medical supplier should be available in the home. All equipment should be inspected on a regular basis, especially hospital beds, infusion pumps, Hoyer lifts, and oxygen tanks. If any equipment is found to be malfunctioning, the client should be instructed not to use it until it is repaired or replaced.

The storage of medications is another safety concern. Medications should be kept in their original containers, unless the client is having medications prepared in color-coded pill boxes. All medications should be stored out of reach of children. Clients receiving home infusion therapy should be instructed on appropriate storage of intravenous medications and supplies.

Infection control measures are taught to all clients regardless of their diagnosis. Clients, families, and caregivers need to know about handwashing, disposal of waste and sharps, cleaning of blood and body

fluid spills, and other general household maintenance. The transmission of disease can be prevented
with adherence to infection control. See Chapter 8 on
Universal Precautions.

Home safety would not be complete without assessing the client's knowledge and ability to seek
emergency help. Emergency numbers should be
placed by the telephone. The client's phone number
should be on the phone in case 911 needs to be
called, and they need to know the number you are
calling from. Emergency contact persons and information should be obtained and kept on file by the
agency. Clients who live alone or have certain medical conditions may need to be assessed for an emergency response system.

It is necessary to document in the medical record
identified safety hazards, teaching done pertinent to
the safety hazards, and the client's response to teaching. Concise and accurate documentation facilitates
better coordination of teaching and care.

EMERGENCY SITUATIONS

The home care nurse needs to know how to recognize
and handle medical and nonmedical emergencies. It
is important to follow agency policies and procedures
for managing emergencies in the home. Unexpected
events can occur that will completely change the
plans for the home visit. Emergencies may be a life-
threatening illness or situations in which the nurse
must respond immediately. Emergency planning and
preparation is very important for the safety of clients
and their families.

Emergencies can happen at any time; therefore, careful planning may reduce chances of serious accidents and help the client deal with sudden illness. Clients with life-sustaining equipment or other electrically powered medical equipment should register with the utility and telephone companies and fire department. Severe weather conditions, such as blizzards, earthquakes, hurricanes, and floods, can be disastrous for anyone, but especially for clients receiving care at home. The nurse must know the agency's disaster or emergency plan.

Some medical emergencies require the nurse or caregiver to call 911 immediately. These are usually life-threatening conditions, such as heart attack or other acute cardiac impairment, respiratory distress, stroke, poisoning, severe burns, and imminent childbirth. Other medical conditions may be less acute but nonetheless require immediate nursing interventions or first aid.

Once the emergency medical system (EMS) has been activated, the nurse should perform appropriate emergency procedures. If there is a caregiver or family member in the home, they should assist with preparing for the arrival of the ambulance. The physician and agency must be notified of the emergency as soon as possible. If the client lives alone, the agency should also notify the emergency contact person.

Nurses who perform cardiopulmonary resuscitation (CPR) should wear gloves and use a protective face shield or mask. It is important to follow universal precautions and adhere to infection control guidelines. Caregivers and family members should also learn CPR through classes offered by the American Red Cross or Heart Association.

There are other possible situations in the home that will require the nurse to intervene, such as cases of suspected abuse, particularly involving children and elderly persons. Nurses are mandated to report to state officials cases of child and elder abuse and neglect.

INCIDENT REPORTING IN HOME CARE

The purpose of reporting incidents is to identify actual or potential situations that may cause harm or injury to clients, nurses, and other home care personnel. It is the responsibility of the home care agency to protect the health and safety of its clients and employees. The nurse must report accidents and other unusual events or situations that pose a liability risk to the agency.

Accidents that may cause injury to clients include falls, medication errors and adverse drug reactions, equipment malfunctions, and treatment errors. Other reportable events include the loss or damage of the client's property and missed visits. Missed visits occur when a scheduled home visit was not made.

Personnel-related incidents include injuries caused by falls, car accidents, violent crimes, and occupational exposures to infectious disease. According to federal and state regulations, occupational exposures to blood-borne and airborne pathogens must be reported. Therefore, agencies must track and provide medical follow-up for all needle stick injuries and exposures to tuberculosis.

Incident reporting is a function of the agency's quality improvement process. All agencies must have a system of reporting and documenting all accidents, injuries, and safety hazards related to the care provided. Incident reports are reviewed by a designated agency administrator for follow-up and management of risks.

CONCLUSIONS

In conclusion, safety precautions need to be followed by all home care nurses and by clients receiving care at home. The nurse must assess for safety and environmental hazards, then implement strategies to prevent injury or accidents. Nurses making the transition into home care must understand the importance of developing skills that will enable them to provide safe care in the community.

7

The Role and Responsibility of Paraprofessionals

Kathleen P. Murtagh, RN, MSN

This chapter discusses the home health aide (HHA), personal care worker (PCW), home attendant (HA), and family-employed substitute (FES). A sample home health aide/personal care worker plan of care and a functional status sheet are included, with guidelines for documentation.

HOME HEALTH AIDE

A home health aide (HHA) is a paraprofessional worker who attends a state-established training program. The program consists of at least 65 hours of classroom lectures and supervised practical training. A registered nurse (RN) observes the worker performing hands-on care for a client within the home setting for a minimum of 15 hours. The individual must complete the classroom instruction as well as the clinical experience before he or she receives a certificate as a certified HHA. After the HHA receives the certificate, he or she must attend 12 hours of in-service education on a yearly basis. Personnel qualifications for an HHA include such factors as commitment to caring for the sick and the ability to read, write, and follow directions. The responsibilities that an HHA can assume are taking a client's temperature, pulse, respiration, and simple record keeping as outlined by an RN. The HHA also can assist a client with transferring from bed to chair or to a wheelchair and can provide a bath, assist the client with dressing, or aid a client in toileting activities.

The HHA is a very important part of the home health care team. At times, the HHA may be the individual that makes the difference as to whether a client remains at home or enters a nursing home. These staff members can be a positive force in a client's life. The HHA communicates vital information to the nurse who visits the home when the HHA is providing care to a client. Reimbursement for an HHA is provided by Medicare, Medicaid, or a client's private insurance company. Reimbursement to a home care agency for HHA services is only provided for a specific period, depending on the client's skilled nursing needs and specific insurance carrier. The usual number of HHA hours Medicare allows is 20 hours per week. If a client only has Medicare and needs additional hours, the client will have to privately hire. If the client has both Medicare and Medicaid or only Medicaid, more than 20 hours of HHA service can be ordered for the client.

If a client needs some assistance with bathing, dressing, or meal preparation, the client is eligible for an HHA 5 days × 4 hours. The client needs to be fairly independent the rest of the time. Depending on the agency, an HHA may be placed in the morning from 9:00 A.M. to 1:00 P.M.; or in the afternoon from 1:00 P.M. to 5:00 P.M. The client is usually given a choice. However, if the nurse believes the client would do better with morning or afternoon help, the nurse should discuss this with the client. If a client needs total help, but a family member is home in the evening and is able to assist, the client may receive 8 or 12 hours each day. If family members are not able to assist, the nurse may need to consider more hours. If the client needs assistance with toileting around the clock, is confused and wanders, needs turning and positioning every 2 hours as to prevent skin breakdown, that client may need two 12-hour workers. If the client needs full assistance with activities of daily living (ADLs), and sleeps at night but cannot be left alone, this client may need 7-days-per-week, 24-hour coverage.

The HHA services must be discontinued by the nurse's last visit. If there are no longer skilled nursing needs, but the client or client's physician believes the client needs continued HHA-type services, the client must make arrangements to privately hire if Medicare or private coverage is the only insurance. If the client has Medicaid and still needs HHA-type services, he or she may be eligible for a PCW or HA.

PERSONAL CARE WORKER

A personal care worker (PCW) attends a state-approved training program that consists of at least 45 hours of classroom education and supervised clinical instruction, which is performed in the client's home. The PCW must complete 6 hours of in-service training per calendar year. Responsibilities include preparing or serving nutritious meals and assisting the client with personal care needs, including bathing, dressing, grooming, and oral hygiene. The PCW also can assist the client with walking and basic transfer activities. A PCW is only placed with a client receiving long-term home care services. PCWs are reimbursed and funded by a state Medicaid budget. The maximum number of PCW hours a client can receive is 42 hours each week, that is, a maximum of 6 hours per day, 7 days per week.

HOME ATTENDANT

A home attendant (HA) is a person who meets the requirements established by a State's Department of Social Services or Department of Health. An HA is able to assist a person at home who is sick, incapacitated, or who cares for someone who cannot be left in the absence of a significant other or caretaker.

The HA can perform household chores such as cooking, laundry, and cleaning. They also can assist the client with feeding, dressing, or bathing. Home attendant services are reimbursed and funded by a state Medicaid budget. The HA hours vary depending on the client's needs.

A client may be receiving HHA services under a Certified Home Health Agency (CHHA) program and may continue to need this type of service after being discharged from the CHHA. If the client is Medicaid eligible or has active Medicaid, the home care nurse may initiate the process for an HA by completing a form called an M11Q. The M11Q outlines why the client needs HA services. The form is sent to the local Medicaid office to be processed. When a client receives HA services, skilled nursing service is not required. When a client is already receiving HA services when admitted to a CHHA program, the HA continues to provide care to the client, and the nurse does not supervise that worker.

If the hospitalized client is Medicaid eligible or has active Medicaid, the client may be "bridged" to a home care agency. This means the client will receive nursing and HHA services under the CHHA. These Medicaid-eligible clients or active Medicaid clients will receive whatever number of HHA hours of service they need along with nursing services until the HA services begin. Once the HA services begin, the CHHA discharges the client. This conversion process could take from 2 to 4 months.

THE ROLE OF THE FAMILY-EMPLOYED SUBSTITUTE

A client or family member may choose to use a family-employed substitute (FES) to perform nursing-level activities. Selection is based on nursing judgment that a nonprofessional person can safely perform this skill without any foreseeable risks to the client or family substitute. The nurse is able to teach tasks that could otherwise be taught to family members.

A home care agency receives a referral for a nurse to teach an FES to perform a specific nursing skill. The FES must be available, agreeable, and capable of learning a nursing skill and performing it safely. A client's significant other or family member privately pays an FES a fee to provide a skill to a client. The home care agency may need to obtain a signed consent form from the client or family member designating the name of the FES and procedure/skill to be performed.

The nurse is responsible to provide the teaching and supervision of the FES. The nurse should continue to visit if there is a skilled nursing need such as monitoring a wound for signs and symptoms of infection.

If the nurse taught administration of oral medications and the FES is competent, the nurse may discharge the client from home care services. The nurse will teach and supervise all skills being performed. The nurse may need to complete a competency checklist, dates of demonstration, dates of return demonstration, and dates goals are achieved. Each time the nurse visits the client, he or she must document on the competency checklist and identify what goal has been met. A copy of the checklist is retained in the client' clinical record. The FES must sign each page of the competency checklist after all goals have been achieved. The FES has no affiliation with the home care agency or vendor agency.

DEFINITION AND CONCEPT OF CLUSTER CARE

Cluster care is a concept designed to provide task-oriented services to a group of clients living in their homes in a designated geographic area. This care is provided in a cost-effective, efficient manner.

Because of state budget cuts, legislators and governmental officials are requesting that home care agencies reorganize the way they deliver home care services without compromising the quality of care provided. Cluster care is a new model of home care, nontraditional in nature. It differs from the traditional model in that, instead of one HHA caring for one client, a group of clients share the services of one worker. The worker performs tasks or specific duties for a group of individuals rather than spending a designated number of hours with one client in his or her home each day.

Requirements for Cluster Care Program

Clients who are recipients of cluster care must live in close proximity. Many times the clients live in a senior housing complex, and support is also obtained from the housing facility. Senior housing units are also popular cluster care sites because many of the tenants living in the apartments are receiving home care services, often from the same home care agency.

Client Criteria

To ensure that a client can participate in a cluster care program, an RN from the home care agency visits the client at home. The RN interviews and performs a nursing assessment to determine whether the client is a candidate for cluster care. The client must be alert, oriented, and mentally stable. He or she must be able to be left alone safely for periods throughout the day and night. The individual must be ambulatory as opposed to bedbound. He or she must also be self-directing and have the ability to summon help in an emergency. Clients who participate in this program cannot be out of the home for extended periods.

Clients also must be flexible and have the ability to accommodate multiple visits from an HHA, depending on the tasks that are scheduled throughout the day. Clients' families and caretakers must be supportive and receptive to this model of home care.

The nurse who performs the assessment must interview the client, formulate a picture of his or her needs, and determine whether he or she is a good candidate for this program. The nurse from the home care agency would also collaborate with the client's physician and inform the physician that the client is going to participate in cluster care.

Requirements for Home Health Aides

HHAs who provide task-oriented services for cluster care clients must possess certain qualifications. They must be mature, flexible, and motivated. They must be experienced HHAs and work in an organized, systematic manner. They must possess a high energy level and have the ability to communicate effectively. They must be able to make appropriate decisions.

Although many HHAs are good candidates for cluster care, many times they must be encouraged to participate. Cluster care workers may earn more per hour because they are responsible for the care of more than one client at a time. A cluster care aide is usually assigned to care for three clients at a time.

Scheduling

After interviewing the client, the nurse assesses the client to determine what types of tasks the client will require based on his or her needs. Schedules are created around the client, not around the HHA. The client is the focal point, and the schedule is built around the client's needs.

The home care agency nurse develops the daily schedule. The schedule lists all of the services the client will require. Often tasks are grouped into categories such as personal care, nutrition, and housekeeping. For example, bathing, dressing, and grooming may be grouped together for the morning hours for each cluster care client. Other tasks such as laundry, errands, and food shopping for the cluster care clients may be scheduled for a block of time during the midafternoon hours.

For organizational purposes and to ensure that time is used in an efficient, effective manner, the aide should become familiar with where the bank and grocery store are located in the neighborhood. Meals may be scheduled according to the client's preferences. If clients are living in a senior citizen housing facility, they may eat lunch together in a common hall or community room.

When creating a schedule, you must take into consideration that a community health nurse may be visiting a client to perform a nursing visit, and time must be allotted for that nursing visit. The client may have physician visits or other scheduled appointments that must be built into the daily schedule for each cluster care client. Creativity and flexibility are two key ingredients needed when developing a schedule to meet the ever-changing needs of the clients.

Staffing Pattern

Most often, two different aides are assigned to care for the cluster care client. The lead aide is the worker who will consistently provide task services for the three clients. However, in the event the lead aide is out sick, on vacation, or an emergency arises and he or she is unable to work, the other aide who is familiar with the clients and their schedules will be assigned to care for those clients.

If the client is receiving services from a certified home health care agency or long-term home health care program, the community health nurse is responsible to supervise the aide once every 2 weeks. They must supervise the aide while he or she is performing a task. They must review the plan of care and schedule with the aide as well as with the client to ensure the tasks are being performed and that the client is satisfied with the services.

The HHAs involved in cluster care must be trained on how to complete their time sheets, because this may be different for cluster care clients. Because this is a new model of care, open communication as well as support for the aides is critical because they are caring for more than one client at a time. The community health nurse and the HHA must work as a team to provide quality-oriented care to cluster care clients.

How to Determine Home Health Aide Hours

When evaluating the number of HHA hours a client requires, you assess the client's needs based on his or her dependence or independence in all ADLs on a 24-hour basis, 7 days per week. During your initial assessment and interview of the client, you must obtain information regarding whether the client has any informal supports, significant others, or family to assist him or her with ADLs on a daily basis:

- If a client needs some assistance with bathing, grooming, or dressing, the HHA may need to assist the client 2 hours per day, 3 days per week. The client may need some assistance with an exercise program but may be independent in transfer activities. The client is alert and able to direct the aide in what type of assistance he or she may need.

- A client may need assistance 5 days per week, 4 hours per day, when he or she requires moderate assistance with personal care, such as a tub bath, showering, and shampooing of hair, or the aide may need to help the client get dressed. The client may be independent in toileting, but may use a urinary device such as a cysto tube, Foley catheter, or external catheter. This type of client is able to direct the HHA. This client may use a personal alarm response system (PERS) if he or she is alone and needs to summon help. This individual may fatigue easily because of the medical condition and may become short of breath during increased activity.

- A client may need from 5 to 8 hours each day if he or she needs the assistance of an HHA to bathe, provide skin care to promote skin integrity, and assist with articles of clothing to dress as well as grooming. This client is safe alone; however he or she uses a PERS for safety reasons. The client is independent in feeding but needs assistance with cooking and meal preparation. The client is independent in toileting but may have an external catheter or may use a commode, bedpan, or raised toilet seat to assist with this activity.

- A client needs 9 to 12 hours of HHA services each day when he or she is alert and oriented and has the ability to direct an HHA but needs a great deal of assistance with bathing, dressing, food shopping, meal preparation, and household chores. The client would need assistance with feeding and may need verbal encouragement to eat during mealtime. The client may have difficulty with transfer activity and may need assistive devices to perform transfers and the assistance of an HHA to transfer from the bed to a sitting position. When the HHA is not present, this individual must have a PERS unit and use it in the event an emergency occurs. The HHA would assist with toileting activities; however, the client may use a commode, bedpan, or urinal or may need some type of Foley or external catheter for toileting.

- A client may require 24-hour HHA services when maximum assistance with bathing, dressing, feeding, meal preparation, and toileting activities is needed. The client may or may not be oriented at all times; however, there may be a significant other who agrees to be involved with this client and give instructions and directions to the HHA who provides care to this client on a 24-hour basis. The significant other or family member may be available if an emergency occurs or a decision regarding the client needs to be made.

  The client who needs a 24-hour HHA may be unable to move in bed because of a medical condition. The HHA would provide skin care and turn and position the client throughout the day to increase circulation to prevent skin breakdown. The client will be dependent on the aide to assist with toileting or using a toileting device.

  The client needs to have a home or apartment that can accommodate the aide and a place for the aide to sleep. The HHA does live in and does not have to wake up more than once during a 7-hour sleep period to provide assistance to the client.

- A client may require two HHAs who work 12 hours each per day because the client's physical care is such that they need maximum assistance around-the-clock both day and night. The client's home environment may not be able to accommodate a live-in HHA, but the client needs total assistance with all ADLs. The client may be unable to move in bed or may be totally dependent on toileting activities. The client may be incontinent of urine and feces and may need the HHA to change diapers, bed linens, and provide skin care to prevent skin breakdown. This client may be confused and disoriented. The client lives alone; however, someone is usually available in the event an emergency occurs or a decision must be made regarding the client's plan of care.

FUNCTIONAL STATUS FORM

The nurse within the home care agency may complete a functional status form to best determine how many hours the client really needs (Display 7-1). A nurse would complete the form, line by line, and determine if the client is independent, needs some assistance, or needs full assistance in the particular function.

This functional status form enables the nurse to obtain and ask the necessary questions regarding how much help the client really needs with ADLs. The nurse must be able to visualize and mentally formulate a picture of the client in the home and get a clear

DISPLAY 7-1. Functional Status Form

Patient's Name: _____ ID #: _____

Functional Status and Level of Independence

Ambulation	Indep. _____	Some assist _____	Full assist _____
Eating	Indep. _____	Some assist _____	Full assist _____
Meal prep	Indep. _____	Some assist _____	Full assist _____
Toileting	Indep. _____	Some assist _____	Full assist _____
Transfer	Indep. _____	Some assist _____	Full assist _____
Dressing	Indep. _____	Some assist _____	Full assist _____
Bathing	Indep. _____	Some assist _____	Full assist _____
Shopping	Indep. _____	Some assist _____	Full assist _____
Cleaning	Indep. _____	Some assist _____	Full assist _____
Laundry	Indep. _____	Some assist _____	Full assist _____

Please circle services needed:

Home health aide   Personal care worker   GSS worker   Private hire

_____ Days × _____ Hours A.M. _____ P.M. _____

V.N. Signature _____   Date _____

© With permission. S. Zang

sense clinically of how much physical help the client needs to be safe at home. Functions include ambulation, eating, meal preparation, toileting, transfer, dressing, bathing, shopping, cleaning, and laundry. For each category, the nurse would determine how much assistance is needed. For the first category, *ambulation,* the nurse would determine whether the client could walk without any assistance or whether he or she needs a cane or walker to ambulate. The nurse would also determine the distance the client could ambulate. The client may need another individual to assist with ambulation, which would constitute full assistance, or may be bed bound or totally wheelchair bound and cannot ambulate at all.

For *eating,* the nurse would determine whether the client could feed himself or himself or requires some assistance such as verbal encouragement to complete the task. The client may need to be fed and then would require maximum or full assistance for this task. The nurse may evaluate whether the client could *prepare a meal* or whether the worker has to gather the food and help the client prepare the meal. The HHA may totally prepare the meal, and then the client needs full assistance in this area.

The client may be totally independent in *toileting.* However, the client may need the worker to accompany the client to the bathroom and partially assist the client with this activity. The client may need full assistance in this area, whereby the HHA takes the client to the bathroom, placing the individual on the toilet, staying with client at all times during toileting for safety purposes, and totally assisting them until they are finished.

For *transfer,* the nurse should document what type of transfer it is. For example, is it sit-to-stand, or wheelchair-to-bed? The client may not need any assistance in this area and would be totally independent in this function. The client may need some help to perform transfer activity, and then the nurse would document "some assistance." If the client needs total assistance, the worker would have to completely transfer the client, bed to wheelchair, or from a standing to sitting position. If the client lives alone and needs full assistance with this activity, 24-hour assistance is indicated.

For *dressing,* the nurse would determine how much assistance the client needs. The HHA may need to help with some articles of clothing, such as buttons or zippers, or the individual may need full assistance, in which the HHA needs to actually put the clothing on and dress the person completely.

For *bathing,* the nurse would ask the client how he or she does this task. Does the person take a tub bath or a shower? Does the client need assistance with turning the water on and testing the temperature to ensure it is not too hot to avoid burns? Does the client need some help with washing his or her back or is the client able to bend down and wash the lower legs or feet? This means he or she can perform some of the activity but needs some assistance. If the client needs full assistance, the HHA would have to perform this activity entirely, that is, to shower or bathe the person totally.

The client may need some help with food *shopping,* whereby the worker would accompany the client to the grocery store and take items off the shelf, wheel the shopping cart around the store, and carry the bags of groceries home with the client. Full assistance with shopping means the HHA may go to the store and food shop alone, bring the items into the client's home, and put them away in the refrigerator or storage cabinets.

For *cleaning*, the HHA may need to provide some assistance to the client in which he or she would help the individual make the beds or mop the kitchen floor or clean the bathroom, because the client could not perform this type of cleaning because of medical problems.

The client may need the HHA to perform light housekeeping, which would include vacuuming, dusting the client's room, or cleaning the entire bathroom because the client cannot perform these activities because of fatigue, weakness, or the amount of energy it takes to perform heavier household cleaning.

Regarding *laundry,* the client may need the worker to help remove sheets, carry a laundry bag up or down stairs, and place clothing in the machine. The client may need full assistance if he or she cannot remove bed linens, wash or dry clothes, or put them away.

After completing each category, line by line, the nurse would determine how many hours the client needs and what type of insurance the client has. The nurse would indicate the type of worker, whether it is an HHA, PCW, or HA. If the client already has an HA, the nurse is not responsible for determining the number of hours the client receives. If the nurse assesses that the HA hours are not enough, the nurse should contact the HA vendor agency and speak with the caseworker regarding the problem.

The nurse receives the Health Care Financing Administration (HCFA) 485, which may already have the prescribed orders for the HHA. This may be because of the client's insurance coverage, whereby the case manager from the insurance company authorizes the number of hours that will be approved. The HHA services may not be ordered on the 485. It may be the responsibility of the nurse on the initial visit to evaluate the client's functional status or determine how many hours are needed or if the hours that were ordered are adequate or need to be changed.

The HHA's responsibility is to only take care of the client receiving services. The HHA is not permitted to perform duties for family members or others living in the home. At times the HHA may be asked to do laundry or clean dirty dishes that are the client's spouse's or significant other's. The worker must communicate this to the nurse, who then discusses it with the client and family member/significant other. The client also may be extremely difficult to care for. He or she may have unrealistic expectations as to what the worker should do.

Many times the client may request a different worker because the worker is not performing the activities the client believes this worker should be performing. The HHA may contact his or her agency and ask to be taken off the case. The client may be requesting heavy-duty housekeeping, such as washing blankets and curtains or cleaning the stove. These tasks are not included in the plan of care, and the nurse may need to discuss this with the client. When this occurs, the home care agency needs to be apprised that the client may be difficult to serve. The nurse should make a home visit to discuss this with the client and family member and also to supervise the worker. At times the nurse must set limits with the client. The nurse must outline each step of the HHA plan of care with the client and family member. At times a written contract has to be implemented if the client continually requests the worker to be changed, or if most of the HHAs cannot remain on the case to care for the client.

If the nurse does visit the client and makes the determination that the HHA needs to be changed, the nurse should contact the agency and request a different worker for the client. Clients can be very demanding, and often the nurse needs to set limits and review and reinforce exactly what the HHA is responsible to do. Over time, the client and HHA may develop a working relationship.

SPECIFIC DUTIES AND FORMATION OF THE PLAN OF CARE

The nurse, on the initial visit to the client's home, performs a nursing assessment and determines whether the number of hours that the HHA is working meets the client's needs. The nurse completes the *plan of care form,* which outlines the specific duties that the HHA/PCW will perform for the client. A sample plan of care that the nurse completes is provided (Display 7-2).

The nurse checks off whether it is an HHA or a PCW assigned to the client. An HHA is used for the CHHA. A PCW or housekeeper (HSK) is the only paraprofessional used for the Long-Term Home Health Care Program (LTHHC).

To determine how many hours a PCW will work, the client's functional status must be determined. Because a PCW can only be provided for a maximum of 42 hours per week, a client needs to be safe at home alone and therefore cannot need full assistance in

DISPLAY 7-2. Plan of Care Form

( ) **HHA**   ( ) **PCW**

_____ Days x _____ Hours   Vendor _____

Patient's name: _____

Address: _____

(Please review plan of care with paraprofessional and update as needed.)

Services to be provided   **Instructions**

Mouthcare: _____

Footcare: _____

Shampoo: ( ) Bed ( ) Sink ( ) Tub _____

Skin care: ( ) Lotion ( ) Massage _____

Nail care: ( ) Fingers ( ) Toes _____

Bath: ( ) Bed ( ) Sponge ( ) Tub ( ) Shower _____

Toileting: ( ) Diaper ( ) Bedpan ( ) Urinal ( ) Commode ( ) Toilet _____

Dressing: ( ) Upper ( ) Lower ( ) Shoes _____

Other: (Specify): _____

Meal preparation: ( ) Breakfast ( ) Lunch ( ) Dinner ( ) Snack _____

Diet (fill in) _____ Fluids (ad lib) _____ Restricted _____

Feed patient _____ Assist w/feeding _____ ( ) Cut food ( ) Prepare tray

Walking _____ ( ) Crutches ( ) Walker ( ) Cane ( ) Guarding ( ) Quad care

Transfers: ( ) Full assist ( ) Partial assist _____

Turning and positioning: ( ) Full assist ( ) Partial assist _____

Range of motion: _____ Active _____ Passive _____

Catheter care (specify) _____

Ostomy care (specify) _____

Measure & record: Intake _____ Output _____

Measure & record: _____ Temp. _____ Pulse _____ Resp. _____ Oral _____ Rectal _____ Auxil.

Medications _____ Assist _____ Remind _____

VN Signature: _____ Date _____

© With permission. S. Zang

transfer activity or toileting. The client may need some assistance with activities such as bathing, dressing, medication preparation, or ambulation. Clients receiving a PCW under the LTHHC Program may receive the worker 3 days × 4 hours, 5 days × 4 hours, or 7 days × 6 hours, depending on how much assistance is need with ADL. A client also may receive housekeeping services under the LTHHC Program.

To evaluate a long-term client for housekeeping services, the functional status form is used. If the client is independent in ambulation, eating, toileting, transfer, dressing, and bathing but unable to do household chores, a housekeeper would be provided. If the client does need some assistance with meal preparation, shopping, cleaning, and laundry, a housekeeper would be provided 2 days × 4 hours each week.

The nurse who completes the plan of care form indicates what vendor agency the worker is employed by. The nurse writes the client's name and address and completes the plan of care form line by line, specifying instructions on the form the worker is to follow while he or she is providing care to the client.

For oral care, the nurse should indicate whether the client has upper or lower dentures or both. If the client washes the dentures with a particular product, the nurse indicates that on the form. For foot care, the worker is allowed to soak the client's feet in warm water and soap. The worker should dry the client's feet thoroughly. If the client is diabetic, the nurse should indicate in the instructions not to cut the client's toenails.

The client should indicate how often he or she would like a shampoo. The nurse should indicate if this is to be done at the sink, or during a tub or bed bath. The nurse should teach and reinforce to the worker the importance of skin care. Lotion would be checked off if the client has very dry skin. Light gentle massage should be performed only if it is not medically contraindicated. If a client has vascular problems, or if there is a history of phlebitis, instructions would be documented not to massage skin. The worker should also soak the client's fingernails in warm water with some soap, and any dirt should be removed from under the fingernail. The worker may cut the client's fingernails and toenails, using the proper scissors. Special instructions should indicate that the nails are not to be cut too close.

On the plan of care form, the nurse should check off the type of bath being provided to the client, based on the client's functional status. The type of bath could be bed, sponge, tub, or shower. If the worker is going to provide a bed bath, the worker should gather all of the supplies, such as basin, washcloth, towel, soap, and drying towel needed for the bath. The bath is usually performed at a specific time during the day or depending on when the client wants this done. The worker should start with the face and work down to the client's feet. The worker should wash each body part thoroughly and ensure that the client is kept covered to prevent the client from getting a chill.

If a sponge bath is given, the worker uses a basin of warm water and soap, and the client is washed with a washcloth. Once again, the client is kept covered to prevent getting a chill. A shower is usually given when a client needs some assistance with bathing. The nurse should indicate under the instruction section that the worker should turn the water on and test the temperature to prevent skin burns.

Under toileting, the nurse should indicate if the client wears a diaper or uses a bedpan, urinal, commode, or toilet. If the client is incontinent of urine, feces, or both, the worker should change the client's diaper on a regular basis to prevent skin breakdown. If a client is bedbound, he or she may need assistance using a bedpan or a urinal. The nurse should indicate whether the client needs assistance using a commode or needs help with toileting.

The client may need help with dressing. Under instructions, the nurse should indicate whether the client needs assistance with putting clothes on or taking them off, or with buttons or zippers. If the nurse checks off shoes, it should be indicated whether help is needed with tying shoelaces.

For meal preparation, the nurse would indicate what meal has to be prepared. If the client is on a special diet, the nurse would review with the client and worker dietary restrictions that should be followed. The worker would cook and prepare the meal for the client. The worker also may be required to prepare a meal for a late lunch or dinner and leave the meal prepared for the client to eat later in the day.

Many clients require special diets, depending on their medical condition. The nurse would include nutritional counseling as part of the visit. If the client is on restricted fluids, the nurse would review with the worker and client the importance of keeping a written record of fluid intake. This would ensure that the fluid restriction was being maintained.

The worker may need to feed the client or assist with cutting food or opening containers. The worker may set up a food tray and sit with the client to ensure that the client eats the meal that was prepared.

Many times a client will only eat if the worker encourages him or her to do so.

The nurse should check off on the plan of care whether the client requires assistance with walking. The nurse should indicate whether the client needs an assistive device such as crutches, walker, cane, guarding, or quad cane. If the client needs the assistance of another person to ambulate, the worker should accompany the client in that activity to ensure that safety is maintained.

If the client needs assistance with transfers, it should be indicated whether it is full assistance or partial assistance. The worker may have to totally transfer the client from one position to another such as from the bed to a wheelchair. If a Hoyer lift, which is a piece of equipment used to transfer a client, is required, the nurse must teach, observe, and supervise the worker using this piece of equipment. If the client needs some help with transfer, the worker may need to provide arm support during the transfer and ensure that the client moves from one position to another safely.

If the client is bedbound or spends a great deal of time in bed, the client may need full assistance with turning and positioning at least every 2 hours. This will increase circulation to bony prominences and prevent skin breakdown. A client also may need minimal assistance moving from one position to another.

For range of motion (ROM) activity, the worker needs to be taught, observed, and supervised. Many times ROM exercises are performed after a bath or in the morning hours. This would be indicated under special instructions.

If a client has a catheter, the nurse would document exactly the type of care that the worker could perform on the plan of care. If a client has a Foley catheter, catheter care would include washing around the catheter site with warm water and mild soap.

The HHA is only permitted to change an ostomy bag. The client usually performs his or her own ostomy care, and the worker is required to either apply the ostomy bag or assist the client in doing so.

The worker may be required to measure and record a client's intake and output. This would be done for clients who are on fluid restrictions. A record is kept by the HHA and reviewed by the nurse each visit.

The HHA may need to assist the client with medications. The HHA is not permitted to administer medications to the client. The worker can bring the medication to the client and remind the client to take it. The nurse can be involved in prepouring medications for the client or setting up a chart. In this way, the HHA can work with the client and ensure that the client takes the medication at the prescribed time.

The nurse must sign the plan of care and date it when it is completed. The nurse discusses and reviews the plan of care with both the client and the worker each visit. The HHA must acknowledge that he or she understands the assignment and communicate this to the nurse. The plan of care is kept in the client's home, usually posted on the refrigerator, and a copy is kept in the client's clinical record in the home care office.

The nurse visits the client and supervises the HHA while he or she is providing care. All care that is taught and supervised is recorded on the progress note.

The HHA's plan of care is modified whenever necessary to meet the needs of the client. A copy of the revised plan of care is placed in the client's home, a copy is sent to the vendor agency for its records, and a copy is placed in the client's clinical record. When a client is receiving skilled nursing services under a CHHA, once the nurse begins to taper the frequency of the visits, the hours of HHA are also tapered.

The nurse begins discharge plans from the first nursing visit. The nurse explains to the client that as he or she becomes independent in care, the HHA will also be needed less and will be tapered. Many times the HHA services and nursing services are tapered and then discharged on the same day.

Unit

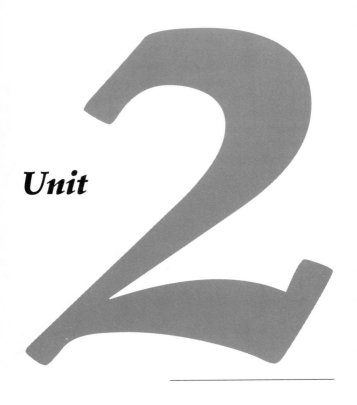

THE HOME VISIT

8

Universal Precautions

Nellie C. Bailey, RN, MS, MA, CS

The importance of protection from and prevention of the spread of infectious diseases such as human immunodeficiency virus (HIV) and hepatitis B virus (HBV) is a public health concern for the nurse, client, and caregiver in home health care. Universal precautions implies that all body fluid is potentially contaminated and should be handled with precaution. The practice of universal precautions is also important because, if the client has HIV/acquired immune deficiency syndrome (AIDS), because of client confidentiality rights, the family and home health aide (HHA)/personal care worker (PCW) might not be aware of the client's diagnosis. Because the prevalence of infectious disease continues to increase, the nurse must be knowledgeable of necessary measures to protect herself or himself and caregivers in the home. This chapter includes specific details, beginning with handwashing and concluding with the disposal of infectious wastes in the home setting. Information presented is based on the Centers for Disease Control (CDC) infection control guidelines.

HANDWASHING

Handwashing is well established as the most effective method of preventing the spread of disease. Handwashing should be the first thing the nurse does, after establishing with the client where the visit will be conducted, before any contact with the client. To ensure adequate compliance, the client and family/caregiver should be instructed in the practice of universal precautions.

First and foremost, the nurse must carry liquid soap and disposable paper towels in the nursing bag. The nurse is responsible for maintaining a clean bag, supplies, and equipment. The agency may provide the bag, supplies, and replacements as needed or the nurse may be responsible for obtaining his or her own bag and supplies. Part of the nursing home visit "bag technique" requires that the soap and paper towels be placed in an outside pocket of the nursing bag, or other convenient location, so that they can be removed while maintaining a clean bag inside. The nursing bag should never be placed on the floor. Instead, the nurse should carry newspaper or paper towels on which to place the bag when in the client's home. All equipment should be properly cleaned before replacement in the bag. Disposable equipment or the client's own equipment should be used whenever possible.

Standard Bag Equipment

disposable sterile and unsterile gloves
4 inch × 4 inch gauze squares
scissors
resuscitation mask
oral thermometers
bottle of liquid soap
bottle of alcohol gel hand cleanser
tongue depressors
roll of non-allergic tape
alcohol wipettes
stethoscope
sphygmomanometer
pen light
tape measure
drug book

To further prevent the spread of infection, it is recommended that the nurse wear minimal jewelry on the wrists and hands. Jewelry with stones or ridges should be removed before handwashing.

Proper handwashing includes applying adequate soap and using friction and continuous running water. Special cleansing should be done to nails and between the fingers. It is also recommended that, after handwashing and drying, the paper towel should be used to turn off the faucet. It is the nurse's responsibility to teach proper handwashing technique to the HHA/PCW and family members. The nurse should also teach the client to wash his or her hands after toileting, after performing personal care, and before preparing food. Handwashing should be performed by the nurse as follows: before beginning each client contact, at the end of the visit, before and after gloving, and after each exposure to any form of contamination. If the nurse is visiting more than one client in the home, such as a mother and baby, hands must be washed between clients.

The nurse never knows when a home will not have adequate hot and cold running water or even a sink that is suitable for handwashing. It is always wise to carry some other type of handwashing supplies for such situations. There are commercially prepared antiseptic towelettes and handwashing products available such as gels or foams. These products come in individually wrapped packets or squeeze bottles and are handy to carry in the nursing bag. They are designed to evaporate after handwashing, thus eliminating drying with paper towels.

INSTRUMENTS

The client's own instruments should be used as much as possible. Instruments such as scissors and clamps from the nurse's bag should be cleansed thoroughly after use. Instruments should be washed with soap and water, wiped with alcohol, and dried thoroughly before replacing them into the nurse's bag. If the client has draining lesions, the recommendation is that the lesion should be covered with a dry sterile dressing. A piece of clear plastic wrap should be placed over the client's extremity before applying the blood pressure cuff. The stethoscope must be wiped with alcohol after each use. If the blood pressure cuff becomes soiled, it should be cleaned with alcohol immediately after use.

Thermometers for oral and rectal use should be labeled and kept separate. The thermometer should be wiped with alcohol after use and placed in a clean dry container. The nurse must use a protective sheath if the thermometer is to be used from the nurse's bag. The sheath should be disposed of according to universal precaution procedures. After use, the thermometer should be wiped with alcohol.

PROTECTIVE EQUIPMENT

Disposable resuscitation masks are to be used for direct mouth-to-mouth contact whenever necessary. The masks might be provided by the home health agency. However, a one-way valve resuscitation pocket mask is another type of emergency protective equipment that the nurse might have in the nursing bag. Generally, the valve and filter must be discarded after a single client use. The mask is reusable and should be washed and scrubbed in warm soapy water, rinsed in clean water, and submerged in a very diluted (1:64) household bleach:water solution, rinsed again, and allowed to air dry. Because there are various types of resuscitation masks that are practical for use in the home, the nurse should check the manufacturer's instruction regarding use, storage, and cleansing of the type he or she will use.

Disposable masks and gloves should be worn during procedures that will potentially generate splashing of blood or body fluids, such as when a client is coughing excessively and is not able to cover his or her mouth; suctioning; irrigation; changing dressings; Foley catheterization; performing fingerstick for glucose monitoring; emptying or checking urinary drainage or other types of body fluid drainage bags; venipuncture; and handling intravenous lines.

In addition, disposable gloves are to be worn when palpating for edema in an area of broken skin or open lesions or cleansing any body orifice. The nurse should remember that after removing soiled bandages/dressings, the gloves must be discarded and changed. The nurse also must be mindful to conserve the client's supplies; therefore, unsterile disposable gloves may be used to remove soiled bandages/dressings. Sterile gloves must be used for cleansing wounds and applying fresh sterile dressings. Disposable gloves should be used also when removing incontinent pads, vaginal pads, or diapers.

The HHA/PCW and family members should also be taught not to use the client's sterile gloves and other supplies unnecessarily, for example, to bathe the client or wipe furniture. The HHA/PCW must be instructed to discard disposable gloves after each use and to use household gloves while performing light housekeeping chores such as dish washing, dusting, vacuuming, or mopping.

Protective eyewear and disposable gowns or plastic aprons are to be worn when there is the likelihood of splashing that will soil clothes or contaminate the face or eyes. Those procedures would include those discussed at the beginning of this section under masks and gloves. This equipment should not be reused. It should be placed in a plastic bag, tied, and discarded after each use.

LINEN

The HHA/PCW and family should be instructed not to shake the linen when making the client's bed. Contaminated linen should not be permitted to come in contact with clean linen, clothing, or other surface areas. The linen should be changed daily and as often as necessary. In addition, soiled linen should be stored separately in a tied plastic bag before washing; soiled linen should also be washed separately in a washing machine in hot soapy water with chlorine bleach added. After washing, the laundry should be machine dried whenever possible. Linen that is heavily soiled should be soaked for 10 minutes in a bleach solution before washing. Linen and clothing that are not colorfast or made of silk wool should be washed in warm water with Lysol® or a similar phenolic disinfectant and rinsed thoroughly. If laundering must be done by hand, washing should be done in the bathroom sink or tub or in a basin. Washing of laundry should not be done in the kitchen sink. Gloves should be worn when washing by hand. The area used should be cleansed with household bleach after laundering is done. The family/caregivers should be instructed to wash their hands after doing the laundry.

SHARPS

In some instances, clients have commercially produced puncture-resistant sharps containers to be used for the disposal of needles, syringes, and other sharps such as lancets and razor blades used in the home. These items should be disposed of immediately after use. Depending on the agency's policy, containers such as a tin coffee can with a lid or the hard plastic detergent, bleach, softener, or cooking oil container are used. All sharps containers must have a lid that fits securely. Needles are not to be recapped, broken, bent, or separated from the syringe. Neither is the syringe to be separated. Instead, immediately after use, the complete syringe unit and lancets are to be placed in the puncture-proof container. Home care agency policy might vary regarding sharps disposal. General guidelines for disposal are as follow: used needles and lancets (sharps) are stored in the puncture-proof container until it is approximately two-thirds full; a 1:10 solution of bleach and water is added; the container is closed, and the lid is taped. The container is then placed in a double plastic bag, tied, and discarded. Clients, family, and HHA/PCW should be taught to keep the container in a discrete place, out of the reach of children, such as in the cabinet under the sink, until it is to be discarded. It is the nurse's responsibility to teach the client, family, and caregiver the procedure for disposal of needles and have them give a return demonstration. Documentation of the teaching and return demonstration are to be recorded on the visit note. Each nursing revisit note should reflect reassessment and the client's, family's, or caregiver's application and knowledge of universal precautions.

SPILLS OF BLOOD OR BODY FLUID

Spills of blood and other potentially infected materials must be cleaned up immediately with a 1:10 bleach solution. The area should then be rinsed thoroughly. Large spills should be cleaned with paper towels or newspaper first, which are discarded immediately, before mopping the area with warm soapy water and bleach. Spills that come in contact with the skin must be washed immediately with liquid soap and running water. These instructions must be taught to the HHA/PCW.

The nurse should also teach the family, client, and HHA/PCW that clothes that are contaminated with spills must be removed immediately and stored properly for washing. Equipment such as the bed frame, side rails, or suction machine that becomes splashed with blood or body fluid should be washed as soon as possible with soap and water and dried thoroughly.

GUIDELINES FOR INCIDENCE OF RISK EXPOSURE

The nurse must be familiar with the agency's policies regarding HBV and HIV/AIDS risk exposure. In today's health care systems, most agencies, including home health care, require that professional staff receive the HBV vaccine or sign a statement of decline. Polices may vary from agency to agency and from state to state. General guidelines require that if the nurse, HHA/PCW, or caregiver has been exposed through splashing into eyes, the area is to be immediately flushed thoroughly with water, the agency supervisor must be notified, and the individual is to be seen by a physician.

Spills onto broken skin surface are to be washed thoroughly with soap and water and rinsed with plain water; the agency supervisor is to be notified, and the individual is to be seen by a physician. The agency might require that the nurse fill out an incident report.

If a nurse incurs a puncture wound or needle stick while caring for a client in the home, the injury should be reported immediately to the appropriate agency personnel. Depending on the agency, that person might be the supervisor or risk manager. The guidelines for the particular agency then will be followed. Some agencies, however, provide HIV and HBV testing free of charge. The nurse then will be referred to the city Health Department or to his or her own physician for precounseling before the HIV test is performed. Some agencies provide free counseling. Postcounseling services also may be provided. Additional procedures also might be included.

The HHA/PCW must be instructed to report any such incident immediately. Because home health care is a 24-hour service in many cities, such incidents can be reported to the weekend supervisor or other designated personnel.

DISPOSAL OF INFECTIOUS WASTE

Disposable gloves must be worn when disposing of waste. Hands should be washed immediately after handling waste. Contaminated and potentially contaminated waste should not be left in the client's home overnight. A waste container lined with two plastic bags, of any color except red, must be kept in the client's room for disposal supplies. In some cities, the sanitation department will not pick up red plastic bags. Small amounts of waste may be properly bagged and discarded at least once daily. Large waste such as all types of catheters, intravenous (IV) lines, large amounts of soiled dressings, drainage bags, and underpads should be bagged, tied, and discarded immediately in the regular outside garbage disposal.

Items soiled with visible blood should be soaked with a 1:10 solution of household bleach before discarding. Liquids such as urine, vomitus, drainage, and feces should be flushed down the toilet. The family, client, and HHA/PCW must be instructed never to pour liquid waste in the sink or in the garbage. They should also be taught to avoid splashing when discarding liquid wastes. Noncommercial punctureproof sharps containers should be stored and bagged as previously discussed and put out close as possible to the garbage pick-up day. Clients should be instructed that clear plastic beverage bottles are not suitable as sharps disposals.

OTHER PRECAUTIONS

Liquid soap should be used in the client's bathroom instead of bar soap. The client and family/caregiver should be instructed to replace towels and washcloths daily. The toilet bowl should be cleansed with full-strength household bleach. The bathtub and sink should be disinfected with a bleach and water solution. Dishes may be put in the dishwasher or should be washed in hot soapy water. Dishes used by the client need not be separated from those used by the rest of the household. The client also should be instructed not to share personal items such as toothbrush, makeup, razor, and razor blades. The toothbrush should be soaked in 1:3 solution of peroxide and water once a week for 15 minutes. Razor blades should be disposed of in the same manner as other sharps.

CONCLUSIONS

Universal precautions are necessary to help prevent the spread of disease. With the resurgence of previously controlled infectious diseases and the development of new ones, these precautions are important for lay persons as well as professionals. If universal precautions are practiced properly, the home health care clients and nursing personnel can be protected from both spreading and contracting communicable diseases.

9

The Role
of the Nurse

Emma Kontzamanis, RN, BSN, MA

Documentation   Conclusions
Case Study

The nurse is an integral part of the delivery and success of home health care. The nurse assesses the client's needs at home and integrates the client and client's support system into the plan of care. Communication of the findings of the nurse's visit enhances the home care process and enables all members of the team to effectively plan to provide needed services. The gamut of services that can be provided includes medical, nursing, physical, speech, and occupational therapy, social work, nutrition, home health aide, laboratory, medical supplies, and durable medical equipment. This collaborative approach to health care ensures that the whole client will be treated.

The knowledge and skills needed to maintain the client safely at home must be taught to the client or caregiver to ensure continuity of care 24 hours a day. Coping mechanisms and the ability to be an active participant in the plan of care should be assessed as well as the living situation and family history. How the client functioned in the past will influence the client's clinical course. For example, if the family assisted the client before the illness, will they be able to assist the client now while they are receiving home care services?

The provision of direct care on an intermittent basis is another component of the nurse's role. Administering parenteral medication, providing wound or Foley catheter care, and physical assessment are examples of direct care. Teaching the client or the caregiver instructions regarding medications, diet, activity, and specific treatments is also direct care.

The nurse functions as a case manager, overseeing the total care the client receives at home, communicating with all disciplines to ensure comprehensive cost-effective care. The nurse needs to assist clients to negotiate the complex health care system. Frequent telephone and written communication allows this to be done. Case conferences among various disciplines may be regularly scheduled. Changes in the client's condition are reported, and changes in the plan of care are discussed and implemented. As the coordinator of services and case manager, the nurse must report abnormal findings or significant changes in client status to the client's physician. The nurse also must order services and supplies as needed. In addition, follow-up on any service delivery or client care problems identified during the visit, obtaining written physician orders for any care plan changes resulting from the visit, and documenting all visit and follow-up activities must be done.

An awareness of client's health insurance coverage is also necessary. The nurse operates within the client's financial framework to ensure that needed care and services are provided. This necessitates frequent communication by telephone or written documentation about the client's clinical course. With the current trend toward increased enrollment in health maintenance organizations (HMO), clients may also have a case manager at an HMO, who is monitoring the efficient delivery of home care services.

The nurse's role as client advocate is perhaps the most important. The firsthand contact and care provided allows the nurse to determine what the client needs at home. The professional judgment exercised must be accurate and comprehensive. The nurse must be aware of community resources that can assist the client. This may be an alternative to the traditional care that clients receive. Various religious and community groups do provide needed home care services free of charge or at a nominal fee. The nurse needs to be aware of services, devices, and resources that will enhance the client's recovery.

DOCUMENTATION

The clear and concise documentation of the nurse's initial assessment and plan of care is necessary to formulate realistic goals and timeframes. Revisits to the client will focus on problems initially identified, teaching needed, and any significant changes occurring between nursing visits. All of the nurse's documentation should convey the client's clinical course and the client's response to the medical and nursing plan of care. These factors will determine the frequency of nursing visits, as well as their duration.

Frequency of care is defined as how often home visits are made to a client in a specified period. Duration of care is defined as the length of time the client receives home care. In collaboration with the physician, the nurse must determine whether the frequency of visits should be changed and when to discharge the client from the agency. The client should be involved in the plan of care, and discharge planning should begin when a client is admitted to the program.

The client record is a tool used to justify reimbursement from third-party payers, such as Medicare, Medicaid, HMOs, private health insurance, or free care. It is a written account of the client's history, status, progress, and the nurse's plan of care. As such, it is one of the factors used in determining the quality of care provided by the home care team.

The terminology used in documenting must be exact and specific. Avoid words such as *chronic, monitor vital signs, observe, reinforce, check, discussed/ stressed, stabilized, plateaued, general weakness, scant/ little, sometimes,* and *tires easily.* Do use *acute exacerbation, measure/assess, reinstruct, performed/evaluated, instructed, responding to treatment, exhausted with exertion,* and describe what client cannot do, use measured amounts, and list specific frequencies (Table 9-1).

The treatments and procedures performed on the nurse's visit must be documented on the visit report. For example: *Visiting nurse (VN) cleansed ankle wound on left (L) leg with normal saline (NS) and applied wet to dry NS dressing.* When an injection is administered, the site must be indicated as well as the disposal of needle and syringe, as agency policy dictates.

Teaching done during the nurse's visit also must be specified. This generally encompasses therapeutic diet, medication regimen, activity level, and treat-

text continued on page 161

Table 9-1
Effective Versus Questionable Documentation

Questionable Documentation	Effective Documentation
At patient's request (may be questioned if patient appears to be directing care)	By request of physician (if accurate; focus on the physician's directing of care)
Chronic	Acute exacerbation or acute episode
Discussed	Instructed, educated
Doing well	Comprehends (state quantitative measurements)
General weakness	Short of breath on exertion, unable to walk without assistance because of poor balance, can only sit up for 30 minutes, chair-bound, bed-bound, hemiparesis
Left home to live with son	Was removed from the home by relatives to more suitable surroundings
No change	Unresolved
Improving	Give details: improving, wound decreased from 2 to 1 cm, continues to need instruction on safe use of walker
No complaints	Identify problems and needs: poor balance, unsteady, able to ambulate only 10 feet without tiring and becoming dizzy

continued

Table 9-1

Effective Versus Questionable Documentation Continued

Questionable Documentation	Effective Documentation
No problem	No problem or no *new* problems
Not at home	Locked door, no answer
Observed	Assessed, evaluated (document specifies)
Reinforced	Continues to need instructions because patient is slow learner because of recent stroke
	Appears to be responding to treatment, unstable, deteriorating
Stable or stabilizing (except at discharge)	Lack of understanding, language barrier, slow learner
Noncompliant	Document specifics of progress (measurements, gradations, and levels); otherwise discharge (especially rehab patients)
No progress	Document specifics of graded progress; if no progress is demonstrated, either discharge patient or place on hold and re-evaluate in a timely manner
Plateaued	
Pulse irregular	Describe pulse: bounding, weak, thready, unequal, skipped beats, bigeminal rhythm
Reviewed	Continues to need instruction because _____ (explain)

Told patient to contact physician (when relates to plan of care)	Registered nurse or therapist contact physician (when relates to performance of skilled care, instabilities, deficits, or significant changes in patient's condition; document all changes)
Accu-check (sugar) readings very inconsistent from one reading to the next	Accu-check (sugar reading, range 220–460 2 hours postprandial)
Ambulates independently, ambulates without difficulty	The ability to ambulate may bring the patient's homebound status into question; therefore, the documentation must clearly indicate what makes the patient homebound and should refer to specific function and affected extremities, upper, lower, or psychological instabilities that render a patient homebound.
Caregiver	Family member, sitter, companion, homemaker (specify if person performs personal care)
Gait steady, gait steady at times	Unsteady gait, poor balance, tremors, vertigo, syncope
Intake poor, poor appetite	Describe exact intake, no solid foods, taking 2,000 cc fluid/day: see attached diet log to be placed in patient's chart
Lack of description of the dimensions and drainage of wound	Wound 14 cm x 9 cm x 8 cm, with serosanguinous drainage saturating two 4 x 4 gauze dressing in 4-hr period (use consistent measurements, either centimeters or inches in accordance with agency policy)

continued

Table 9-1
Effective Versus Questionable Documentation Continued

Questionable Documentation	Effective Documentation
Monitored	Evaluate, assess
Supervised	Evaluate, instruct
Repeated instruction	Patient/family unable to give return demonstration of previous instruction, requiring additional education/instruction
Low sodium taught	Began teaching on 2-g sodium diet (give specific aspect taught)
Diabetic diet taught	Began teaching on 1,200-cal ADA diet (give specific aspect taught)
Insulin injection given	Nurse administered 15 units NPH insulin subcu. right deltoid area; patient tolerated procedure well

© With permission. MJGC Orientation Manual

ments performed. The nurse focuses on helping the client gain as much independence as possible at home. The teaching of knowledge and skills allows this to happen. For example, *VN taught aseptic technique to client's wife* or *VN instructed client in medication dosage, action, and side effects* are ways that the nurse should document teaching.

The short-term and long-term goals established on the initial visit must be clear and consistent with the plan of care. Goals are formulated based on the needs identified by the nurse. They chart the course of the client's care at home and are reviewed and evaluated on an ongoing basis. Short-term goals need to be specific, timeframed, and measurable: *Client will verbalize two side effects of digoxin in 1 week* or *client's wife will demonstrate aseptic technique in 2 weeks* are examples. Long-term goals indicate what the end result of home care should be for the client. They generally reflect where the client will be on discharge from home care. They should be realistic, measurable, and in line with the client's anticipated clinical course: *Client will ambulate independently with walker* or *client's neighbor will be independent in Foley catheter care* are examples of long-term goals. See Table 9-2 for examples of improper goals and effective goals.

Visits to the clinic or to the client's physician need to be noted by the nurse. Asking when appointments are scheduled enables the nurse to obtain this information. The nurse does not usually visit on the day the client is scheduled to see the physician, unless the visit is not related to the specific care the nurse is providing. If the client is going to the cardiologist, and the nurse is performing wound care, the nurse visits on that day, because the cardiologist

text continued on page 166

Table 9-2
Improper Versus Effective Treatment Goals

Improper Goals	Effective Goals
Patient's abdominal distress will be resolved.	Patient will describe 3 comfort measures for relief of abdominal distress by 2nd visit.
Patient and family will demonstrate basic understanding of medical and dietary regimen. Patient will be compliant with medication regimen. Learn medications and side effects.	Patient will identify each medication by either name or action and describe no less than 2 precautions for each one by 4th visit. By 2nd visit, patient/significant other will construct accurate/safe system for dispensing medication according to time/dosage.
Patient will remain free from seizure activity.	Patient/significant other will describe 3 symptoms of and interventions for seizure activity by 1st visit.
Patient will remain well nourished and hydrated. Good nutritional status. Learn 1,800-calorie low-sodium diet.	Patient/significant other will construct a 3-meal sample menu in keeping with prescribed diet by 5th visit. Patient will list preferred/allowed foods to incorporate daily diet plan by 4th visit.

Patient will remain safe and comfortable in home environment. Elimination of safety hazards in the home. Patient will remain free from diabetic crisis complications.

Sacral wound heals without complications. Promote healing of wounds. Wounds will remain free from infection. Maintenance of infection-free status.

Patient/significant other will implement 3 measures to enhance enviornmental safety by 2nd week of service.
Patient/significant other will describe symptoms of acid/base imbalance and describe emergency treatment plan by 2nd visit.
1. Efficiency of present wound care regimen will be assessed every 2–3 weeks.
2. Family will list/describe 3 signs/symptoms of wound infection by 4th visit.
Patient/family will describe 3 measures to promote wound closure by 6th visit.
Patient/family will demonstrate all aspects of proper wound care by 2nd week of service.

© With permission. MJGC Orientation Manual

DISPLAY 9-1. Sample Case Study

Date: _____ Patient's Name: _____ Case Number: _____

Procedures/Treatments Performed: _Cleansed incision on left thigh with soap and water. DSD applied._

Teaching Done:

1. Pt./wife taught signs/symptoms of CHF and emergency measures to take if patient exhibits any signs/symtoms.

2. Pt./wife taught signs/symptoms of wound infection.

3. Pt./wife taught 2 g Na+/150-mg cholesterol diet.

4. Pt./wife taught action, dose, and side effects of medications.

5. Pt./wife taught measures for home safety.

Short-Term Goals With Timeframes:

1. Pt. will state 3 signs/symptoms of CHF by 1st visit.

2. Pt. will state 2 emergency measures to take for CV/CP decompensation by 1st visit.

3. Pt. will state signs/symptoms of wound infection by 2nd visit.

4. Pt. will be able to identify foods high in sodium and cholesterol after 3rd visit.

5. Pt. will be knowledgeable regarding medication schedule by 1st visit.

6. Pt. will be knowledgeable regarding medication purpose, dose, and side effects by 4th visit.

Long-Term Goals:

1. Pt. will have stable cardiac status.

2. Pt. will maintain compliance with diet and medication regimen.

3. Pt. will maintain safety in the home.

Clinic/MD Appointments: To Be Scheduled

Coordination: Telephone call to M. Jones, NCC to report initial visit findings.

Date: _____   Next Revisit Date: _____

V.N. Signature: _____   Date: _____

© With permission. S. Zang

would not be changing the dressing. The nurse also must ask what happened when the client saw the physician.

Changes in the plan of care must be verified with the physician and reported to the nurse coordinating the client's care. All documentation related to client visits and coordination must be signed and dated by the nurse. Visit documentation must be submitted within specified timeframes.

Case Study

The following case study is presented to illustrate how the nurse should document:

A 65-year-old man with a diagnosis of coronary heart disease (CHD) was admitted to the hospital for coronary artery bypass surgery. He also has a secondary diagnosis of congestive heart failure (CHF). Four days after surgery, he was discharged to his home. The physician has ordered the nurse to visit to assess his cardiac status and surgical sites. He must be taught a 2-g sodium, 150-mg cholesterol diet, and use of his medications, which are digoxin and lasix.

See Display 9-1 for a sample initial form using this case study.

CONCLUSIONS

The role of the nurse in home care is unique and diverse. Provision of direct care focused on the client's physical, social, and psychological needs is one component of the role. As the coordinator of services and case manager, the nurse oversees the total care of the client. In collaboration with the physician, the nurse implements the plan of care as frequently and as long as needed. An awareness of the client's financial coverage enables the nurse to assist in developing the plan of care.

As client advocate, the nurse ensures that the client receives the care and services needed. Inherent in the role of nurse is the ability to plan, problem solve, make decisions, set priorities, and take appropriate actions. A sound knowledge base in the biological, physical, social, and behavioral sciences is needed. Effective interpersonal skills and the ability to communicate orally and in writing are essential skills for the nurse.

10

The Initial Visit

Sheryl Mara Zang, RN, MS

This chapter discusses the initial visit. It is during this visit that the nurse is able to use everything that has been discussed in the previous chapters. Our roles as providers of direct care, coordinators of services, and client advocates are addressed. A sample page of an initial form and appropriate documentation also are covered in this chapter.

PREPARATION FOR THE INITIAL VISIT

In preparation for the initial visit, you need to become familiar with the Health Care Financing Administration (HCFA) 485 or physician's orders and any history or comments written about the client. A discharge planner may or may not have seen the client, so the 485 may or may not be complete or accurate. The 485 will give you the information to assess the timing and prioritizing of the visit. If the 485 tells you that the client is an insulin-dependent diabetic, you want this to be one of your first cases seen. It also tells you the medication, frequency, and services that were ordered. This gives you your baseline to see if any other services are needed.

The next contact with the client is through the telephone. This is the time that you tell the client to get all the medication (prescription and nonprescription), insurance cards of both the client and the spouse, the names, addresses, and phone numbers of the physicians involved, and the hospital discharge papers ready for the visit. Verify the address, cross streets, and apartment number at this time. Safety guidelines for planning a visit should be used, making sure you know exactly where you are going. The client should be given a 2-hour timeframe when you plan to visit. If you are delayed longer than the 2-hour timeframe, the client must be contacted.

Before seeing the client for the first time, it is necessary to have all of the initial forms that need to be filled out and completed. The type of forms needed may vary from agency to agency. Always have extra initial forms available in case a mistake is made. The initial visit is when the nurse meets the client for the first time. The client may have been on the program before, but if the client is rehospitalized for a certain number of days, a new referral is needed. When you meet the client, introduce yourself and the agency you represent. It is important to always find out who answers the door and who is in the home. This way you know how involved the person should be in the visit and plan of care, and the level of privacy and confidentiality that is needed. A very important part of the initial visit is to find out who the client lives with, their health status, and their readiness and willingness to be involved. It is always the decision of clients how involved they want family members to be. Family members also have the right to decide how involved they want to be. You do need to tell the client that the services provided may be for a limited amount of time, and family members may need to become more involved or other arrangements may need to be made at a later date.

Being in a client's home is different from seeing the client in the structure and routine of a hospital or clinic setting. The client usually sets the tone of the visit, and the environment of the client's home also structures the interview. Ask clients where they would like to conduct the visit. Most nurses feel comfortable conducting the first part of the visit in a room with a table and chair, and you can suggest this to the client.

Consent forms should be signed before the actual visit is started. Various documents such as the health care proxy and Patient's Bill of Rights may need to be reviewed by the nurse and signed by the client. The type of health insurance that the client has should be reviewed at this time. It determines the services that the client is eligible for. The financial status is also determined, because clients may be eligible for programs they are unaware of. This is also the time to check the client's medications. Begin by checking each medication the client takes with the medication listed on the 485. If there are any discrepancies found, discuss it with the physician. If the physician wants the client to take only what is on the 485, make sure the client understands this. If the physician agrees to the changes that were found in the home, make sure the 485 reflects these changes or that an interim order or modifier is sent to the physician for a signature. A copy will go in the client's record until the original is signed by the physician. When you check each medication, do teaching about the need, action, and side effects of each medication and discuss with the client that individual medication teaching will be done at each revisit.

CONDUCTING THE VISIT

The initial visit includes taking a detailed history and doing a complete physical assessment. The physical examination is usually performed in the client's own bedroom. Infection control practices are used at all times. Ask the client where you can place the nursing bag, and place it on a barrier. Ask where you can wash your hands, and use your own soap and paper towels. Remove all equipment needed from the nursing bag for the visit and place it on a barrier. If a home health aide (HHA) or home attendant (HA) is very involved in the client's care, usually a client with complex medical needs or long home health aide hours, ask the client if the HHA/HA can be present during the examination. If a client has a diagnosis of human immunodeficiency virus (HIV)/acquired immune deficiency syndrome (AIDS), confidentiality needs to be maintained. If the client has made the diagnosis known, the HHA or the HA could be involved in the teaching about medication, diet, and each system as it relates to the client's diagnosis. The client who is more independent should choose whether to have aides or attendants present for all or part of the examination. You also may have to perform some procedure or techniques as per physician orders. During the initial visit, assess if the client will be able to learn how to perform it himself or herself or if a family member is able to learn.

During the physical assessment, address each body system and how it relates to the client. Using your agency's initial form is a good way to organize and focus the visit and address each system. Because many of the forms have check-off boxes and fill-ins, it is recommended that as much of the form as possible be completed in the home. If a body system is not related to the diagnosis and the client is asymptomatic, still do teaching about complications to observe for and when to notify the physician. The client's response to teaching guides how you plan your visit frequency and discharge outcomes. This is the time to assess any factors that interfere with the client's ability to comply with the plan of care. If someone has a diagnosis of asthma or bronchitis and is smoking, address the diagnosis, but you also have to find out why the client smokes and why he or she has not stopped. Realize that you cannot always change a client's behavior, but you have to teach them the reasons why they should try to modify it. Assess the role that culture and religion play and how this affects the client's health practices and incorporate it into the plan of care.

Cultural and religious beliefs that have been a part of a client's life are stronger than some new health practices that the client has to learn. There may be some adjustments needed. Any change that does affect the physician's orders has to be discussed with the physician. If the physician becomes aware of any interfering factors, the physician could modify or change the treatment plan.

Family dynamics play a major part during the initial visit. Clients are facing a new situation that they may not be prepared for. A client may have been admitted to the hospital with a nonhealing vascular ulcer, underwent vascular tests, received intravenous (IV) antibiotics, and the client's outcome was a below-knee amputation. This is a very new experience for the client. The client went into the hospital and is now nonambulatory with a whole new way of life to learn. The role that clients have played in their family will change.

If the client happens to be the household bread-winner and will be unable to work, the whole family structure will change. The family will also feel the change if it is the homemaker who is now impaired. Family members are thrown into new roles, which they may not want to assume or cannot assume. Families have a history all their own. Respect the family dynamics and realize that this situation may or may not change the way family members feel about each other. Assess the situation and find out what roles they will play and what services can be ordered to make sure the needs of the client are met.

When there are many family members involved, it is important to ask the client which family member will be the spokesperson for the rest of the family. Family members have many different opinions and different ideas for their family member. If there are many different opinions, the nurse must be consistent and reinforce that decisions be made among the family, and that the nurse will continue to speak with the designated family member about family decisions.

The initial visit is the time when you assess the level of understanding of the client and family's perception of his illness. If a client is diagnosed with new-onset insulin-dependent diabetes and thinks that he or she will need insulin for only a short period, much teaching is needed. Full family involvement may be needed in the teaching about the disease process, preparation of meals, and complications to observe for. The nurse needs to assess the client's and family's readiness to learn. Teaching about one aspect of the disease at each revisit will give the client and family a chance to incorporate it into their lifestyle. It is very important to have a clear understanding of the client's perception of his or her diagnosis, because the frequency of visits needs to reflect this. When you schedule visits, make sure that the client will be safe between your visits. Plans for frequency of visit and plans for discharge begin on the initial visit. The nurse will plan with the client to visit more frequently in the beginning and taper the visits as the client and family progress toward goal completion.

The client you are meeting may be completely different at home than in the hospital. A client may have been confused, bedridden, and completely dependent for all activities of daily living (ADL). Based on a hospital assessment, a physical therapist and a 24-hour HHA was ordered. When the nurse met the client, he or she saw a completely different person. The client at home lives in a studio apartment. She became completely familiar with her surroundings and oriented. She was able to ambulate the short distances in her apartment without problems. She was able to perform her own ADL, needing some assistance with bathing, shopping, and laundry. The nurse felt comfortable in reducing the HHA to 4 hours per day, and the physical therapy evaluation revealed no need for additional physical therapy visits. The initial visit is the time when additional services can be ordered or reduced if not indicated. These changes can only be made in consultation and verification with the physician.

When you enter a client's home, you are seeing the client in his or her own environment. This is truly the meaning of home care. You must always respect the way a client chooses to live. When you assess the environment, involve the client and discuss with them what you are looking for. Check that there are no safety hazards and that the apartment is well ventilated in the summer and well heated in the winter. If you find problems, you must plan for intervention at that time. Do this by having the client or family member take responsibility, or initiate a referral to a social worker. Always follow up at revisits to see if any progress was made or if additional services or community supports are needed. Check the corridors to make sure that the client can easily ambulate with a walker or maneuver a wheelchair. It is at this time that you may make suggestions in rearranging furniture to create a clear path. If the client is bed bound and the bed is located in the back of the house, you may suggest that the client be moved into a room that is more accessible to family members and company. Before ordering any bathroom equipment, make sure it is appropriate for the bathroom the client has.

Depending on insurance coverage, clients must be aware of any expenses they will have to pay. Clients have the right to refuse any supplies or equipment they have to pay for, even though the nurse believes it is indicated. When you instruct a client in diet restrictions and nutritional intake, ask permission to look in the refrigerator and cabinets to make sure there are adequate amounts of appropriate food. If you see that the food in the client's refrigerator and cabinets is not adequate, assess the problem. It may be that the client was hospitalized and a family member removed the perishable and spoiled food. It may also be attributable to economic hardship or because the client is not able to go to the store to purchase food. At this time you assess for services needed. Community programs such as Meals on Wheels or senior centers may be the solution. Clients may be in financial distress although they are not eligible for Medicaid or food stamps. Family members may not be aware of this. You may want to discuss the findings of the initial visit with family members, but you can only do this with the client's permission.

Coordination with the physician is done at the initial visit. Discuss the findings of the visit, verification of the medication or any change in medication or treatments that were found in the home, or any new services or supplies needed. You also may coordinate with family members, vendors, and supply companies. If a client has private insurance with prior approval needed for home care services, at this time you determine who the contact person is for the insurance company and coordinate the services.

Discharge planning begins at the initial visit. You have learned about the client as your visit has progressed. You have learned what role family members and community supports play in the client's daily life. It is at this time that you assess if long-term planning is needed or the client will be able to manage independently after discharge from the program. If the client's diagnosis is complex, and the client has many skilled and unskilled nursing needs, you have to assess if there are any services that you can provide or plan for at this visit. The major role of your visit is to help the client successfully incorporate their new diagnosis or health needs into the home setting. You are their first contact at home, and your positive outlook and therapeutic approach will make their adjustment an easier one. Understanding the client's needs and planning for realistic goal achievements is what you need to accomplish during the initial visit. The following guidelines should help in filling out the form (Display 10-1).

Display 10-1. **Sample Initial Visit Page**

Date:_____ Patient's Name:_____ Case Number:_____

Address:_____

Apartment Number:_____ D.O.B.:_____

Phone Number:_____ Allergies:_____

Physician:_____ Phone #:_____ Specialty:_____

Address:_____

Second Physician:_____ Phone #:_____ Specialty:_____

Address:_____

Insurance: Medicaid #:_____ Medicare #:_____ Other #:_____

Managed Care:_____ Frequency of Visits:_____

Primary Diagnosis (S):_____

Secondary Diagnosis (S):_____

Aware Of Diagnosis: Yes_____ No_____ Explain:_____

Medical History (Onsets):_____

Surgical History (Onsets):_____

History of Alcohol Abuse:_____ Drug Abuse:_____ Cigarettes:_____

MSW Referral Needed:_____

Family History—Members in Household and Their Ages:

Name   Age   Any Health Problems

Name of Emergency Contact and Phone #:_____

Is Pt. Able to Participate in Plan of Care?_____

Is Family Member Able to Participate in Plan of Care?_____

Is Inside of Home Free of Hazards?_____

Is Outside of Home Free of Hazards?_____

Is Apartment or Home Suitable for Living?   Yes_____   No_____   Please Specify:_____

Advance Directive/Bill of Rights/Health Care Proxy/Reviewed with Patient?   Yes_____   No_____

Language Spoken:_____   Interpreter Needed: Yes_____   No_____

V.N. Signature:_____   Date:_____

© With permission. S. Zang

SAMPLE OF AN INITIAL VISIT PAGE

Date

The date should be within 24 hours of the client's discharge from the hospital. There are times when a client is seen on the same day of hospital discharge. Examples are when a client needs twice-daily insulin or wound care and has had the morning dose or treatment in the hospital and needs the evening dose or treatment at home. A client may receive a hospital pickup, and the nurse needs to visit to supervise and write the plan of care for the HHA. The nurse may not visit within 24 hours if the client requests that the nurse make a visit on a different day or the client is seen by the physician on that date. Documentation must reflect the reason.

Client's Name

Always verify with the client the correct spelling and check to see that this is the name on the client's insurance cards. If a discrepancy is found, changes need to be made on all of the client's records.

Case Number

This is the identification number that the client is given on entry to a home care program. It could be called an ID number or entry number. It needs to always be filled in to ensure that visits are correctly accounted for and that the note is filed into the correct chart.

The reason this number is so important is that many clients have the same name, and this helps to distinguish them.

Address and Apartment Number

Always verify that the client's address and apartment number are the same as is written on the referral and the 485. Always make sure changes are corrected on all documents.

Phone Number

Always verify that the phone number is correct, and make appropriate changes as needed. If there is no phone number listed, discuss with client whether there is a family member or neighbor that the nurse can contact if there is any change in the time or date of the visit. Assure client that anything confidential will not be discussed.

Allergies

The nurse needs to discuss with the client if there are any allergies to medication or food. The 485 or referral packet may not reflect this area, so it is important to discuss this with the client and make the necessary changes on all documents.

Physician/Phone Number/Specialty

During the initial visit, the nurse needs to discuss with the client if the physician listed on the 485 is going to follow his or her care at home. At times, the physician in the hospital who signed the discharge papers and

485 is not going to follow the client at home. You need to know which physician will follow the client and sign orders for the client. If a client has complex medical needs and will be seen by many physicians, you need to document the specialty of the physician so that the appropriate orders are signed by the appropriate physician. It is important to get the correct spelling of the physician's name, address, and phone number so that new orders can be verbally verified, and written orders can be sent for a signature. If the physician listed is not correct, always make sure that changes are corrected on all documents.

Secondary Physician/Phone Number/Specialty

If a client has complex medical needs and is followed by different specialists, you need to fill in this area. The primary care physician should be made aware of the client's different medications if it was not ordered by him or her.

Insurance

It is necessary to check the client's or spouse's insurance coverage on the initial visit. If a client has managed care, please document who the contact person is and when the next contact for authorization is needed.

Frequency of Visits

This usually reflects what is ordered on the 485. If the nurse believes that a change in frequency of visits is indicated, this should reflect the change for a 9-week period, and the physician orders should reflect the new frequencies needed.

Primary Diagnosis

This is usually the diagnosis that the client was admitted to the hospital with. If you do a full physical assessment and find that there is a skilled nursing need or diagnosis that necessitates a change in frequency of visits, please discuss this with the physician and change the diagnosis to justify the change in frequency. An example of this would be a client with a diagnosis of Parkinson's and a stage III decubitus ulcer that was discovered on initial visit. Visit frequency ordered for the diagnosis of Parkinson's was two times per week. The frequency for treatment for the ulcer is daily. To justify daily visits, the diagnosis needs to be stage III decubitus.

Secondary Diagnosis

Once again this may be written on the 485, but the nurse needs to discuss with the client if there are any other medical conditions. The nurse should carefully review the medication list, because each medication that the client is taking should correspond to a diagnosis.

Aware of Diagnosis

The nurse needs to always start with the question, "Are you aware of your diagnosis?" or "Do you know what is wrong with you?" This helps to assess if the client is aware of the diagnosis. If the client tells you,

"I have a growth and they removed it all," and you have a diagnosis of terminal cancer on the 485, you should document what the client said. The actual diagnosis does not have to be told to the client, but all teaching should address the systems involved. The nurse needs to find out what the physician has told the client and relay the client's perception of his or her diagnosis to the physician. This part of the form needs to be filled out carefully so that a covering nurse will understand if client is aware of his or her diagnosis.

Medical History

The nurse should ask the client for his or her medical history. If a diagnosis of cancer of the stomach 1989 was on the 485, the nurse could ask the client if he or she ever had problems with his or her stomach. This also gives you an awareness of the client's understanding of the client's health history. If you know that the client had a heart attack in 1991, the nurse should ask if the client ever had heart trouble or a heart attack and formulate a baseline from that. If a client is not responsive and family members are the historians, the nurse should ask the same type of question. With a diagnosis of AIDS, in some states, confidentiality does not allow us to talk about the diagnosis with other family members.

Surgical History

The nurse needs to fill this in and include it in the plan of care if it is indicated.

History of Alcohol/Drugs/Cigarettes

This needs to be discussed with the client and documented. If client answers no, you could fill out this form by writing *client denies*. If client admits to use, you need to incorporate it into the plan of care. If a client denies and you suspect abuse, this needs to be documented. Example: *Client denies smoking cigarettes but his breath smelled of smoke and ashtrays were filled in his room.* This needs to be addressed again on revisits.

MSW Referral Needed

You must document the reason a social worker referral is needed.

Family History/Members in Household/Ages

Ask the client who lives in the house and their ages. You also need to find out about any health problems or infectious diseases. During this time, do a family check for tuberculosis, asking if any family member has a cough, fever, or chills. Knowing the ages and any significant health problems of family members helps with the plan of care and goals for the client.

Emergency Contact and Phone Number

At times, you need to locate the client and cannot reach him or her by phone or by visit. The emergency phone number should be someone who lives close by or knows the routine of the client. A long-distance relative may be the contact person listed, but you should ask for a local emergency contact. At times, the spouse with the same address and phone number is the contact. In addition, you should ask for another local contact person.

Is Pt. Able to Participate in Plan of Care?

If the client can be involved in all aspects of care, you would document that the client can participate in the plan of care. If the client cannot, you need to document why. At times, the client may be independent in some aspect of his or her care but cannot participate in other parts. If a client is able to self-administer medications correctly but cannot do a treatment or procedure, it needs to be written in this space. You need to document why a client cannot participate. Example: A client may not be able to do wound care because of the location of the wound or poor manual dexterity.

Is Family Member Able to Participate in Plan of Care?

If a client is not able to participate in some aspect of care, assess whether family members can. At the initial visit, it may be hard to evaluate if the family member will be able to do it. If the family member does show interest, you can document that. Example: *Client's wife is willing to learn to care for wound* or *client's wife shows no interest in learning wound care.* This helps with formulation of goals.

Is Inside of Home Free of Hazards?

We assess the environment for safety, making sure the pathways are clear. You assess for proper heating and ventilation. If there is an unsafe situation, discuss it with the client or family and find out if it is something that they can fix or take care of. If not, a social worker referral is needed, because emergency housing may be indicated, or you may need to send the client back to the hospital.

Is Outside of Home Free of Hazards?

You also need to assess the outside of the home for safety. The same guidelines for family involvement or appropriate referrals must be followed.

Is Apartment or Home Suitable for Living?

If there are hazards found inside or outside the home that place the client in an unsafe situation, you need to remove the client from the environment. You should document why the environment is unsafe, the interventions you implemented, and the referrals you made. You can never leave a client in an unsafe situation.

Advance Directive/Bill of Rights/Health Care Proxy/ Reviewed With Patient?

You are responsible for reviewing these forms with the client. If the client does have any of these forms active, such as a health care proxy or a do not resuscitate (DNR) order, you need to get a copy of these for the client's record.

Language Spoken/ Interpreter Needed

If an interpreter is needed or used, you must document the language that the client speaks. You should also document who the interpreter is.

All forms need to be signed and dated.

11

Physical Assessment of the Home Care Client

Arlene Pericak, RN, FNP-C, MSN

General Appearance
Vital Signs
Heart
Nervous System
Mental Status and Speech
Vision
Hearing

Peripheral Vascular System
Skin
Musculoskeletal System
Elimination
Gastrointestinal System and
    Nutrition

This chapter discusses physical assessment of the client. Although good physical assessment skills are essential in diagnosing, this cannot be accomplished without a thorough history. The nurse needs to ask the client what the major concern or problem is that he or she is experiencing at this time. This may or may not be related to the diagnosis. Obtaining the main concern will help focus on what assessment skills need to be performed. For example, if the client reports a fall in which he or she hit his or her head, it is important to ask some pertinent questions. These might be: Do you have a headache or are you vomiting? If the client answers yes, the nurse will need to perform a thorough neurologic assessment. The nurse also needs to ask questions that will give a clear organized account of the events that led to the fall. These might be: Were you dizzy or did you lose your balance? This helps to focus on the systems that need further evaluation.

GENERAL APPEARANCE

The nurse should first assess the environment and the space where the client will be examined. Ensure that the lighting is adequate and the client is comfortable. The nurse would start by looking at the client and asking: How does this client look in general? Is the client overweight or underweight? Does the client look sick? Does the client look pale? How is the client breathing in general? Is the client in distress? Is the client ambulating? Does client look depressed? Is the client well kept? Sample forms for taking a thorough history are shown in Displays 11-1 and 11-2.

VITAL SIGNS

After you take an overview of the client and are able to say that the client is in no acute distress, you would begin with the vital signs, starting with the temperature. An oral thermometer is inserted bulb first under the tongue for 3 to 5 minutes. Do not use an oral thermometer in a child younger than age 5 years or an adult with respiratory or cognitive impairment. An oral temperature should not be taken after a client has just finished smoking or drinking hot or cold beverages. A rectal thermometer can be used with a small amount of lubricant. The thermometer is inserted 4 cm and left in place for 3 minutes. Use a rectal thermometer when an oral thermometer is contraindicated. An axillary temperature can be used. An electronic thermometer will speed up all of these methods. Be sure to use an oral thermometer for oral temperature only and a rectal thermometer for a rectal temperature only. Ear probes work quickly but are not to be used if a client has ear pain.

Next you take client's blood pressure (BP). Always assess and document if there is a reason not to take the BP, such as postmastectomy, cerebrovascular accident (CVA), or if the client has a dialysis shunt. Before you get alarmed about a BP finding, be sure you have elicited a history about past BPs, including medication the client is taking. Assess the clients arm size, because cuffs that are too short or too narrow may give falsely high readings. Using a regular-size cuff on an obese arm may lead to a false diagnosis of hypertension. The nurse as well as the client should be in a comfortable position when the blood pressure is being taken. Be sure to have the cuff on properly: use the arrow to point toward the brachial artery. Try to have the client's arm rest on a table. A loose cuff will result in an abnormal reading. It is important to take BP in both arms to assess a pressure difference of more than 5 to 10 mm Hg.

If there is a pressure difference of more than 10 to 15 mm Hg, this may suggest obstruction on the side with the lower pressure or arterial compression.

text continued on page 196

DISPLAY 11-1. **History-Taking Form**

Date: _____ Patient's Name: _____ Case Number: _____

B/P (R) _____ Pulse(A) _____ Temperature(O) _____ Respiration _____ Lungs (Anterior) (R) _____ (L) _____ (WT)

(L) _____ (R) _____ (R) _____ (Posterior) (R) _____ (L) _____

(A) _____

Circle all that apply:

CNS: LOC: Alert   Lethargic   Other _____   Orientation: Person   Place   Time

Mood/Beh: WNL Irritable Restless Nervous   Headache: N Y Location: _____ Frequency: _____

Dizzy? N Y Tremors? N Y Seizures? N Y Numbness? N Y

Comments and teaching: _____

CP: SOB: At rest? N Y After activity? N Y Describe: _____

Orthopnea? N Y   # Of pillows needed for sleep: _____

Endurance: Poor Fair Good   Oxygen: _____ L/min.

Cough? N Y Productive? N Y Describe: _____

Chest pain? N Y Describe: _____

Palpitations? N Y   Angina? N Y   Cyanosis? N Y

Edema? N Y Location: _____   Measurement: R _____ L _____

Pacemaker? N Y Rate: _____

Comments and teaching: _____

Vision: Glasses Contacts Glaucoma Cataracts: R/L Extraction: R/L

Pupils: Right Left

Reactive to light _____

Equally respond _____

Follows point _____

Hearing loss or changes: _____ Hearing aid: Right _____ Left _____

Vascular: Pulses Present or Absent

Popliteal (R)_____ (L)_____ Skin turgor: Good Fair Poor

Posterior tibial (R)_____ (L)_____ Varicose veins: Y N

Pedal (R)_____ (L)_____ Toes: Abn Normal

Capillary refill (R)_____ (L)_____ Nails: Abn Normal

Skin color: _____

Comments and teaching: _____

V.N. Signature: _____ Date: _____

©With permission. S. Zang

DISPLAY 11-2. **History-Taking Form**

Date: _____ Patient's Name: _____ Case Number: _____

GI:

Diet: _____ Fluids: _____

Teaching Needed: _____

Appetite: WNL: _____ Fair: _____ Poor: _____

Nausea: N Y Vomiting: N Y Comments: _____

Musculoskeletal:

Distance pt. can ambulate: _____ Pain: N Y Relieved with: _____

Devices used: _____

PT referral needed: _____

GU:

Voiding WNL: _____ ABN: _____ Nocturia: N Y Pain: N Y Hematuria: N Y

Suprapubic tube: N Y Last changed: _____ Size Foley/Balloon: _____

Foley catheter tube: N Y Last changed: _____ Size Foley/Balloon: _____

Comments and teaching: _____

Bowels:

Frequency of bowel movement: _____   Description of stool: _____

Ostomy site: _____

Type of appliance: _____

New ostomy: N _____ Y _____   Date of surgical procedure: _____

Patient able to learn: N _____ Y _____

Comments and teaching: _____

_____

_____

V.N. Signature: _____   Date: _____

©With permission. S. Zang

The nurse should take the client's BP in different positions if the client has a history of taking antihypertensive medications, prolonged bed rest, fainting, dizziness, or anemia. A decrease in systolic pressure of 20 mm Hg or more and with a history of the above could indicate orthostatic hypotension. If BP is high, diastolic greater than or equal to 90 mm Hg, and the systolic greater than or equal to 140 mm Hg, and this is new for the client, retake the BP later in the visit. If BP remains elevated, it is vital to assess the effects on the eyes and the cardiac, neurological, and urinary systems.

Next, take an apical and radial pulse together to check the heart rate. Do not use your thumb. When checking the radial pulse, count it for a full 60 seconds. Irregular rhythms should be evaluated, because beats that occur earlier can indicate atrial fibrillation and frequent premature contractions. You also might note if a rhythm is irregular but regular for this client. Note if there is a pattern to the client's irregular pulse. Notify the client's physician of any changes not noted on previous visits. Describe the changes in rate and rhythm.

Respiration is measured by observing rate, rhythm, and depth. A normal rate is between 14 and 20 breaths/minute.

Cardiopulmonary

The following questions are essential in assessing the respiratory system: Is the client short of breath (SOB)? Is this a condition the client has had? If it is, ask if it is worse. Ask if the client is SOB at rest or after an activity, and whether this is a change. Notify the physician if the client has a new onset of SOB, if the symptoms are worse, or if there is a chronic history of SOB that has never been reported. Does the client experience orthopnea (ability to breathe only in an upright position)? Report to the physician if this is a new symptom, if it is chronic and has never been reported before, or if it is worse than before. How is the client's endurance? If the client is on oxygen, always instruct safe use. Evaluate how often oxygen is being used and if the client is comfortable. Report any changes or new findings to the physician. Lastly, does the client have a cough? If there is a change in the client's cough—for example, productive cough, new cough, or chronic cough—that was never assessed by the physician, report these symptoms.

The respiratory system would be the first on your list if you suspect any respiratory distress. Always start inspecting the respiratory system of the client with the client's clothes off of the chest. Do not try to listen under the client's clothing. Clothing can interfere with lung assessment. Observe for any asymmetry, deformities, or abnormal retractions. The client should have both arms crossed in front of the chest with hands resting on opposite shoulders.

Posterior chest palpation can be evaluated by placing your hands (thumbs up) on the lower back (level of the 10th ribs). After the client takes in a deep breath, look to see if your hands remain symmetrical. If your hands are asymmetrical, suspect pulmonary disease.

Tactile fremitus is when you place your hand on the client's chest and back and ask the client to say "ee." The increase in transmission of tactile fremitus (spoken words louder and clearer) could mean a consolidation, as in pneumonia. Conversely, a decrease in transmission of tactile fremitus (spoken words not louder and clearer) could indicate the presence of air or fluid, as in pneumothorax and pleural effusion. Tactile fremitus areas are shown in Figures 11-1 and 11-2.

Percussion is done by placing your index and middle fingers of your dominant hand on the areas shown in Figures 11-3 and 11-4. Tap these fingers with the middle finger of your other hand. You can elicit a resonant sound over a lung, a tympanic sound over the stomach, a dull sound over the liver, and a flat sound over the thigh.

Use this technique to tap two times in one location and then move to the next area. Percuss the posterior chest in 5-cm intervals. There are seven bilat-

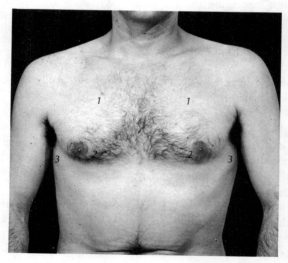

Figure 11-1. Locations for feeling fremitus.

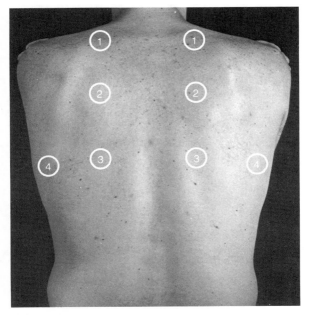

Figure 11-2. Locations for feeling fremitus.

eral percussion spots on the posterior thorax. Compare from side to side. Percuss the anterior chest in 5-cm intervals, comparing both sides. There are bilaterally six spots beginning above the clavicle and two spots laterally.

Auscultation is listening to lungs. Auscultate the chest, front, and back and do not forget the lateral sides. Remember that the right side has a right upper lateral, right middle lateral, and a right lower lateral. The left side has a left upper lateral and a left lower lateral. Always auscultate from side to side and from top to bottom, comparing one side with the other.

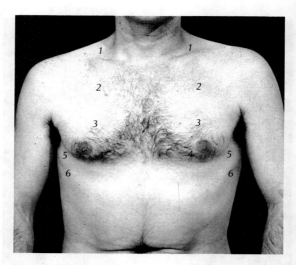

Figure 11-3. Locations for percussion and auscultation.

If there is a different sound in the right or left lungs, further evaluation is needed. When listening to breath sounds, use the diaphragm of the stethoscope. Ask the client to take deep breaths through the mouth.

You might hear abnormal sounds: crackles (rales), wheezes (rhonchi), and pleural rubs. Crackles can be compared to rubbing hair next to your ear, usually heard during inspiration. Crackles are heard in cases of pulmonary edema and congestive heart failure. Wheezes are most commonly heard in asthma. They have a high-pitched musical sound. You can visualize the air squeezing through the narrow bronchi. A pleural rub, which is a grating sound, may indicate inflammation of the pleura.

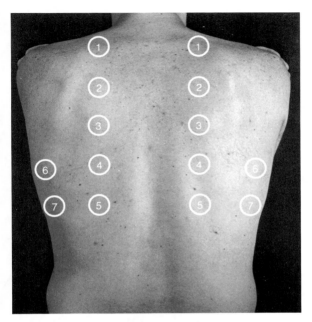

Figure 11-4. Locations for percussion and auscultation.

HEART

One way to assess clients' endurance is to walk with them, have them take a few steps, or have them do a simple activity. The following are essential questions when assessing the cardiac system: Does the client have chest pain? If yes, allow the client to describe it in his or her own words. If chest pain is not relieved with rest or if the client looks cyanotic, call 911 or the physician immediately. Does the client have palpitations or any symptoms of angina? Discuss with the physician if the client's chest pain is not relieved with medication or if it is a new symptom. Does your client have edema? If yes, compare both legs. If this is a new finding or if it is worse, discuss with physician. Measure leg circumference in the same location for both legs and carefully document measurements. Apply pressure to assess for pitting edema; document the location. Lastly, be sure to ask if the client has a pacemaker. Report any irregular rates. The heart rate should be monitored when vital signs are taken. A normal heart rate is 60 to 100 beats/minute. A fast

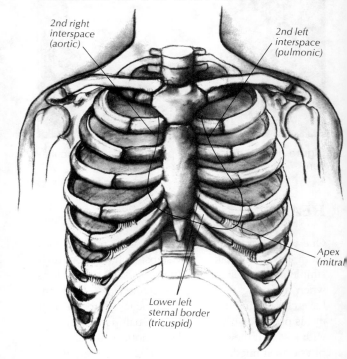

2nd right interspace (aortic)

2nd left interspace (pulmonic)

Apex (mitral

Lower left sternal border (tricuspid)

Figure 11-5. Heart areas.

heart rate is over 100 beats, and a slow heart rate is below 60. If any extra beat or irregularity is noted while monitoring the client's vital signs, the nurse should do a more complete cardiac assessment.

Auscultate the heart in the areas described below: aortic (right second interspace), pulmonic (left second interspace), tricuspid (at or near the left lower sternal border), and the mitral (cardiac apex). A complete assessment includes using the bell and the diaphragm. Listen very carefully for S1 and S2: S1 is the first heart sound, and S2 is the second heart sound. S1 is usually louder than S2 at the apex, and S2 is usually louder than S1 at the base. If you do hear murmurs or extra heart sounds, try to locate the areas where you identify them and discuss this with the physician (Figure 11-5).

NERVOUS SYSTEM

If the client admits to headaches, dizziness, tremors, seizures, or numbness, a complete history and assessment are needed. If these are new findings that have not been reported to the physician, evaluate when they began, how often they occur, and whether the client does anything to relieve them. When a client describes a symptom such as a seizure, make sure that you are both describing the same thing. Safety measures are taught, and all findings need to be followed up with the physician. Ask the client if other family members are aware of the symptoms or ask if family members have seen the client have a seizure or tremors. Assess whether these could be side effects of medication. If there is anything that would indicate immediate intervention, have the client seen by the physician or send the client to the emergency room. Feelings of numbness or seizure activity may need immediate intervention. If you notice lethargy, disorientation, or change in mood and behavior in the client, a neurological assessment is certainly needed, but always be alerted that follow-up with a mental health provider may be indicated.

MENTAL STATUS AND SPEECH

The components of mental status include evaluation of a client's level of consciousness. Note the client's posture, motor behavior, dress, grooming, and personal hygiene. A slumped posture and deterioration in grooming could be a sign of depression. Bizarre motor behavior could be a sign of schizophrenia. Facial expressions could alert you to anxiety, apathy, anger, elation, and depression. Be astute to the client's manner, affect, and relationship to persons and things. This could rule out paranoid behavior as well as tell you if you are dealing with an angry or hostile client. Assess the client's speech pattern. Are you hearing circumlocutions (a roundabout way of expressing something) or paraphasia (words that are malformed) in their speech, as noted in aphasia disorders? *Aphasia* refers to a disorder of language itself.

Expressive aphasia is generally not clear-flowing speech. Speech is slow, with few words and laborious effort. Comprehension is good. Naming of objects is impaired, although clients recognize objects. Reading comprehension is good, but writing is impaired.

Receptive aphasia means language is fluent, often rapid and effortless. However, sentences may lack meaning, and words may be malformed. Speech may be totally incomprehensible; naming, reading, comprehension, and writing all are impaired. In receptive aphasia, the client cannot understand what you are saying. In general, the client communicates by giving and receiving information. It is important to assess the client's level of understanding and possible learning needs to see if he or she will follow health care instructions.

Thought and perceptions as well as memory and attention should be assessed if you suspect an underlying psychiatric problem or limited learning. Note if the client has abnormalities in sensory or motor function. For example, does the client have hemiparesis (the weakness of one side of the body) or hemiplegia (paralysis of one-half of the body)? Evaluate this by having the client squeeze two of your fingers as hard as possible and not let go. If the client has abnormalities in sensory function, note what the abnormality is, for example, pain or numbness. Touch and sensation can be tested with a cotton ball and a paper clip. Have the client close his or her eyes. Ask the client to tell you when he or she feels the cotton ball. Go from side to side on the client's face. Do the same with a dull and sharp edge of the paper clip. Notify the physician of abnormal findings.

VISION

In the home, near vision can be checked by using reading material held 13 inches from the client. Have the client use his or her glasses; chart if glasses were used. For gross vision assessment, simply allow the client to read from a newspaper. Document if the client uses contact lenses, has a history of glaucoma, or has an artificial eye. If visual problems are noted, find out when the client last saw an ophthalmologist. Check for pupillary reaction to light. Use a circular motion and, starting outside the client's field of vision, quickly shine your penlight. The pupil should quickly constrict. In acute glaucoma, the pupil is mid-dilated and fixed. Have the client see an ophthalmologist right away if this is detected. Using oblique lighting, inspect the cornea for any opacities. A cataract is an opacity of the lens. Document if cataracts are present. Notify physician of any abnormalities.

HEARING

Check hearing by whispering to the client from 1 to 2 feet away, and have the client cover one ear at a time. If there is a deficit, note if it is in the right or left ear. Document any losses or changes. Ask if the client has a hearing aide, and do they use it? Does the client and or client's family believe that the hearing aide is working properly? Document any findings of the left or right ear and notify physician.

PERIPHERAL VASCULAR SYSTEM

Arms

As always, start with inspection. Edema of an arm with prominent veins could suggest venous obstruction. Assess radial and brachial pulse.

Legs

Note skin turgor, varicose veins, and any abnormalities in the client's toes and nails. Inspect the skin for any discoloration and or venous enlargement. Inguinal nodes should be assessed for lymphadenopathy. Check pulses in both extremities. Observe for differences. The popliteal pulse is assessed by feeling behind the knee with fingertips of both hands. The knee should be slightly flexed and leg relaxed. The posterior tibial is felt by curving your fingers slightly below the medial malleolus of the ankle. The pedal pulse is felt by feeling the dorsum of the foot. Pain, numbness, or tingling could be the result of sudden arterial occlusion caused by embolism or thrombosis. Seek medical attention immediately if the limb is cold and pale and pulse is absent. Coldness of a leg suggests inadequate arterial circulation. When assessing edema of the legs, take special time to note pitting edema. Is the skin thickened? Are there any ulcers or changes in pigmentation? Is the foot itself edematous? Lastly, compare the legs and note if the edema is bilateral. If edema is present, measure the circumference of the leg and note measurements. Be sure you document exactly where you measured the circumference. A leg can be edematous because of chronic venous insufficiency or thrombosis. Thrombosis will present with a pale, swollen, and painful leg. A positive Homan's sign is calf pain when the foot is dorsiflexed. This could be suggestive of thrombosis.

SKIN

This is the first system you would assess. Observe the client's skin throughout the examination. Look at the color of the skin. Document if you note an increase or decrease in pigment, redness, pallor, cyanosis, rashes, or yellowing of the skin. Palpate the skin. Note moisture, texture, mobility, and turgor. Pinch a piece of skin and release it. A decrease in motility indicates dehydration or edema. Notice any moles that might be irregular or discolored. Ask the client if the mole has changed in color and size. If there has been a change in the mole, measure it in centimeters and refer the client for an evaluation. The nails and hair are a part of the skin evaluation. Spoon nails (concave nails) could indicate iron-deficiency anemia. Beau's lines (indentations in the nails) could indicate an acute or chronic illness. Hair assessment includes looking for lice and noting alopecia.

MUSCULOSKELETAL SYSTEM

To start this assessment, watch how far the client can ambulate. Does the client use any devices to ambulate? If so, assess the devices. Does the client have pain? Does anything relieve the pain? Lastly, does this client need a referral to a physical therapist?

Assess the strength of all the muscles. Start from head to toe, always comparing one side with the other. For clients who are bed or chair bound, have them pedal push or attempt to step on the gas of a car. To assess tremors, have the client hold the arms upright, or ask the client to reach for something. Inspect to assess muscular atrophy. Muscular atrophy could be seen in muscular dystrophy, motor neuron disease, disuse of the muscles, rheumatoid arthritis, and malnutrition. Impaired strength indicates paresis. Weak resistance of the thumb could indicate carpal tunnel syndrome.

ELIMINATION

Is the client voiding within normal limits? A decrease in urine output in 24 hours is abnormal. Always assess the fluid intake before getting alarmed. Ask about nocturia, pain on urination, or hematuria. If the client answers positive for nocturia, ask if this is new. Be sure the female client with positive hematuria does not have her menses. If positive hematuria, consult the physician to obtain a urine culture. If the client has a suprapubic tube or a Foley catheter, document the last time the catheter was changed, the size of balloon, and the size of the Foley. Always document the teaching done and what teaching is still needed.

Bowels

Ask about frequency of bowel movements. Describe the stool. Be sure to have the client explain what diarrhea and constipation means to him or her. You might need to reassure the client that his or her bowel pattern is a normal variant. If client has an ostomy, document when the client had the surgery. Note the type of appliance and if it is working well for the client. Document the teaching and client response.

GASTROINTESTINAL SYSTEM AND NUTRITION

Ask about the client's meal routine. Describe the client's meal pattern. This is particularly important if you are doing diabetic teaching. Does client have three meals a day and snacks? Are fluids adequate? Does client understand diet restrictions? Is nutrition teaching needed? How is the client's appetite? Any nausea and or vomiting? How much are they vomiting?

Before inspecting the abdomen, the client should empty his or her bladder. Have your client lay flat (supine) with hands at the side. Visualize the abdomen into four different quadrants: right upper quadrant (RUQ), left upper quadrant (LUQ), right lower quadrant (RLQ), and left lower quadrant (LLQ). Inspect first to look for exaggerated or unusual pulsations of the abdomen, which could be suggestive of an aneurysm. LISTEN before touching the abdomen to assess bowel sounds in all four quadrants. Bowel sounds may be increased because of diarrhea or early intestinal obstruction. Bowel sounds may be decreased or absent in the presence of an ileus and if the client has peritonitis. If you do not hear bowel sounds, you might not be listening long enough in all four quadrants. Listen again. If the client complains of abdominal pain, looks uncomfortable, and you can not hear bowel sounds, consult with the physician. A flat and upright radiograph of the abdomen may need to be ordered.

Next, percuss the abdomen. This helps to evaluate any possible masses. Tap the abdomen lightly. If a mass is found, evaluate whether it is solid or fluid filled. When you percuss the abdomen, you will hear different sounds. Over the liver area it is usually a dull sound; over the abdominal area it is usually a tympanic sound. Talk to the client as a distraction while assessing the abdomen. Watch the client's facial expressions to help assess pain or tenderness of the abdomen.

Light palpation is first, followed by deep palpation of the abdomen. This can be done by pressing down lightly on the abdomen with your fingers together. Use one hand on top of the other hand. Palpate with a light dipping movement, moving from quadrant to quadrant. A deeper palpation is needed to define any masses and to elicit pain.

It cannot be emphasized enough that a complete history precedes a complete physical assessment of the client. This chapter includes forms that need to be filled out on the initial visit. The nurse should carefully compare the forms with each system review presented in this chapter. This will help guide you in focusing your initial visit and doing a complete physical assessment.

12

The Revisit

Sheryl Mara Zang, RN, MS,
and Marilyn Tillim, RN, BSN

Using the Findings of the
    Initial Assessment
Conducting the Revisit
Family Involvement and
    Long-Term Planning

Guidelines for
    Documentation and a
    Revisit Form
Guidelines for the Revisit

This chapter discusses the revisit. The revisit is either
a follow-up to an initial visit or a follow-up to other
revisits. At times, the revisit is made by the nurse who
is coordinating or following the case, or a float nurse
who happens to see the client for that one visit. This
chapter focuses on what is involved at the revisit, and
a sample revisit note with appropriate documentation
is included.

USING THE FINDINGS
OF THE INITIAL ASSESSMENT

In preparation for the revisit, the nurse needs to become familiar with the completed initial assessment
form. This gives the history, a baseline for vital signs,
and other significant findings. It also guides the nurse
in planning for goal achievement. If this is a client
who has already been revisited, the nurse needs to be

familiar with the last few revisit notes. It will help to see what medications the nurse focused on, any significant findings, what teaching was done, and the client's response to teaching. The nurse needs to be familiar with the Health Care Financing Administration (HCFA) 485, because this helps in planning the visit frequency. If this is the first time seeing the client, the nurse needs to see the 485 to be familiar with the physician's orders.

When you plan your route for the day, prioritize your revisits and leave time for an emergency situation or a new initial client you may have to visit that day. Telephone the clients first thing in the morning before you make any visits. This way you are aware if they have any medical appointments, have a preference for a time they like to be seen, or if there is a home health aide in the morning or afternoon who needs to be supervised. If you see a client daily and you know what time you will be there the next day, you can let the client know at the previous visit.

CONDUCTING THE REVISIT

During a revisit, the nurse and the client are usually more relaxed. The client has already been oriented to agency policies and has a better understanding of what to expect. The nurse who saw the client before also feels more comfortable because he or she is familiar with the client and the client's surroundings. During the initial visit, the nurse was able to obtain the client's history, and a complete physical examination was done. The nurse was able to examine each system, get a baseline of vital signs, and document abnormalities. The nurse was able to get a picture of how the client is coping with the diagnosis and the impact of the diagnosis on his or her lifestyle. Teaching was started, and the level of readiness to learn was assessed. The level of understanding of the client's diagnosis and willingness to accept medication and diet restrictions also were assessed. It was during the initial visit that goals were set up by the nurse and client. Timeframes for achieving goals were established. The focus of the revisit is to assess how the client is responding to treatment, how the client is functioning at home, and whether the goals that were planned on the initial visit are realistic and achievable.

Begin each visit by asking the clients if they have any concerns or changes in their health since last seen by the nurse. This will help you to find out the client's chief complaint or concerns at this time. It may or may not be related to the diagnosis or affected system, but there may be teaching or further evaluation needed.

Another question to ask is whether the client saw the physician since the nurse's last visit. If so, the nurse can further assess if there were any new findings or any change in medications or treatments. The nurse should follow-up with the physician to discuss the findings and verify any change in medication or treatment. If the nurse knows that the client is due to see the physician, the nurse should send a letter or a change in order form so the physician may communicate any treatment changes to the nurse.

Even though you may feel more comfortable with the client, continue to conduct a very professional visit. At each revisit, practice universal precautions and infection control. You must do a complete set of vital signs and a full systems review. While in the home, you should try to fill in as much of the progress note as possible. It helps you to focus the visit and address each system. Focus your teaching on each system and how it relates to the diagnosis. Even if the client has no symptoms relating to a system, still address it and teach complications to observe for. If a client has a diagnosis of peptic ulcer disease, and you do a cardiopulmonary assessment that shows no abnormalities or significant findings, you still should instruct what to do if the client has complaints of chest pain or shortness of breath.

Continue to monitor the clinical picture. If the client was diagnosed with a new illness or disease, continue to monitor the client's acceptance. If the client's symptoms and vital signs are stabilizing, evaluate if nursing visits can be tapered. You need to make sure that the client is safe between visits and that the client has a very good understanding of medication and diet restrictions.

Continue to monitor if the client can maintain this level of safety with fewer nursing visits. If the condition has been unstable, you need to use all our skills to find out why. Has the client been adhering to the diet restrictions? Has the client been taking the prescribed medication? Ask the client very specific questions, such as, "What did you eat for supper last night?" You also could have the client write down what he or she eats. The client's understanding of the diet restrictions may be different from what you thought he or she understood.

Ask very specific questions regarding medication compliance. You must make sure that the client understands the correct dose and the right times to take prescribed medication. If you assess that the client has a good understanding of his diet and medication and he or she is compliant, you need to continue to evaluate.

Examine each symptom the client is concerned with and see if it is related to the diagnosis or if it is a new symptom related to some other disease process. Continue to visit as indicated, making sure that the client's level of instability is monitored closely. Follow-up with the physician to discuss the findings of the visit, to see if any change in medication or treatment is needed, and to obtain an order for extra visits or an increased frequency of visits if needed.

If there is a procedure or technique ordered, continue to evaluate if there is potential for the client to learn to do the procedure or treatment independently. You always need to consider the client's acceptance of the disease. If a client is a new insulin-dependent diabetic and accepting of the diagnosis, involve the client in every aspect of the teaching. On the revisit, you need to see what the client knows, how much has been retained from the previous visits, and how ready the client is to learn at this visit.

When you formulate a plan of care for a diabetic client, focus on each aspect of diabetic management. When the client masters every aspect, the nurse documents this and can begin to taper the visits at that time.

There are some situations in which you continue to visit daily. If the client lives alone and has a sacral wound with packing needed, the nurse needs to continue daily visits because the client cannot care for it independently because of the location. When you visit daily for some type of treatment, you must carefully document why the client cannot do it independently. An insulin-dependent diabetic may manage every aspect of care, but because of Parkinson's disease, cannot independently fill syringes or administer insulin. You should discuss with the physician that an occupational therapist may be indicated, and you need to evaluate for the use of assistive devices. You need to document that the client cannot independently fill or administer insulin at this time because of shakiness of both hands and poor manual dexterity.

An important role that the nurse plays is the role of case manager and coordinator. You need to be aware of the different disciplines involved so that you can instruct the client to follow through on what he or she was taught. Involve the home health aide (HHA) in the teaching, and make sure that the plan of care for the HHA reflects this.

If you are a coordinator of care and the client needs continued services, including physical therapy (PT), occupational therapy (OT), or social work, you need to know the frequency planned so that the recertification and the 485 reflect this. Evaluate whether any other disciplines need to be ordered. You need to be aware of when the other disciplines are planning to discharge the client. Your coordination with the disciplines as well as with the physician needs to be documented. Coordinate with the physician any change in the client's condition, any additional services needed, any change in frequency of visits, and any discharge of services. Also coordinate with private insurance companies if prior approval for visits is needed.

If a client receives home visits for a procedure or treatment, you are responsible for making sure that the client has the appropriate supplies needed. When you order supplies, you should order at least a 2-week supply. Also evaluate whether any equipment is needed on each revisit.

You have to discuss with the client and family members that home care is short term. The client is admitted to a certified home health agency because the client has a skilled need. The client and family need to understand that when the client reaches the maximum rehabilitation potential or no longer has skilled nursing needs, all home care services will be discontinued. The nurse needs to reinforce this at each revisit and continue to plan for discharge on an ongoing basis. When the nurse tapers the visits as goals are met, the HHA also should be tapered.

The client and the family need to understand that the client cannot remain on the program just for HHA services. The exception to this may be when the client is Medicaid eligible and awaiting HA conversion.

FAMILY INVOLVEMENT AND LONG-TERM PLANNING

You need to continue to assess how involved family members or significant others are with the client. The situation that you saw at the initial visit may be very different at this time. Many family members who gladly took on the responsibility of caring for the client may be overwhelmed or feel that they cannot continue to be the caregiver.

The other extreme also may exist. A family member who at first was overwhelmed with the responsibility and did not want to assume care may now be more comfortable and willing to assume more responsibility. The most important thing you need to convey at the visit is that the communication shared between the nurse, client, and family should be open and honest. The plan of care has to be mutual and reevaluated at each visit. You need to look at the whole picture and see what is working and what is not working.

Home care may not be for everyone. If a client is completely dependent for all activities of daily living, and both the family and the aides feel overwhelmed, a nursing home may be an alternative. You need to discuss this openly and honestly with the family. A social worker referral may be indicated at this time for long-term planning. If the family is willing to do more, you can help them to organize their day, prioritize the client's needs, and to make sure they get proper rest periods also.

You also act as the client advocate and see if there are any community services available to assist the client and family. You also need to encourage clients and family members to join support groups. Each revisit should take you closer to discharge. You need to carefully assess whether the client is meeting the goals set out on the initial visit. If you assess that this is a client who still has many teaching needs or is clinically unstable and needs close monitoring, you need to recertify this client and continue to visit until he or she can be safely discharged.

Clients may never be clinically stable. You meet them at a weakened state, either with a chronic illness, with a new diagnosis, or recovering from a surgical procedure. The goal here is to teach the importance of the prescribed medications, diet restrictions, and to suggest lifestyle changes that will have a positive impact on the client's health. If these goals are met, you need to discuss the clinical findings with the physician and see how much longer a client should be revisited.

You have to accept that a client's instability may be a part of his or her life, and continued monitoring may no longer reflect skilled nursing needs. Make sure that this type of client understands complications to observe for and when to follow up with the physician or call 911.

GUIDELINES FOR DOCUMENTATION AND A REVISIT FORM

You always need to ask yourself, "Why are we seeing this client?" Your answer needs to include skilled nursing needs. Your documentation for a revisit also needs to reflect this. When documenting on a revisit note, each revisit note must stand alone, independent of the other notes. Medicare or private insurance companies may want to see the notes of specific revisit dates. The notes must reflect physical findings, teaching or instructions given, client's response to teaching, complications to observe for, and when to notify the physician or 911.

If you are visiting to perform a procedure or technique, you need to document why the client or family member cannot do it. Each revisit note must have appropriate documentation. A revisit note is shown in Display 12-1.

GUIDELINES FOR THE REVISIT

Date

The date of the revisit should match the frequency ordered on the 485. If a client is not able to be seen on that date, a narrative note should be written for the client's record.

text continues on page 224

DISPLAY 12-1. **Revisit Note**

Date: _____ Patient's name: _____ Case number: _____

Address: _____

Primary diagnosis: _____ Secondary diagnosis: _____

HHA Name: _____ Agency: _____ Follows POC: Yes _____ No _____

HHA PCW Supervised in

Medications–Reviewed for Dose: _____ Action: _____ Side Effect: _____ Pt. Compliant: Yes _____ No _____

Specific medication taught/Patient's response: _____

B/P (R) _____ P(A) _____ T(O) _____ (R) _____ Lungs (Anterior) (R) _____ (L) _____ (WT) _____

(L) _____ (R) _____ (Posterior) (R) _____ (L) _____

(A) _____

GI: Diet: _____ Fluids: _____

Teaching needed: _____

CNS: L.O.C.: Alert Lethargic Other _____ Orientation: Person Place Time

Mood/Beh: WNL Irritable Restless Nervous Dizzy? N Y

Headache: Location _____ Frequency _____

Comments and teaching: _____

CP: S.O.B. at rest? N Y After Activity? N Y Describe: _____ Edema? N Y

Orthopnea? N Y # Pillows: _____ Cough? N Y Productive? N Y Describe: _____

Endurance: Poor Fair Good

Chest Pain? N Y Describe: _____ Palpitations: N Y
Comments and teaching: _____

Ambulatory status: _____ Devices used: _____
Teaching needed: _____

Skin: Turgor: WNL Poor Fair _____
Ulcer areas: _____
Measurement of ulcers: _____
Drainage: _____
Odor: N Y Redness: N Y Swelling: N Y Pain: N Y Other: _____
Assessment of Pt./Pt's concerns and symptoms and response to teaching: _____

Procedures performed/Care given: _____

Equipment/supplies in home: _____
Supplies/equipment: Needed & ordered: _____
Coordination: Follow-up with: _____
Change in plans or goals: No _____ Yes _____ Specify: _____
Revisit date: _____ Frequency: _____ Change in frequency: _____
M.D. Visit: _____
V.N. Signature: _____

© With permission. S. Zang

Client's Name/Address/Case Number

These items should all be filled in completely to assure that visits are accounted for and that notes are filed correctly.

HHA Name/Agency/Follows Plan of Care/Supervised in

HHA supervision is part of the nurse's role. Ideally, the plan of care is written with the client, the HHA, and the nurse. The plan of care should be very specific to the client, and the supervision of the HHA needs to be very specific and match what is on the plan of care. If there are any changes in the client's status, they need to be reflected on the plan of care and the HHA needs to be supervised.

Medications

This part of the form needs to reflect a specific medication that is taught and the client's response to teaching. Medication teaching should include doses, actions, and side effects. If the client does not adhere to the medication schedule, you need to document the reason and the intervention and follow-up that you did.

Vital Signs

Blood pressure should be taken in both arms. Apical/radial pulse should be monitored at the same time. Temperature should be taken at every visit. Lung sounds should be documented. If a client has a scale, the weight should be recorded. If the client has no scale, document that client has no scale. If the client knows his or her weight, document *client states* and the weight.

GI/Diet/Fluids/Teaching Needed

Specific diet and fluid restrictions need to be documented. Teaching done at each revisit and client's response need to be reflected. If client does not adhere with diet or fluid restrictions, document why and the intervention and follow-up that you did.

CNS/CP/Comments and Teaching

Both of these systems contain a number of very specific assessment questions. It is advisable to use the revisit form in the home and to complete as much of it as possible during the visit. If any abnormalities are found, the nurse should do a more detailed assessment and document the specific teaching and intervention that was done and the client's response to teaching.

Ambulation Status/Devices Used/Teaching Needed

Document the status of how the client ambulates and any device used. If there is a change in the client's ambulation status, document it and any intervention or follow-up that you did. If the client changes from using a cane to using a walker, it must also be reflected on the HHA plan of care.

Skin

See Chapter 21 on skin and wound care for measurements and proper documentation.

Assessment of Client, Client's Concerns, and Response to Teaching

This narrative part of the revisit note should focus on any abnormalities found at the revisit or any new concerns or problems that the client has had since last seen by the nurse. Be specific if a client is showing any instability. Documentation should include teaching related to the primary and secondary diagnosis and any abnormalities or new findings. It should include the client's response to teaching. If a family member is involved in the teaching, document it. The narrative should give a picture of how the client is progressing toward goal achievement. If any extra visit or change in frequency is indicated, this is where you would justify the reason.

Procedures Performed/Care Given

This part of the documentation should include the exact procedure or treatment performed. Examples are wound care, Foley insertion, and injections administered. Example: *Visiting nurse filled and administered Lente insulin, 12 units, into client's left upper arm. Syringe properly disposed of as per agency policy.*

Equipment/Supplies in Home

All equipment that the client uses, such as a glucometer, wheelchair, or walker, should be included. All

supplies that are used for client's treatments or procedures should be listed.

Equipment/Supplies Needed and Ordered

All supplies and equipment needed should reflect the
client's status and the care he or she is receiving. All
equipment and supplies ordered must have a physician's order.

Coordination/Follow-Up With

Be very specific when documenting who you spoke
to. Document the date, the person's complete name,
and the outcome of the conversation. Include telephone calls to the physician, family members, other
disciplines, vendor agencies, or supply companies.

Change in Plans or Goals/Specify

Be very specific, because this may justify a reason for
a change in frequency. If a client's status changes and
it is documented in the narrative, it should be addressed at this time with new plans or goals.

Revisit Date/Frequency/ Change in Frequency

This should match the 485 unless a change is indicated.

M.D. Visit

Document any planned physician appointments. If a
client has a planned physician appointment for the

same reason that you see the client, you cannot visit on that date.

Example: If you provide postoperative wound care to a client who just had surgery, and the client will see the surgeon that day, you cannot visit.

All forms need to be signed and dated.

13

Recertifying a Client: The Sixty-Day Summary

Anne Delores Kelly, RN, MSN

REASONS FOR RECERTIFICATION

When a client is admitted to the Home Health Agency, the client is referred to as being certified to receive home care services. Certification is embodied in the signed Physician's Plan of Treatment/Health Care Financing Administration (HCFA) 485. Not only does it give the home health agency the authority to provide care and services as ordered in the 485; it also gives the agency the authority to bill third-party payors, both public and private, for services provided by the agency. A certification is effective for a 60- to 62-day period. This applies to both Certified Home Health Agencies (CHHA) and to Long-Term Home Health Care Programs (LTHHCP). Recertification simply means certifying again, that is, continuing service to the client. On recertification, a new 485 is required, with revised goals, plans, and services to reflect the current status of the client.

To determine the appropriateness of recertification, the nurse needs to reevaluate the client against the criteria for certification. Reevaluation of the client is a dynamic and continuous process that occurs throughout any given service period. For the purpose of this chapter, we take that process and capture it at that point when recertification is pending. We look at the client from a number of viewpoints. Our reevaluation review examines the following:

A systems summary of the client status

Each interdisciplinary service and paraprofessional service

Goal achievement of the client to date

A projection of revised goals and plans

Physicians orders at the onset of service and modifications made to these

Orders within the service period

Consideration must be given to the limitation on service reimbursement by specific insurers. Medicare and programs that model Medicare criteria for home care services generally focus on acute problems. Extension of service beyond a certain timeframe for a given diagnosis or client situation will be questioned. For instance, a client with a diagnosis of hypertension whose orders are limited to a daily antihypertensive drug and a sodium-restricted diet would be expected to achieve goals within a 60- to 62-day period, or even faster. For Medicare clients, the homebound status of the client must be clear. Clinical documentation demonstrating the skilled need, the skilled interventions, and an effective client response support the recertification of the client. A client may not meet the requirement for service reimbursement from a specific payor such as Medicare, yet may meet the criteria for recertification. In such a case, billing for service is transferred to an alternate source, such as Medicaid, private pay, or free care. An example may be a client who no longer needs skilled care as defined by Medicare, but needs a weekly pre-pour of multiple medications. The client is unable and has no available support person to provide this care.

Reasons for recertifying a client are summarized further in this chapter and illustrated by case examples. First, however, we take a look at the aspects of review just noted. It is through the integrated review of these aspects that a determination can be made to pursue recertification.

SYSTEMS SUMMARY

When we admit a client to a home health agency, a comprehensive assessment of all systems is performed. This full assessment not only provides baseline data that define the client status, but it also provides the measure used to determine status changes throughout the service period. A basic assessment includes health history, physical examination, cognition, nutrition, mobility, safety, sensory function, and activities of daily living (ADL) function. The client's psychological status, social network, home environment, financial status, educational level, and current perception of his or her health status all have significant bearing on realistic care planning. Assessment helps us also to identify factors that will support or compromise the client's course.

Beyond the initial assessment, continued assessment defines progress, regression, or new problems. Although a diagnosis-focused assessment may be adequate on selected visits, the value of taking a broad view as you evaluate the client is important. Many home care clients have one or more secondary diagnoses compounding the primary problem. Many are treated with multiple medications. The physiologic changes in the aging client create additional risks. Medical treatments aimed at relieving one set of problems may, through their adverse side effects, create new ones.

The recording of findings in objective, measurable terms will serve to measure more precisely the degree of existing symptoms or the degree of progress made in symptom management. This systems summary conducted by the nurse provides information pertinent to decisions regarding recertification. It does not, however, stand alone.

INTERDISCIPLINARY COORDINATION

A client may be receiving more than one service through the home health agency. In such a case, the approach to client care must be an interdisciplinary team approach. This mode is in contrast to multiple disciplines each providing care from an isolated view of the client's need. With the team approach, care planning is coordinated throughout the service period. Goals, though focused by each specialty service, are integrated for the maximal benefit to the client.

The paraprofessional is also an integral member of the home health team. Consider the following examples of an integrated approach to client care:

• The occupational therapist (OT) is working with a hemiparetic client on dressing and grooming activities. The nurse directs the aide to provide step-by-step coaching rather than actually dressing the client as instructed by the OT.

• The physical therapist (PT) communicates to the nurse coordinator that a client's lack of motivation during the therapy sessions may be caused by difficulty in coping with a changed body image. The nurse, on receipt of physician's orders, modifies the initial plan of treatment to include a medical social worker (MSW), who will assess emotional factors impeding the progress of this recent amputee.

GOAL ACHIEVEMENT AND REVISED GOALS AND PLANS

At the onset of home health service, client-centered goals are established. Goals should be realistic, given the individual client circumstances. They should be stated in objective measurable terms. A predicted timeframe for the achievement of each goal is part of the goal or outcome statement.

In certain home care programs, or for certain client situations, goals that focus on maintenance of the client or prevention of complications may be acceptable. For example, a client on an LTHHCP may receive services aimed at maintaining the client at his or her current medically stable state or preventing complications from his or her chronic illness or disability. However, for Medicare and Medicare-modeled services, the goal focus is on resolution of acute problems. In these Medicare-type services, generally when medical stability of the acute problem and learning prescribed treatments for its management are achieved, the client is discharged from service. Otherwise, the client may be considered for recertification. The long-term client, however, may be considered for recertification with maintenance continued as a goal in the next period of service.

Goal statements may be generic in nature. That is, they are applicable to a broad range of diagnoses. Examples of generic goals:

- The client will verbalize understanding of the disease process within X weeks.
- The client will accurately identify and administer medications as prescribed within X weeks.
- The client will demonstrate understanding and compliance with prescribed diet within X weeks.

Goal statements may be individualized according to a particular client's circumstances. Examples of individualized goals:

- The client will ambulate independently on level surface using a straight cane within 9 weeks.

- The client will explore two referred community agencies within 3 weeks.
- The client will demonstrate accurate measure of prescribed insulin and safe self-injection within 4 weeks.
- The wound bed will granulate 60% within 9 weeks.

The nurse coordinator ascertains, from each involved discipline, goal achievement to date. For the unmet goals, it is determined whether they can be achieved in an extended but finite period. Have new problems developed that are appropriate to home care service interventions? If so, what revised goals and plans will address these new problems? In examining the rehabilitation services, has the maximal potential been reached by the client? If the client is at a maintenance level, rehabilitation therapy is considered by Medicare to be no longer reasonable and necessary. However, establishing and teaching a home maintenance program can be acceptable on a short-term basis.

The nurse looks at achievement of nursing goals. What progress has the client made in gaining knowledge of a disease and its management? How accurate and safe is the client in performing prescribed procedures? In addition, the nurse examines all the areas that have impacted on the client's ability to perform personal care and ADL. Has the client regained independence totally or in part? Has dependency decreased to the point that informal caregivers can now assist the client? For a client who no longer requires personal care assistance, aide service is no longer appropriate and should be discontinued. A client who needs assistance with shopping and house cleaning may be referred to a housekeeping service. A client anxious about being alone may benefit from companion or telephone reassurance service and can be referred to such services.

PHYSICIAN ORDERS AND MODIFICATIONS WITHIN THE SERVICE PERIOD

Communication between the service providers, primarily the nurse coordinator and the physician, should occur throughout the service period. The frequency of the communication is dependent on the status and the course of the client. The nurse needs to report adverse symptoms as they occur. The physician may alter the treatments or medications. The physician may order more frequent visits for assessment of the client's response to treatment changes. The physician may want more frequent assessment but be conservative regarding change in treatment because of a client's history of adverse drug reactions. The nurse would also communicate to the physician a delayed response to a prescribed treatment. For example, a wound shows no sign of healing within the expected 4 weeks. The nurse requests medical reevaluation of the wound and the treatment modality. A wound may have progressed to the point that the current treatment is no longer appropriate. The nurse would inform the physician of this and may recommend a change of orders from daily normal saline solution wet to dry dressing to every third day application of a hydrocolloid dressing.

As recertification is pending, the nurse reviews with the physician the client's progress made, continued needs, and revised goals and plans. Current medications, diet, treatments, and activity restrictions as well as ongoing service needs are verified. The nurse receives verbal orders from the physician to continue home care service. These verbal orders for recertification are transcribed in written form, generally on the 485 form, and forwarded to the physician for signature.

SUMMARY OF REASONS FOR RECERTIFICATION

It is through the integration of all of the features discussed that the nurse coordinator determines the appropriateness of the client for recertification. The basic consideration and determining factor is the continued need for skilled service.

The following examples illustrate this "skilled" need:

- A client who remains medically unstable and requires skilled assessment on an intermittent basis with frequent nurse–physician coordination for treatment adjustments
- A client who needs further teaching to manage the medical treatment plan effectively
- A treatment or procedure that cannot be performed by the client because of its complexity or because of the condition of the client
- A client needing a therapy program for restoration of function; the client has demonstrated progress in the past, and further progress is anticipated
- A client requiring a home exercise program to be set up and taught to the informal caregiver

- A client requiring insulin injections when varied approaches to teaching self-management have been unsuccessful, and there is no available caregiver to provide this care on a daily basis

Case Studies

A 74-year-old woman has diagnoses of hypertension, arteriosclerotic heart disease, and arthritis. In the current period, the client experienced fluctuating blood pressure. She was receptive to treatment and teaching. Intolerance to prescribed medications occurred, which necessitated several readjustments by the physician. She remains homebound. The goal for the client is to stabilize her blood pressure within satisfactory limits without significant adverse effects. Nearing the end of her certification period, she is started on a new antihypertensive agent.

The client is appropriate for recertification. She remains medically unstable. An active treatment plan continues, and the client is cooperative, making the plan potentially effective. Her homebound status meets Medicare standard as well.

An 86-year-old woman was admitted to the home care program after a colostomy for a benign bowel obstruction. She has done remarkably well in learning colostomy care, with the assistance of her daughter, who lives nearby. Through a course of trial and error, she has identified foods better tolerated and adjusted her diet accordingly. In other areas she remains in good health, except for developing cataracts. She keeps appointments with her internist and ophthalmologist on a regular basis. The client tells the visiting nurse that it is her visits that keep her going.

This client is not appropriate for recertification. At this time, acute problems are resolved. Colostomy care, once taught, is not a skilled procedure. There is every expectation that, with physician visits and her daughter's involvement, any new problems will be noted. If the need for skilled service arises in the future, she can again be referred to the home health agency.

A 68-year-old man has a diagnosis of cerebrovascular accident with left hemiplegia. At the onset of home care service, he experienced a number of problems necessitating frequent nursing visits for skilled assessment, as well as teaching. The nurse instructed about a sodium-restricted diet, medication management, and understanding signs and symptoms of decompensation and what to do if they occur. In addition to nursing visits, he has had physical therapy and a home health aide. The aide assists him with his prescribed exercise program in addition to bathing and other ADL. As the end of the initial certification period approaches, the nurse reflects that objective signs have been stable within the last few weeks. The client has done well in learning about his condition and how to take his medication and comply with his diet restrictions. He remains limited in transfer, ambulation, and ADL ability. The therapist reports that he has made significant progress in these areas and expects that he will regain even more function.

This client is appropriate for recertification. His therapy program continues to be restorative. Nursing goals are achieved, however, and skilled nursing is not a necessary service in the recertification period. Because personal care and ADL needs continue, home health aide service will be continued. Although federal regulations allow for supervision of the home health aide by the physical therapist, most home health agencies require through their policies that home health aide supervision be provided by the nurse. Nursing visits would then be included on the recertification orders. Visits made by the nurse for the purpose of home health aide supervision are not billable to Medicare. Review of prior teaching and home health aide supervision, by Medicare definition, are not skilled services.

A 90-year-old client has made a nice recovery after a hip fracture. Both the physical therapist and the nurse find no further reason to continue. The medical social worker has evaluated the client for long-term planning and has referred her to agencies for ADL/instrumental ADL (IADL) assistance. The client is not willing to use her savings to pay the current rate for private help. Because of her age and the possibility of a fall in the future, she requests that the home health aide, at least, be allowed to continue.

This client is not appropriate for recertification. Without a need for skilled professional service, aide service cannot be continued. Despite age and potential for risk, no significant threat to health and safety exists. Discharge planning communicated with the client, her family, and the physician is the appropriate course of action.

WRITING A 60-DAY SUMMARY

When a client is discharged from the home health agency, a discharge summary is written. This summarizes the client's course of treatment from the start of care date to the last date the client received service from the agency. When a client is recertified, a summary is written that reflects the preceding 60-day period. Each agency may have a specific form for this purpose. Some forms may be set up to accommodate use as either a 60-day summary or a discharge summary. Though the forms may differ from agency to agency, certain content is generic to all.

Generally, a 60-day summary should include the following:

Client identifying information

Physician

Diagnosis

Service period being summarized—from the initial date of the current service period to the date 60 days from this initial date

Goal achievement to date—Goals are noted as met or unmet. For unmet goals, a reason is noted

Client status through the service period should include: vital sign range, systems review, significant parameters as relevant, such as blood glucose, wound measurements and description, significant changes, that is, progress, regression, and new symptoms or problems. Also included are adjustments to the plan of care in response to client changes and factors affecting the client's response to the plan of care

text continued on page 244

DISPLAY 13-1. 60-Day Summary Form

Patient's Name: _____

Address: _____

Physician: _____ *primary physician – name and address* _____

Diagnosis: _____ *primary diagnosis; secondary diagnosis* _____

60 Day _____ X _____ Discharge _____ Period of service: *initial date of* To: *date 60 days from initial date of*

_____ *current certification period* _____ *current certification period* _____

Vital sign range – within the certification period

B/P: _____ ARP: _____ R: _____ T: _____

Status of goal outcomes:	Met	Unmet	Reasons unmet
Understands and complies with medication	*For each listed goal*		*For any unmet goal note reason.*
Understands disease process	*check if met or unmet.*		
Understands s/s of infection			
Understands diet restriction			
Understands when to notify MD			

Changes in medication/treatment/diet within the past 60 days: *Note any changes or modified orders made within the* *current certification/recertification period. Changes may include additions, deletions of medications or* *treatments or change in dosage, frequency, route of administration. Changes in ordered services should also be in-* *cluded.*

HHA: _____ Days X _____ Hours Note number of days per week and hours per day for home health aide ser-vice during the period.

Supervised in: Note assigned tasks HHA was instructed and supervised in during the service period.

Change in HHA plan of care: Note any change in plan of care during the service period. Include change in assigned days, hours, and/or tasks.

Review of systems/Status of goal achievement over 60 days: Summarize client status during this period to include: system review, significant findings, objective measures as pertinent, e.g., blood glucose, abdominal girth, wound measurements and description (stage or thickness, exudate, margins, etc.).

- significant changes, i.e., progress, regression/deterioration, new symptoms or problems

- adjustments to plan of care in response to changes

- factors affecting client response to care plan

Plans and goals for the next 60 days: Note revised goals and plans for each discipline projected for the next recertification period.

Reason for discharge: N/A

Coordination: Note coordination activities during the service period with physician, therapist, medical social worker, community agencies, informal caregivers.

V.N. Signature: _____ Date: _____

©With permission. S. Zang

Services provided, that is, specific disciplines, paraprofessional and ancillary services
A projection of revised goals, plans, and services for
the recertification period

In conclusion, recertification looks at the recent
past to determine the future home care service appropriateness for a given client. Because recertification
orders should be physician signed and received by
the agency at the start of the recertification period, review of the client should be initiated 10 to 14 days
before the start date of the new period of service.
When coordination and reevaluation of the client's response to treatment and goals occur on an ongoing
basis, this review need not be too complex or too time
consuming. Once the determination is made to recertify the client, it is actualized by the following:

Obtaining verbal physician orders
Completing a 485/Physician Plan of Treatment
Completing a 60-day summary

In addition, some agencies may require revision
of other documents to update the client record. These
may include the Home Health Aide Plan of Care and
a Medication/Treatment listing. The challenge of
home care is to use the time we have with the client
most efficiently toward goal achievement. Individual
client factors affect the rate of progress a client will
make in a 60-day period. Through recertification, we
continue to use our professional skills to move a
client on a continued path toward goal achievement.
Display 13-1 is a sample 60-day summary with
guidelines for completion.

14

Discharge From Home Care

Sally A. Sobolewski, RN, MSN

Planning for a Discharge   Documenting the Discharge
Criteria for Discharge

Discharging the client from nursing care is a concept familiar to most nurses. This topic is taught in nursing education, as well as during the orientation the nurse receives when beginning employment. Although there may be aspects pertaining to discharge that are fundamental to the process regardless of the client care setting, discharge from home care is distinctly different in several ways.

In home care, the nurse collaborates with the client, family, and physician to determine the client's needs and then designs a plan that will lead to the achievement of identified goals and outcomes. Unlike other settings in which the nurse may only be *informed* of the client's discharge, in home care it is most often the nurse who is responsible for evaluating the client's readiness for discharge. Because the purpose of home care is to enable the client to become independent in the management of his or her health condition, the knowledge the client therefore requires can be vast, exceeding what is needed in the days and weeks immediately after hospitalization. The nurse must anticipate possible situations the client will face in regaining and maintaining his or her level of health. Before the nurse considers client discharge from home care, the client needs to understand what complications to look for and how to handle them, the progression of the illness and the related lifestyle changes, and how to basically manage their care to prevent rehospitalization.

Another difference for the nurse in the approach to client discharge from home care involves managing the cost of care. Home care nurses make decisions about the effectiveness of care in relation to its cost. This is done through careful analysis of cost in relation to its benefit in meeting the client's desired health outcome. This degree of accountability, or fiscal responsibility, is unique to the practice of home care and unparalleled in other settings of nursing practice. Home care nurses are expected to be able to objectively decide what needs are able to be addressed effectively in the home care setting and constantly evaluate the established plan. It is possible that the client's needs do not diminish, or improve, in which case the nurse must exercise fiscal responsibility by identifying that home care is no longer the appropriate level of care for the client. For instance, a client who requires a steadily increasing number of home health aide hours to be maintained in their home may actually exceed the cost of placement in a nursing home. Identification of such situations and conducting the extensive planning associated for alternate plans often require intricate and detailed work and may not be readily received by the client or family.

Finally, discharge from home care requires that the nurse involve the client and family members. One of the key benefits of practicing in home care is that the client is seen in his or her own environment. Such an awareness gives the home care nurse a great deal of information concerning what it means for the client to make a lifestyle change or carry out a particular treatment. Oftentimes treatments or care that are perceived by health care providers to be simple and routine may actually be complicated and unreasonable in light of other family needs and demands. To succeed in helping the client achieve independent care, it is necessary to openly discuss what assuming care management means to the client and family if the goals are to be achieved. This allows the family to decide what is unrealistic and gives the nurse the opportunity to negotiate the plan. Without the mutual support of the client and family, it is difficult to ensure a successful discharge. Involving persons within the client–family system in ongoing care needs also creates support once the nurse is removed from the situation. The nurse needs knowledge, skill, and practice to appropriately, safely, and effectively complete the discharge process. The remainder of this chapter discusses how to plan for the client's discharge, criteria for discharge, and how to document a client discharge in home care.

PLANNING FOR A DISCHARGE

The statement, "Discharge planning begins on admission," is the foundation on which the home care nurse builds a plan of care. There are several good reasons for introducing discharge on the initial home visit.

The first home visit is the time in which the nurse establishes a rapport with the client and explains the services available in home care, as well as their limitations. Clients often have questions concerning the frequency and duration of the service. They may have been told, or perceived, that once admitted to home care, they would receive care indefinitely. It may come as a surprise to the client or family member that home health care is usually related to an episodic illness and has a finite focus. Knowing the client's perceptions and expectations about service helps the nurse to respond and provide a clear definition about home care and its duration. The client should be made aware of what criteria guide the nurse in determining service. Not only is this a part of each client's rights, but ultimately, such a forthright approach in providing information assists in allowing the client to view the nurse as one who shares information openly and honestly.

Another reason to initiate discharge planning on the initial visit relates to that of timing. Often, immediately after a hospitalization, the client is more amenable to discussing a plan for recovery or adjustment to the new condition. This readiness allows the nurse to introduce the notion of eventual independent management. Even if it is not possible to establish an entire plan, this discussion can be useful in motivating the client to participate in prescribed activities.

The plans for discharge must include discussion with the client and family. Asking questions and listening to their ideas for managing care, expected outcomes of care, and real or perceived obstacles to their participation allows the nurse to tailor a mutually acceptable plan of care. This discussion is used in the assessment of the client's beliefs about illness, meaning of care, and level of family involvement. It will guide the nurse in the diagnosis of problems that must be addressed to achieve client outcomes and discharge. It is important that the nurse understand that discharging the client is a process that must be initiated early to allow time for a suitable plan to be developed and implemented.

The nurse must also bear in mind that a client may be insured by a company whose timeframes for outcome achievement may be less than what the client requires. For instance, a managed care program may authorize two visits to teach a newly diagnosed insulin-dependent diabetic client how to inject insulin. However, if the client has extensive visual impairment and residual hemiplegia from a previous stroke, it may take longer for the nurse to help the client achieve the goal. Those limitations should be acknowledged on the initiation of care to plan for the most effective use of the home care admission. This will have special bearing on the discharge plan, causing the client and nurse to scrutinize it closely for feasibility. Priorities will need to be established to ensure that the client has attained completion of the most significant outcomes before expiration of payment.

If the insurance company will not allow for continued visits, and the nurse assesses that the client still has skilled nursing needs, the manager of the home care agency needs to be informed. The client's safety is the major concern. Alternate plans might need to be discussed.

CRITERIA FOR DISCHARGE

Ideally, a client is discharged from home care when the goals or outcomes of care are met. There are times when the client is discharged from home care when this does not occur. There can be a number of reasons for this, many of which are not related to the nurse's ability to develop or implement the plan of care. For instance, the client may refuse care or move to another location, or the client's physician may not agree with the need for the continuation of services. Also, third-party payers have criteria that may be unique to specific coverage plans, which may dictate discharge from home care service. All home care agencies have policies and procedures that address such circumstances. The nurse should be familiar with how to access this information within the agency. This discussion is limited to the most frequent reasons for discharge from home care.

"Client Is Medically Stable"

The client's medical stability is a very frequent reason for discharging the patient from home care and is an outcome that would be expected and desired for all clients. As an expected outcome, this means that when the client is stable and has no further skilled nursing needs, the reason for home health care ceases. Very often, the nurse is performing care leading to other outcomes, such as independence in performing a specific skill, or learning about how to manage other aspects of care. When there are other needs that the nurse is addressing, it may be possible to continue in the care. Even in such instances, once the client has achieved a stable physical status, this introduces the possibility of the client being able to move to an alternate level of care for achieving unmet outcomes. For instance, the client referred to home care after a hospitalization for newly diagnosed insulin-dependent diabetes may achieve stable blood glucose levels and be ready to return to work before having fully learned all aspects of their diabetic self-care management. This may necessitate the nurse arranging for the client to have the remainder of this teaching completed in a group class at a local hospital after the client's work hours or, if the reimbursement criteria does not require the client to be homebound, the nurse may arrange to visit the client on weekends or before or after working hours. This may not need to be done, however, if the same client needs only one or two additional visits to complete the teaching and will remain home from work for an additional week.

"Client's Family Can Assume Care"

This criterion is both a reason and a possible solution for helping a client to achieve discharge from home care. A client may not be able to perform all of the care required. Nurses should be aware that the client, as well as the family members, may have varying feelings related to carrying out client care-related activities. It is important to hear these concerns to identify the best approach to helping the client and family agree to assuming care. The family may decide that they will participate so that the client can remain in the home setting. The nurse will then teach family members or significant others to assist with ongoing needs. Discharge can only take place when the client's family or significant other can assume care.

"Client Not Willing to Participate in the Plan of Care"

There are times when even the client who engages in the development of the plan of care may withdraw from participation. This can take the form of active resistance, such as the client who openly speaks of an unwillingness to learn or perform certain behaviors. The resistance may also be of a passive nature, in which the client verbalizes an agreement with plan of care but does not, for example, carry out planned treatments, "forgets" to take medication, or does not follow through with making arrangements for medical care. There can be many reasons for a client to decline participation in the plan of care. The nurse must explore the meaning of the behavior and its cause with the client. Most often the behavior stems from a problem that may require an alteration or addition to the plan of care to help the client regain interest in participating. For instance, "forgetting" to take medication may have its roots in the client's lack of financial resources, which could be addressed through a referral to a social worker. It may also be attributable to the onset of depression about the illness and would need to be discussed with the physician for appropriate referral and treatment.

It is not uncommon for the nurse to feel frustrated by the client's lack of participation in care. However, this should not be the basis for discontinuing service. Failure to explore the reasons for client's participation and alternate methods of enlisting the client's cooperation could be considered abandonment by the nurse.

If all attempts to involve the client have not succeeded, the nurse must speak with the client about possible discharge. The client must be told what the consequences of lack of care could mean to his or her health. The nurse should also offer to help the client make other arrangements for care on discharge from the home care agency if the client desires.

In the course of this entire process, the nurse should be communicating with the client's physician and any significant family members. All conversations about discharge because of the client's lack of participation in the plan of care must be documented in the client's record. Some home care agencies may have policies that would require that the client be sent a letter with the reason for discharge as a way of allowing the client an opportunity to reconsider their decision.

Other Reasons for Discharge

There may be other reasons for which the client is discharged from home care. Many agencies have categorized the most frequent reasons for discharge and list them on a form for easier completion by nurses and for purposes of data collection. The nurse can indicate the reason by simply entering a code or checking a form.

Examples of such reasons include: client not stable (hospitalized), client refused further service, client moved to alternate level of care (nursing home/hospice/rehabilitation center), client moved (cannot be found), physician does not consent to sign orders, or client died. As previously noted, a home care agency may have different policies and procedures related to the reason for discharge or the client's disposition at the time of discharge. The nurse should be familiar with the specific issues in his or her home care agency.

DOCUMENTING THE DISCHARGE

Once the client is discharged, the care is not complete until the appropriate documentation has been done. The contents of a client's discharge documentation are dictated by regulatory bodies overseeing home care, as well as the policies and procedures of the specific home care agency. Basically, the paperwork consists of a discharge summary and the documentation of the achievement of the client's goals or outcome as a result of the home care admission.

In most cases, part of the documentation requires that the nurse write a narrative note, usually related to the summary of the client's length of stay. Sometimes this is in the body of the client record, or it may be located on a separate form. Many home care agencies use some form for the nurse to record the attainment of client goals, often in the form of a checklist. A completed discharge summary is shown in Display 14-1.

Documenting Outcome of Care

The ultimate goal of home care is to help the client or family member to become independent in self-care management. Independence in self-care management is usually achieved by meeting outcomes that fall into one of three categories: knowledge, skill, and physical status. This means that during the home care admission, the nurse usually finds that the plan of care and its associated interventions are designed to help the client learn information (knowledge), perform treatments or behaviors (skills), or achieve a stable physical status.

The goal statements in this example of the discharge summary are primarily related to knowledge (client understands medication, disease process, infection, diet restriction, and when to notify the physician). The only skill listed is related to medication (client complies with medication). The physical status is reported by listing actual ranges of vital signs, in which the nurse determines if stability has been achieved.

Some home care agencies have listed the most frequently selected outcomes for clients and printed them for the nurse to check. This example calls for the nurse to complete such a checklist by responding to *met* or *unmet*. For those outcomes that have not been met, the nurse must supply a reason. As with client discharge, there may be a number of reasons that a particular outcome has not been met. For example, an interruption in care such as rehospitalization may result in the plan of care not being fully implemented, and hence, outcomes remain unmet.

Sometimes, the nurse will find that the outcomes were unrealistic for a particular client. Again, this would result in an unmet outcome. Unmet outcomes are not to be regarded as nursing failures. It is important that the nurse record the status of the client outcome honestly. Accurate information about the client's admission can be of assistance if the client is readmitted to the home care agency at a later date and can possibly shape future approaches to care.

The summary of care in the example is also aided by the prompting statements on the form. For instance, the nurse is able to report changes in medication, treatment, and diet; review the body systems; describe any paraprofessional care that may have

DISPLAY 14-1. **Discharge Summary Form**

Patient's Name: _____

Address: _____

Physician: _____

Diagnosis: _____

60 Day _____ Discharge ___X___ Period of service: _when case opened_ To: _date of discharge_

Vital sign range: _If a 60-day summary was already done, VS range should just be from date of new recert to D/C date. If a recert was not done, VS should be from date of opening to D/C date._

B/P: _____ ARP: _____ R: _____ T: _____

Status of goal outcomes:	Met	Unmet	Reasons unmet
Understands and complies with medication	___	___	_At time of discharge most needs are_
Understands disease process	___	___	_met. If the need was not met document_
Understands S/S of infection	___	___	_why and what was done, e.g., "Patient_
Understands diet restriction	___	___	_not compliant with diet although he/she_
Understands when to notify MD	___	___	_understands negative implications of_
			not complying. M.D. aware."

Changes in medication/treatment/diet within the past 60 days: *If recert was already done, only unmet changes from the last recert to date of discharge should be documented. If recert was not done, changes from initial visit to discharge are documented.*

HHA:_____ Days X_____ Hours_____

Supervised in: *Not applicable as HHA is already out at end of discharge.*_____

Change in HHA plan of care:_____

Review of systems/Status of goal achievement over 60 days:_____

*Review of each system is done at time of discharge.*_____

Plans and goals for the next 60 days:_____

*Not applicable with discharge.*_____

Reason for discharge:_____

Coordination: *Document who you spoke to. Physician must be notified of status of discharge.*

V.N. Signature:_____ Date_____

©*With permission. S. Zang*

been provided; and elaborate on the activities designed to achieve the goals.

Again, each home care agency offers the nurse a different approach to capturing this information. It is important that the nurse acquire the ability to do this in a succinct manner, especially if the format is solely narrative. The discharge summary (Display 14–1) should tell the client's story in an encapsulated fashion.

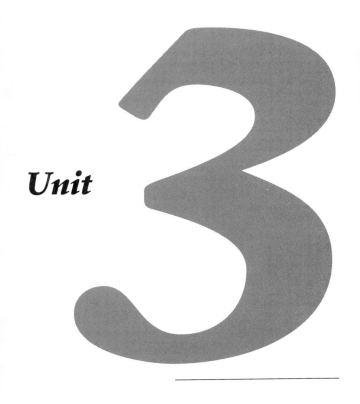

Unit

3

CLINICAL
CHALLENGES

15

Medication Management in the Home

Gale O. Surrency, RNC, MA

In the home care setting, the nurse is the most frequent observer of the medication regimen. It is the nurse who, during a home visit, discovers the need to validate a medication discrepancy, and who reports adverse symptoms, changes in the clinical status, or therapeutic responses to medication therapy. It is often the home care nurse who initiates the call to the pharmacist or physician to begin the interdisciplinary communication necessary to stabilize the client at home or make the referral to the appropriate emergency medical treatment site. After this intervention, other members of the health care team may be called on to assist the client. The social worker may be required to facilitate financial access to obtain the necessary medication supply, or the nutritionist may be needed to explain and plan dietary management in relation to drug therapy.

NATURE AND PATTERN OF MEDICATION CONSUMPTION

A review of the literature and clinical practice experience shows that over-the-counter (OTC) nonprescription drug consumption is increasing among a cross-section of the population. This, in conjunction with prescriptive drug treatment for a variety of multiple and chronic diseases, produces an ideal environment for adverse drug interactions to occur. Consumption of OTC medication without the knowledge of the physician also poses a threat to the medical treatment plan. Many individuals do not know how to read, do not read labels carefully, or fail to read and follow label instructions. Some OTC medications contain combinations of drugs and or nutrients that would be therapeutically contraindicated for specific disease entities. Another common and long-standing behavior is to take both prescription and OTC medications according to how one feels. When symptoms decrease, treatment may stop or be erratic. If symptoms recur or increase, medication intake may resume or dosage may be doubled without consulting the physician.

TYPES OF NONADHERENT BEHAVIOR

Nonadherence can be broadly defined as failure to adhere to prescribed instructions regarding the use of medications. Many factors influence the client's ability to manage a self-administered medication regimen. The home care nurse must perform a thorough assessment to determine why there is often failure to adhere to the treatment regimen. However, once the tendency or risk factors are identified, the nurse must endeavor to understand the motivating behaviors behind nonadherence. This knowledge then becomes the building blocks on which interventions can be designed to assist the client in adapting more positive adherence patterns.

Omission of the Medication: Omission occurs when the client fails for various reasons to take the medication. This may happen as a result of a conscious overt decision or may be attributable to other extenuating circumstances.

Taking Medication at Incorrect Times: Taking medication at the wrong time may or may not cause significant clinical problems, depending on the action and duration within the body. A situation wherein deviation from intended use could prove adverse would be the client who takes insulin after, as opposed to before, meals.

Excessive Consumption of Medications (Overdosing): Excessive consumption occurs when either the frequency or dosage of the medication is increased by the client. This can result in organ dysfunction or skewed laboratory results.

Premature Discontinuation of Medication: Premature discontinuation occurs when the client stops taking the medication before the prescribed course of treatment is completed. This may arise in antibiotic, steroid, or chemotherapy treatments, when the client experiences either improvement or worsening of symptoms.

Failure to Fill Prescriptions: Failure to fill prescriptions results when the client does not follow through in obtaining the prescribed medication. Thus, treatment is never initiated. Symptoms or conditions may exacerbate, and medical personnel may be led to believe that treatment is ineffective.

RESPONSIBILITY OF THE HOME CARE NURSE IN MEDICATION MANAGEMENT

Information from the baseline data and continuing assessment is incorporated as part of an ongoing plan for successful medication management in the home. This systematic approach ensures the gathering of pertinent data, conserves time during the home visit, and assists in the prioritizing of learning needs.

The following discussion outlines the responsibilities of the home care nurse.

Prepare the client before the visit by asking that all medications be gathered together and made available for review. You need to see *all* the medications the client is taking.

It is important to do a complete assessment of prescription as well as OTC medication found in the home. Also be alert and discretely observe the home for any medications that may be overlooked or not brought forth initially by the client. Any evidence of hoarding or stockpiling of medication can be explored, and you should review safety precautions and dangers relative to this behavior.

Take a thorough and accurate history of medication patterns from a reliable historian. This can be the client or the primary caregiver. In some instances, this may be a paraprofessional. Although paraprofessionals are not allowed in some states to administer medications, they often do accompany clients to medical appointments and cue and assist self-directed clients with positioning and preparation for medication administration.

Ask the client to read the labels on each medication bottle. If the client cannot read, ask him or her to describe how he or she knows one medication from another and why it is being taken. If you detect problems in literacy levels, it should be carefully noted in the teaching plan.

Examine each container and ask the client to verbally describe, in lay terms, intended action, side effects, duration, dosage, and frequency. Always ask the client for this information, rather than volunteer instructions up front. In this way, discrepancies can be identified more readily.

Instruct client to keep medications in original containers. If client is unable to open childproof bottles, the client should request easy-open bottles from the pharmacy.

Teach medication therapy in small segments. Start with the most therapeutically indicated ones and then move on to the supplements, vitamins, and so forth. Teaching should be done in a quiet atmosphere with adequate lighting and seating, and there should be no distractions such as radio or television.

Explore with the client special instructions and precautions relative to each medication. Some important points in this area would be: sustained-release capsules, how to guard against megavitamin intake, nutrient/drug interactions and foods that block absorption or effectiveness of the medication, medications that should not be altered, for example, crushed, broken, or put into foods. In addition, the client should receive instructions regarding missed dosages, sick days, travel, or vacation planning in relation to medication therapy.

Check containers to see if medications have been prescribed by the same physician and filled at the same pharmacy. If more than one physician or pharmacy is involved, determine whether duplicate medications exist, especially under different brand or trade names. If a problem is discovered in this area, the client and physician of record must be notified immediately. The primary physician must then provide orders for the appropriate treatment plan. In the event the client's condition is such that there are two physicians involved, both physicians must be aware of and agree to a mutual plan of care. The home care nurse is then responsible for the coordination of the teaching plan.

Explore past and present accounts of drug, food, or environmental allergies. Ask the client to describe any unusual, untoward effects to any therapy, no matter how subtle or overt the symptoms.

Examine containers for expiration dates and changes in color or consistency of medication.

Evaluate the regimen in terms of relationship between prescribed medication and appropriate medical diagnoses, excessive or questionable dosage levels, excessive duration of treatment, therapeutic effects, and expected outcomes of drug therapy.

Identify and verify medication discrepancies between physician order, what was found or not found in the home, dosage, and frequency variations.

Carefully evaluate the therapy in relation to other chief signs and symptoms or problems the client may be experiencing, such as bowel, bladder, or upper or lower gastrointestinal complaints.

Identify physiologic dysfunction in terms of swallowing, eating, or malabsorption syndromes, which interfere with ingestion and drug metabolism in the body.

As-needed medication regimens should be evaluated to determine what symptoms generate the need to take which medication. Instructions should be given as to how to stay within safe limits and those side effects that would denote overuse and toxicity.

Explore potential for use of home remedies. Cultural and ethnic mores come into play here very strongly in some homes. Precautions and dangers of these practices must be tactfully discussed.

Social habits should be assessed, including alcohol and nicotine intake. Illegal drug use must be explored. All of these substances could adversely impact the therapy and clinical status of the client.

Evaluate mental acuity and capacity to determine client's potential for safe self-administration. Do a baseline assessment, and continue to do this at each visit to determine if gradual toxic side effects are occurring.

Review, in layman's terms, basic drug interaction in the body starting with absorption, distribution, metabolism, and excretion. It is crucial for the client to understand how various factors can affect each phase of metabolism and thus alter the therapeutic effects of the regimen.

In efforts to control cost, clients may skip dosages, share, or take medications prescribed for someone else. Safety precautions and dangers regarding these practices must be explained.

Check for unfilled prescriptions and determine how long the client has been without the medication. Observe for adverse clinical symptoms and notify the physician of findings immediately.

Ascertain how client obtains medication refills. Include a discussion of financial resources and transportation arrangements and assess their impact on regimen. Identify methods to decrease cost both for medication expenditure and trips to the pharmacy or hospital for prescription refills. Perhaps the client is paying out of pocket for the medication. Encourage the client to explore with the primary physician opportunities to substitute the less costly form of the medication or OTC vitamin supplement, whenever it is therapeutically feasible. Prescription refills also can be obtained in a variety of ways, which may decrease trip expenses. Some pharmacies provide free delivery services. Various senior citizen, other community groups, neighbors, or friends may be willing to provide errand services. Prescription refill trips also may be combined with other chores. In addition, some insurance plans offer mail-order medication plans for a nominal fee or free of charge. If a financial problem is noted, a social worker referral may be indicated.

Complete a learning needs assessment as a prerequisite to establishing a client education plan. Start by assessing the client's potential for learning, then go on to validate the current knowledge base regarding diagnoses and relationship to present medication therapy.

During this process, you also must identify barriers to learning, for example, age, literacy, illness/disease process, cultural diversity, and cognitive, affective, or psychomotor dysfunction. Accurately identify and promptly address sensory, psychomotor, or mental acuity deficits, make the necessary referrals to the appropriate discipline, and include the interventions for that discipline in the overall plan of care.

Design an individualized client education plan. Use of the nursing process and nursing diagnoses to identify actual and potential problems assists in developing a plan that is client and family focused. Each visit, you should identify essential content that must be learned or reinforced. Plan the steps so that the client and family achieve success as they progress toward the goal of independence. Continually evaluate interventions and client outcomes, then modify strategies as indicated.

Encourage full caregiver participation by more than one support person, if available. This provides backup as well as respite for the primary caregiver.

ADAPTIVE DEVICES TO FACILITATE SELF–MEDICATION MANAGEMENT

No plan of care could be implemented without appropriate supportive educational tools and adaptive devices. The nurse plays a key role in selecting the appropriate adaptive device to meet the needs of the client. This task is undertaken after thorough client, home, and learning needs assessments. Following is a selected description of such devices that can be incorporated into the home care teaching plan:

Visual aids, such as written charts, flash cards, pictograms, and medication clocks

Color-coded pill boxes with electronic or battery timers to alert the client or announce medication schedules

Prepour pill boxes and containers for liquids. Oral medication is prepared for up to 1 week at a time by the nurse and placed in closed pill boxes, or containers for liquids. The boxes or containers are labeled for each day of the week. Color-coded combinations of the containers can be used to prepour oral medications for up to four times a day.

Automated medication dispenser. This system allows the nurse to prepour and program the unit to dispense medications at a predetermined time, along with an instructional screen menu detailing how the medication should be taken. Medications are placed in a cassette, which is then loaded and locked into a computerized unit. The unit is then programmed by the nurse to dispense medications at a predetermined interval. A buzzer sounds, and a drawer opens to deliver the necessary medication.

Prefilled syringes. This is a common method employed for the client who is independent in insulin administration, but lacks either the visual, mental, or motor skills to accurately draw up insulin. The nurse makes scheduled home visits, performs the necessary assessments, and prefills syringes. The prefilled syringes are then stored in the refrigerator in a covered container for use each day by the client. Magnifiers that snap onto insulin syringes are useful for visualizing the lines on the syringe. There are also insulin vial holders with magnetic backs that attach to metal surfaces. It holds the vial while the client draws up the insulin. There are also visual center aids that help center the needle correctly to penetrate the vial.

Needle-free injector system. This lightweight, easy-to-use needle-free insulin injector system eliminates the discomfort of repeated needle injections and is very useful for children.

Medical alert bracelets and necklaces, although not considered as adaptive devices, do serve a very useful purpose. Individuals with seizures, cardiac disease, diabetes, or other life-threatening conditions wear these alerts to identify their medical emergencies.

In addition, there are various devices for visually handicapped client to assist in self-administration of medication. The local organizations for the blind or visually impaired as well as surgical supply companies can provide more information.

DOCUMENTATION

Medication management documentation serves to identify learning and knowledge deficits after a thorough needs assessment. Documentation also outlines the teaching and learning plan, interventions, and expected outcomes and details progress toward these goals. Teaching plans should be clearly outlined, and documentation must include data that illustrate that the plan meets the needs of the client.

Important Points to Remember in Completing Documentation Relative to the Plan

- Frequency of visits, physician orders, and medical and nursing plan must support the teaching needed.
- Identify new or changed medications and related interventions.
- Describe knowledge, skills deficits, client limitations, and barriers to learning. Explain how the teaching and nursing plans address all of these areas.
- Describe responses to teaching and need for additional or ongoing teaching.
- Clinical record should reflect evidence of a complete physical, socioeconomic, environmental assessment, problem identification, and follow-up interventions.
- Initial assessments and medication histories should provide key information to assist the nurse to identify, observe, and evaluate the client's status. It also establishes a baseline for future visit comparisons, evaluation of responses to

teaching, and progress toward goal accomplishment.

• Reassessment or follow-up visits should reflect continuation of observation and assessment of the client's status, identification of factors that necessitate modification of the medication regimen, and overall plan of care.

• Documentation data must identify quantifiable goals, initial and ongoing needs for skilled services, or readiness for discharge.

• There must be clear evidence of care coordination, and notification to physician regarding changes in client status, medication regimen, or adverse effects to treatment. Communication with other disciplines and referrals to community resources also must be included in the clinical record.

MEDICATION PROFILE

Although the home health agency may have written policies regarding medication management, there must be a mechanism for the nurse to record the medications included in the regimen. Various formats exist, but most agencies use some type of medication profile to satisfy this purpose.

The basic content of the profile consists of client identification demographics, that is, name, medial record number, address, listing of medications, including dosage, route, frequency, start and discontinuation dates, allergies, an area for updating the profile, and an area for the signature of the nurse. Some preprinted profiles also identify medications by category and list side effects and contraindications. The profile should include prescription and nonprescription medications.

During the visit, the nurse assesses responses to medication therapy and uses the profile as a basis for teaching and obtaining a complete picture of medication ingestion. The profile also serves as a useful tool for other nurses and assists in care, coordination, and communication with the primary physician. The client should be instructed to always take an updated list of medications to the physician. Changes should be made from that list.

Up to this point, the discussion has centered around independent self-administration of medications by the client. The question remains, what about the client who requires total or partial assistance with management? The nurse must design appropriate interventions to include available caregivers to fulfill this role. Various options can be explored. If there is a continuing need for skilled nursing care, medication administration and management can be incorporated into aspects of the home visit. Alternative support systems such as family, friends, or neighbors can sometimes provide the necessary supervision and assistance. Sometimes a combination of an adaptive device and intermittent supervision by a caregiver establishes a safe method for management. The final decision ultimately becomes client specific, and requires collaboration between all health care team members.

16

Tuberculosis in the Home

Nellie C. Bailey, RN, MS, MA, CS

Factors That Contribute to the Spread of Tuberculosis

Factors That Put People at Risk for Tuberculosis

Home Health Care Admission Requirements

Responsibilities of the Home Health Nurse

Conclusions

As homelessness and poverty continue to plague our society, tuberculosis remains prevalent and at epidemic levels in some sectors of our urban populations. Included in this chapter is an overview of factors that contribute to tuberculosis (TB), factors that put individuals at risk for TB, and specific criteria for admitting clients with TB for home care services. This chapter also discusses the United States Department of Health and Human Services (US-DHHS) and Centers for Disease Control (CDC) guidelines and recommendations for the management and control of the spread of TB.

Although policies regarding guidelines for the management and control of TB in home health agencies may vary from agency to agency and state to state, the general recommendations are mandated by the US-DHHS and the CDC. Emphasis in this chapter is placed on the responsibilities of the home health nurse providing care to clients with TB, their families, and caregivers, for example, home health aide (HHA) or personal care worker (PCW).

FACTORS THAT CONTRIBUTE TO THE SPREAD OF TUBERCULOSIS

Tuberculosis is a bacterial infection caused by *Mycobacterium tuberculosis*. TB is spread by the airborne route, and the respiratory system is the portal of entry. The most frequent site of infection is the lungs. However, miliary or extrapulmonary TB may be present in other sites, such as organs, meninges, blood, bones, and liver.

To provide adequate and appropriate care in the home to clients with TB, it is necessary for the nurse to have an understanding of the factors that contribute to the spread of TB and put individuals at risk for TB. One of the main factors that causes the spread of TB is overcrowding, with poor ventilation or lack of ventilation. If the client with TB lives in a home situation that is overcrowded, then the members in that household are at risk for contracting TB. This includes the HHA, PCW, and family members who have to spend long periods in the environment. Overcrowding could mean six people living in a one-bedroom apartment, four people living in a studio apartment, or a family living in a shelter that houses multiple groups. Whatever the situation, the nurse's primary concern is to provide the care that is prescribed while keeping in mind the need to prevent spreading and contracting the disease.

The nurse may have to provide wound care, give an injection, or teach well baby care in any of these situations. Ideally, the client with TB should have a private room with a door that can close, and the supplies needed for client care should be left outside the room. This is an ideal situation that does not exist in most of the homes the nurse visits.

FACTORS THAT PUT PEOPLE AT RISK FOR TUBERCULOSIS

Many of the clients that the home health nurse visits could potentially be at risk for TB. Also, it is prolonged contact with a client with active TB that puts individuals at risk for contracting the disease. Clients with inactive TB are not infectious and cannot transmit the disease. The characteristics that put individuals at risk for TB include:

- Poor immune system
- Poor nutrition
- A chronic debilitating condition
- Substance abuse
- Increased stress
- Advanced age

The home health nurse has many clients with these characteristics in a regular caseload, such as young children, clients with acquired immune deficiency syndrome (AIDS)/human immunodeficiency virus (HIV), terminal cancer, chronic alcoholism, clients who are poor, and the frail elderly. It is important for the nurse to know that such characteristics put these individuals at risk for TB and that certain precautions must be taken when providing care to them.

HOME HEALTH CARE ADMISSION REQUIREMENTS

The guidelines that home health agencies establish for admission of clients with TB for service are based on the strict recommendations established by the US-DHHS and the CDC. The guidelines are adopted by the state health departments and communicated to the home health agencies in each state. As mentioned earlier, the policies may vary from agency to agency and state to state, but because the guidelines are mandated by the U.S. federal government, similarities may exist. It is important for home health nurses to be familiar with the criteria for their respective states and to follow the policies of the home health agency where they are employed. Nurses should also know that with treatment and a healthy immune system, TB in the client can be rendered inactive. An individual can also carry the TB disease and not have the disease themselves. This type of inapparent infection can only be detected through a tuberculin skin test.

When screening a client for acceptance for home health services, the nurse should know that a positive test usually indicates that a person has been infected with TB. It does not necessarily mean that the person has the TB disease. It should also be pointed out that some clients might have been given bacillus Calmette-Guérin vaccine at some point and will therefore have a positive TB test. If the TB test is positive, the CDC requires that other tests such as chest radiograph or sputum sample be taken to see if the person actually has TB.

The requirement is that clients with active TB should be noninfectious before being eligible for home care services and that verification of the client's noninfectious status must be provided to the agency that is to provide the services. Admission criteria also requires that the client with a diagnosis of active TB must have been receiving TB drug therapy for at least 2 weeks before admission, and that the client shows clinical signs of improvement that have been verified by radiograph and other clinical symptoms such as changes in the characteristics of the sputum or resolution of the cough. In addition, the client must have documentation of the following: at least three acid-fast bacillus smears on 3 consecutive days, and that the client is adhering to the medication regimen and routine medical follow-up evaluations. Agencies also may have policies that would permit them to admit clients who require home care services but do not meet all of the above-mentioned criteria. Admission of such cases will be determined on an individual basis by the agency. Therefore, before recommending or referring a client with TB for home health care, the nurse should contact the home health agency to verify its policies.

RESPONSIBILITIES OF THE HOME HEALTH NURSE

As discussed in a previous chapter, the Health Care Financing Administration (HCFA) 485 is the plan of treatment that provides the nurse with the client's diagnosis, medications, and other pertinent information. It is on the 485 that the nurse will find the diagnosis of TB and the primary site.

One of the most effective ways of preventing the spread of tuberculosis is an awareness of the client's diagnosis. Although universal precautions should be practiced with all clients, it is pulmonary TB that is of primary concern. The special respiratory precautions will vary depending on the agency policies and on the basis of a single- or multiple-drug-resistant type of TB. However, the recommendation is that special precautions should be maintained for up to 3 weeks once a client is on medications. It is during the initial visit to the client's home that the nurse will get a picture of the client's environment and living conditions and determine if overcrowding is a problem with the particular client and how it can be handled. The nurse must be prepared to follow the protocol of wearing a mask.

Although the client might have been in a hospital where isolation precautions, including the wearing of a mask, were practiced, the client at home might not expect this to continue. Therefore, it is extremely important for the nurse to be aware of this possibility and address it on the initial visit. The nurse has to be very sensitive to the client and family needs and be able and prepared to handle the situation professionally but as gently as possible.

The nurse must have masks that cover the nose and mouth as part of the nursing bag equipment. Many agencies provide such protective equipment for clients and caregivers. Remember, in addition to providing care, another important objective is to prevent the spread of the TB.

Respiratory Precautions

Part of the nurse's assessment must include adequate assessment of the client's home environment. The environment should be assessed for any signs that would promote the spread of the disease, such as overcrowding and poor ventilation. The nurse will probably not be able to get a family of four out of the one-bedroom apartment on the first visit but will be able to begin to teach the client and family/caregiver measures to improve the ventilation in the apartment, such as opening windows periodically during the day.

If it is determined that inadequate housing is the situation, a referral should be made to the social worker. The client and family/caregiver should also be taught other respiratory precautions, such as to use tissues during episodes of coughing, sneezing, or laughing and proper disposal of those tissues. The nurse should assess if used tissues are lying around on the floor, table, or other furniture. If the apartment is cluttered or overcrowded, this would mean that the nurse must use careful discrete observation techniques to note any improper tissue disposal. The client should be taught to never expectorate into the wastebasket. Also, contaminated tissues should not be left in the home overnight but should be discarded in a lined wastebasket and removed from the home at the earliest convenience. The nurse also must teach the client and family/caregiver to wash their hands with soap and running water after handling contaminated tissues.

When caring for the client with TB, masks that cover the nose and mouth are to be worn during suctioning and administration of aerosolized treatments and for at least 24 hours after the treatment if the caregiver must remain in the client's home. It is the nurse's responsibility to teach the client and caregiver these precautions. The disposable 3M mask is one type used in the home. The high-efficiency particulate air filter respirator is also recommended by the Occupational Safety and Health Administration and the CDC, although its use is not widespread in home care. The caregiver must also be taught that the mask should be worn once and discarded, because it is not effective after 5 minutes because of moisture accumulation.

As was discussed in Chapter 7, the average block of time a HHA/PCW is in the home is from 2 to 8 hours. However, if the HHA/PCW must be in the home during the time the client with TB receives aerosolized treatment, and the client does not have a room with a door that can close, the HHA/PCW must wear a mask and must change it when moisture accumulates. In the case in which the client has a private room and is independent in self-administering the prescribed treatment, it will not be necessary for the HHA/PCW to remain in the same room. Once the HHA/PCW has assisted the client with preparing and setting up the treatment, the client can then be left alone in the room while the treatment is in progress. After the treatment is completed and the HHA/PCW has to go back into the client's room to help disassemble and clean the equipment, the HHA/PCW must wear a mask. An adequate supply of masks should be part of the supplies provided for the client. The HHA/PCW should also ensure that windows are opened to provide adequate ventilation of the environment during and after the treatment. In the case of active TB, the HHA/PCW is usually only required to remain in the home for 2 hours to provide the care that is needed.

Medications

The client with TB will be on drug treatment for a prolonged period (usually for a minimum of 9 months). In addition to teaching about the medications and assessing for therapeutic and side effects, the nurse also must check the client's medications to ensure that they are being taken as directed. The nurse must visually check the oral medication every visit, counting pills if nonadherence is suspected. Many agencies have a policy that if a client is not adhering to the medication regimen, that client will have to be referred to the local department of health for closer monitoring. Nursing visits can be increased or tapered, depending on the client's level of adherence to the regimen. The client must be instructed never to stop or alter the prescribed medication regimen, even though he or she is no longer experiencing symptoms. If the client or nurse suspects some type of adverse reaction to the medication, the physician should be notified at once to avoid any disruption in the treatment regimen. Medications should also be checked for drug interactions. Clients who are taking oral contraceptives and rifampin and rifabutin, for example, should be informed that these drugs reduce the effectiveness of the oral contraceptives. The client would therefore need to use an alternative form of birth control. If a client becomes pregnant, the physician must be notified.

Nutrition

Adequate nutrition is essential in the treatment of TB. Good nutrition helps to rebuild healthy cells and tissues, strengthen the immune system, ensure adequate bodily functions, and foster protection from exacerbation of the disease. Although the food pyramid and the basic four food groups are two guidelines used in selecting a healthy nutritious diet, clients have different religious and cultural dietary practices. Therefore, the nurse should assist the client with selecting nutritious menus that are in keeping with his or her dietary practices and any dietary restrictions the client might have to follow. A balanced diet that contains adequate complete protein, which comes from meat, poultry, fish, and dairy, is recommended for the client with TB. If the client has limited finances or no refrigeration, nonperishable foods such as powdered (dry) milk, peanut butter, and canned tuna are also good sources of protein. The client who does not eat meat usually has other sources of protein such as dry and canned beans and peas, soy, and tofu. Whatever the dietary practices, the nurse must work with the client during food selection. Assessment of the client's eating patterns for signs of anorexia is essential. Adequate fluid intake is also a part of the nutritious diet. Fluids assist body functions as well as facilitate adequate absorption of medications and elimination.

Activity and Rest

Adequate rest, exercise, and good personal hygiene also help to promote red blood cell production and prevent infection. The client should be encouraged to engage in exercise such as walking around the apartment, and to perform other activities, such as light housekeeping, as tolerated. If the client is experiencing fatigue, scheduled rest periods and pacing of activities should be encouraged by the family/caregiver. The client should also be instructed by the nurse to avoid overexertion and strenuous activity, such as heavy cleaning. Proper hygiene includes daily bath or shower, shampoo, and oral hygiene. The nightgown or pajamas, towels, and bed linen should be changed every few days and when necessary.

Vital signs should be checked on each nursing visit. The client's own thermometer should be used and left in the home. The client should be instructed to purchase a thermometer, if one is not in the home. Thermometers for oral and rectal use should be labeled and kept separate. The thermometer should be wiped with alcohol after use and placed in a clean, dry container. The nurse must use a protective sheath if the thermometer is to be used from the nurse's bag. The sheath should be disposed of according to universal precaution procedures. After use, the thermometer should be wiped with alcohol. The client should be instructed to take his or her temperature every evening at a specified time and keep a record for the nurse to review. Eight o'clock P.M. is usually recommended. Tylenol® may be prescribed whenever necessary for a temperature above 100°F.

The client also should be assessed for signs and symptoms of exacerbation of the TB, such as night sweats and persistent weight loss. If signs and symptoms are present, this must be documented, and the physician must be notified. The client would need to have further medical evaluation. A record of the client's daily weights also should be kept. Instructing and encouraging the client to keep all scheduled clinic appointments is also a part of the nurse's responsibility.

In addition, it is the nurse's responsibility to assess and evaluate the HHA/PCW and family members for early signs of TB. This assessment would include observing for any signs of malaise, persistent cough of more than 2 weeks' duration, and complaints of night sweats, anorexia, weight loss, or hemoptysis. If the HHA/PCW or family members have symptoms, the nurse should refer them to their primary physician or to a local hospital emergency department. If it is determined that either of the individuals has become infected, the state health department must be notified by the diagnosing physician.

CONCLUSIONS

The management and control of the spread of TB is as important in the home as it is in acute care settings. The home health nurse plays an important role in this process. The nurse is responsible for the quality of care not only for the client but also for the family and caregivers. In addition to preventing the spread of TB to others, the nurse must use appropriate measures to avoid contracting the disease. Although home health nursing involves the provision of services to clients and families in their residence, the prevention and spread of infectious disease is beneficial to the community at large.

17

HIV: Considerations for Home Care

Joan Schmidt, RN, MS/MPH

Health History and
    Assessment
Health Teaching
Disease-Specific
    Recommendations

Case Study and Care
    Planning Exercise

Working with persons who are infected with the human immunodeficiency virus (HIV) challenges all nursing skills. The nurse must deal not only with the physical manifestations of a complex disease process, but also with a variety of psychosocial issues. This chapter provides a basic understanding of the essential assessment parameters and interventions for persons with HIV who are receiving home care services.

It is important to remember that the spectrum of HIV infection encompasses a range of individuals, from those who are HIV positive but asymptomatic, to those who have been diagnosed with acquired immune deficiency syndrome (AIDS). To the general public, AIDS is one disease entity, but health professionals need to understand that the list of AIDS-indicator diseases includes more than 20 different opportunistic infections (OIs) and specific types of cancer. Some AIDS-indicator diseases attack certain body systems; others can disseminate. Other problems, such as candidiasis and herpes simplex, are not considered AIDS-defining illnesses, but they can be exacerbated in the presence of HIV infection. Figure 17-1 provides an overview of the most common AIDS-associated conditions and the systems affected.

Nursing interventions change depending on which conditions have been diagnosed and the systems involved. As the life expectancy for persons living with AIDS (PLWAs) increases, it is not uncommon for them to have multiple infections in different body systems. In addition, the nurse needs to be aware that HIV itself affects the functioning of the neurologic and gastrointestinal systems, resulting in problems such as memory loss, peripheral neuropathy, or malabsorption.

HEALTH HISTORY AND ASSESSMENT

As a home care nurse, you will find that clients with HIV infection fall into different categories: (1) those who have been diagnosed with AIDS; (2) those who are HIV positive; and (3) those who are at high risk for HIV infection but not yet tested. Let us start with the person who is referred to home care with a diagnosis of AIDS.

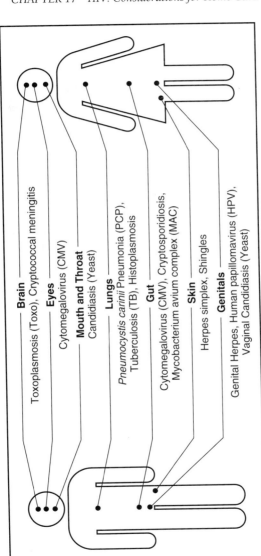

Figure 17-1. Infections linked to AIDS. (Adapted from NIH Publication No. 93-3324, 1993. Bethesda, MD: U.S. Department of Health and Human Services.)

When taking a health history from a PLWA, ask: Do you know what infections you have had? Some clients will be able to name specific OIs, such as PCP (*Pneumocystis carinii* pneumonia). Others may not be able to name the infection, but they will be able to state the nature of the problem using layman's terms. For example, few clients will be able to state they have disseminated *Mycobacterium avium–intracellulare* (MAI), but they will tell you they have "a bacteria in the blood." If a client is unable to give a complete history, contact the health care provider to fill in the gaps.

In addition to assessing the AIDS-indicator diseases, assess the client's knowledge of HIV disease itself. The key measure of immune function is the T4 helper cell count, also known as the CD4 count. T4 lymphocytes are the targets of HIV infection. A normal T4 count is 600 to 1200 per cubic millimeter (mm^3) of blood (Casey, 1995). Persons with HIV infection may be healthy and asymptomatic for years, but as the T4 count drops, the danger of opportunistic infection increases. Clients with HIV infection receive the AIDS diagnosis when they develop one of the opportunistic infections, certain cancers, wasting, dementia, or when the T4 count reaches 200 or less (CDC, 1992).

The current T4 count gives you important information about the status of the client's HIV infection. The nurse needs to know the T4 count both for persons with AIDS and for those who are HIV positive. Clients' awareness of their T4 counts varies widely. Some clients keep careful records of all their T4 results; others may be disinterested in or fearful of the results, especially when the count keeps declining. Clients need reassurance that the T4 count is only one indicator of their overall health. Other factors, such as nutrition and a positive attitude, influence quality of life and prognosis. If the client is unaware of the T4 count, explain its importance and why the health care provider should supply this information.

Knowing the T4 count helps to ensure that the appropriate therapies will be considered. It is now recommended that clients receive prophylactic medications to prevent certain OIs (CDC, 1995a). All clients who have had PCP *or* who have T4 counts of 200 or less need prophylaxis to prevent PCP. Trimethoprim-sulfamethoxazole (TMP-SMX; Bactrim®, Septra®), dapsone, or pentamidine aerosol are used for PCP prophylaxis. When the T4 count reaches 75 mm^3, patients need MAI prophylaxis with rifabutin. If the client is not taking the appropriate prophylaxis, ask whether this has been discussed. If not, contact the health care provider regarding prophylaxis.

Taking a complete health history from persons with HIV means delving into two areas that may cause discomfort for both the nurse and the client: sexuality and drug use. It is reported that 92% of adults who have been diagnosed with AIDS in the United States contracted HIV through either unprotected sexual activity or the sharing of contaminated injection equipment (CDC, 1995b). Recipients of contaminated blood products account for only 3% of reported cases.

As a nurse, you need to identify a client's risk behavior to provide appropriate health teaching about risk reduction. Ask questions about sexuality and drug use in a matter-of-fact, nonjudgmental manner: "Do you know how you were infected with HIV?" If a client admits to intravenous drug use, ask whether the client is still injecting or in recovery. Active injecting drug users need teaching about the multiple hazards of using dirty injection equipment (see section on Health Teaching). All persons with HIV need to be asked about sexual activity and their knowledge of safer sex practices, to prevent both the spread of HIV and exposure to different strains of HIV and other sexually transmitted diseases (STDs).

In addition, a complete medical and surgical history should be taken. Injecting drug users often have a litany of health problems resulting from the use of contaminated injection equipment, such as hepatitis B, endocarditis, and renal disease. If the client has preexisting liver or kidney disease, this will complicate the use of many medications (Ungvarski, 1994). Unprotected sexual activity exposes an individual to a multitude of STDs. STDs such as herpes have periods of exacerbation and remission; in the presence of HIV infection, outbreaks of herpes are common. Women with HIV who are also infected with the human papillomavirus (HPV) have a higher risk of cervical dysplasia and, consequently, cervical cancer (CDC, 1990).

Some clients may be reluctant to discuss either their AIDS diagnosis, their risk behaviors, or both. Such reluctance may stem from denial, guilt, shame, or fear of judgment. A client with PCP may insist that he or she is HIV positive and not diagnosed with AIDS. If your client is evasive or reluctant to give information, do not probe. Instead, concentrate on building trust while offering health teaching and information on symptom management. Once you develop rapport with the client, he or she may be able to discuss sensitive subjects.

It is also important to provide privacy while taking the history and during the assessment. Clients may be reluctant to disclose information with family members present, especially when family members have not been told the AIDS diagnosis. Always ask clients whether they wish to have others present during the interview; if not, politely ask significant others if they could wait in another room.

For persons who are not diagnosed with HIV, you may uncover information about risk behaviors during routine health histories. If the client has a history of STDs or injecting drug use, ask whether he or she has ever been tested for HIV. Explain that a positive antibody test does not mean that a person has AIDS. Clients who are interested in HIV testing should be referred to the local AIDS hotline to find out about the testing sites in their area. To find the number of your local AIDS hotline, call the National AIDS Hotline, 1-800-342-AIDS.

After the health history, the nurse needs to conduct a complete review of systems to determine current symptoms, their effects on functioning, and health teaching needs. When you identify positive symptoms, ask whether this is a new symptom or a long-standing problem. For example, if the client has oral candidiasis (thrush), ask how long the client has had it, what therapies have been ordered, the client's adherence to therapy, and whether the thrush is responding to treatment. Because PLWAs may have numerous symptoms that require nursing intervention, you will need to prioritize them. The person with thrush, for example, needs instructions about mouth care before you address nutrition.

Depending on their degree of physical or cognitive impairment, PLWAs may need assistance with activities of daily living (ADL), assistive devices, or both. Clients may be reluctant to accept ADL assistance, insisting that they can still function independently. Although it is important for you to encourage maximum independence and participation in ADL, you also must consider the potential for injury, especially when judgment is impaired. If a client refuses to accept needed ADL assistance, document this and notify the physician.

Medication teaching is one of your essential roles as a home health care nurse. Like all clients, PLWAs need to know the rationale for each medication and the possible side effects. Be sure to ask about allergies. PLWAs may be taking medications for the HIV infection itself, plus medications for the prophylaxis or treatment of OIs. See Table 17-1 for a list of the antiretroviral medications that are currently approved by the Food and Drug Administration (FDA).

OIs can never be cured; they can only be suppressed with medications (CDC, 1995a). Each time a new OI is diagnosed, more medications will be added to the regimen, making compliance difficult. It is a good idea to recommend a system to enhance medication compliance, such as the use of a prepour box. These boxes, which are available in pharmacies, are labeled with the days of the week and the times to take the pills.

It is not uncommon for PLWAs to stop medications for a variety of reasons: (1) because of side effects; (2) because they are asymptomatic and think the medication is no longer needed; or (3) because the medication regimen is too complicated (Schmidt, 1992). All PLWAs need to be told that if medications for OIs are stopped, the person risks a flare-up of the infection. Clients who wish to stop medications should be instructed about the possible consequences of their behavior. The health care provider should also be notified that the client has stopped medication.

Table 17-1
FDA-Approved Medications for HIV Infection
(As of December 1995)

Medication	Side/Adverse Effects
Zidovudine (Retrovir, formerly known as AZT)	Anemia, leukopenia, neutropenia, changes in platelet count, anorexia, headache, insomnia, nausea, fever, malaise, myalgia, hyperpigmentation of nails (bluish-brown bands), rash, taste alteration
Didanosine (ddI, Videx)	Peripheral neuropathy, pancreatitis (abdominal pain, nausea and vomiting), diarrhea, cardiomyopathy, anemia, granulocytopenia or leukopenia, thrombocytopenia, hepatitis, skin rash, itching, seizures, headaches, dry mouth
Zalcitabine (ddC, Hivid)	Peripheral neuropathy, joint pain, fever, skin rash, myalgia, ulceration of mouth and throat, leukopenia, neutropenia, pancreatitis, gastrointestinal disturbances, headache
Stavudine (d4T, Zerit)	Peripheral neuropathy, hepatotoxicity, headache, anemia, nausea
Lamivudine (3TC, Epivir)*	Headaches, malaise, fever, nausea, diarrhea, anorexia, abdominal pain or cramps, neuropathy, dizziness, insomnia, nasal symptoms, cough, skin rashes, musculoskeletal pain
Saquinavir (Invirase)*	Diarrhea, abomdinal discomfort or pain, headache, weakness, musculoskeletal pain

*These medications are not approved as monotherapy. The FDA approved the combination therapy 3TC/AZT. Saquinavir should be taken with either AZT or ddC.

Sources: United States Pharmacopeial Convention Inc. (1995). USPDI Vol. I (15th ed.). Rockville, MD: Author; Hoffman-La Roche, Inc. (1995); Glaxo Wellcome, Inc. (1995).

The next area to assess is nutrition. Good nutrition has a positive impact on both quality and quantity of life for PLWAs. But nutrition may be thwarted by a variety of factors: (1) HIV can directly affect the functioning of the gastrointestinal (GI) tract, leading to malabsorption; (2) the person may have a GI infection; (3) the medications may cause GI upset; or (4) the person may lack the energy or financial resources to cook nutritious meals (Hoyt & Staats, 1991).

The first step is to ask the person what he or she has eaten for the past 24 hours. Assess whether the diet has sufficient protein and calories from a variety of sources. Small, frequent feedings are the best way to ensure adequate intake. GI symptoms that interfere with nutrition, such as nausea and diarrhea, should be addressed with appropriate medication therapy and teaching about which foods may relieve or aggravate the symptoms. The Nutritionists in AIDS Care (NIAC) publish a comprehensive teaching booklet called "HIV: Fight Back with Nutrition." This colorful, easy-to-read booklet offers information on increasing protein and calories, plus tips on effective ways to cope with nausea, diarrhea, and mouth sores. Copies of this booklet may be obtained by calling the American Dietetic Association, 1-800-366-1655.

If a lack of energy is interfering with nutrition, consider placing a home health aide (HHA) for shopping and cooking. Because paraprofessional placement may be limited by insurance coverage, another option is a referral to a community AIDS organization that provides friendly visitors or meals-on-wheels. If finances are a problem, make a social work referral to ensure that the client is receiving all possible entitlements such as food stamps.

Social supports are an essential part of home care assessments, but for PLWAs, household situations may be nontraditional. Clients may be estranged from their families because of sexuality or drug use. Family members may not be aware that a client is gay and lives with his partner. Because HIV is sexually transmitted, the nurse needs to inquire about the HIV status of sexual partners. If a woman with HIV has children, she may have passed the virus to them while pregnant or breast-feeding, so ask about the children's HIV status and whether they have been tested. Household members who are HIV positive should be referred for follow-up care. Whatever the composition of the client's family, HIV is a family disease that affects everyone who is involved with the client. The nurse should become familiar with the services of the local AIDS organization to be able to refer individuals for counseling or support groups.

A Word About Confidentiality

It is very important to know the confidentiality laws of your state regarding the disclosure of the HIV/AIDS diagnosis. Laws may prohibit you from disclosing the diagnosis without the client's signed authorization, even to family members and HHAs. Always ask the clients if their significant others know the diagnosis and whether they want them to be told. If family members or HHAs ask you, "What's wrong with the person?" you can tell them the nature of the infection, such as pneumonia or a brain infection. If they press you for more information, explain that you are not permitted to discuss the client's condition further, but they are welcome to ask the client. Clients need reassurance that confidential information will not be disclosed without their authorization. When a client's refusal to disclose is causing tension and household conflicts, suggest a mental health referral for counseling.

HEALTH TEACHING

Having completed the health history and assessment, proceed with essential health teaching. Comprehensive health teaching for persons with HIV not only improves quality of life, but it also can reduce the development of new infections and repeated hospitalizations. Health teaching should focus on the following areas: (1) information on HIV infection and any diagnosed AIDS-indicator disease(s); (2) symptom management; (3) measures to prevent infections and complications; and (4) psychosocial issues (Flaskerud, 1995).

All persons with HIV should have an understanding of how HIV destroys the immune response. Persons with AIDS need teaching about any diagnosed infections or cancers. The National Institute of Allergy and Infectious Diseases (NIAID), a division of the National Institutes of Health, has developed teaching booklets on HIV and the most common OIs. These booklets are written in a simple, easy-to-read format in English and Spanish. They can be ordered by calling the National AIDS Information Clearinghouse, 1-800-458-5231.

A study to identify the home health needs of adults with HIV found that the most frequently reported symptoms were dyspnea, weakness, fatigue, pain, ataxia, cough, skin lesions, and memory deficit (Hurley & Ungvarski, 1994). Clients need concrete, practical information on symptom management. For example, the client with fatigue or dyspnea needs instructions on pacing of activities. Nursing notes should reflect the client's response to teaching and whether the intervention was effective.

All home care clients and their caregivers should be instructed about the importance of universal precautions (see Chapter 8 on Universal Precautions). Although HIV transmission to household caregivers is rare, caregivers have been infected after mucocutaneous exposures to blood or other body substances (CDC, 1994). Caregivers should be instructed about the proper use of gloves, handling of laundry, cleaning of environmental surfaces, and disposal of waste and sharps. Persons with HIV should be instructed not to share razors or toothbrushes. The CDC National AIDS Information Clearinghouse publishes a brochure, "Caring for Someone with AIDS: Information for Friends, Relatives, Household Members, and Others Who Care for a Person With AIDS at Home." This brochure can be ordered in English and Spanish by calling the Clearinghouse at 1-800-458-5231.

The importance of good handwashing cannot be overemphasized. Good handwashing is especially important before food preparation, after handling raw meat, fish, poultry, and eggs, and after using the bathroom. Utensils and cutting boards should be washed thoroughly after any contact with uncooked foods. Food safety guidelines can help to prevent certain OIs, such as salmonella and toxoplasmosis. Clients and caregivers should be instructed to cook all meat, fish, poultry and eggs until well done. Emphasize the dangers of eating raw seafood, raw or undercooked eggs, and unpasteurized dairy products. All fruits and vegetables should be washed thoroughly before eating. Because of recent reports of U.S. water supplies that have been contaminated with *Cryptosporidium,* the CDC now recommends that persons with T cell counts of 200 or less drink water that has been boiled for 10 minutes. Food and water safety guidelines should be followed when traveling here in the United States and also when traveling abroad.

Mouth and skin care are essential to alleviate problems and preserve integrity. Clients should use a soft toothbrush to reduce trauma to mucous membranes. Because commercial mouthwashes contain alcohol, clients should be advised to rinse their mouths with a solution of 1 pint water and 1/2 teaspoon each of salt and baking soda. For skin care, clients should be advised to shower with a mild soap and apply moisturizing lotion. Clients should be taught to check their mouths for thrush or sores; skin rashes or lesions should also be reported to their health care provider.

HIV infection and medication therapy may affect the hair texture and result in hair loss. Instruct clients to shampoo less frequently with a mild shampoo, such as baby shampoo.

Wearing a shower cap at night will reduce hair loss caused by friction on pillows. Recommend a cap, hat, scarf, or a wig as ways to camouflage hair loss.

If the client is sexually active, instruct in safer sex guidelines. Barrier precautions such as latex condoms should be used for vaginal or anal intercourse or oral sex on a man; dental dams should be used for oral sex on a woman. The female condom now provides an alternative to the male condom. Clients who engage in anilingus (oral stimulation of the anus) should be warned about the risk of contracting a GI infection.

Dental dams may also be used for anilingus. Clients also can be informed about activities that do not involve the exchange of body fluids, such as dry kissing, hugging, massage, or masturbation.

Persons with HIV may have questions about procreation. Counseling about reproduction should be presented in a nonjudgmental manner. Women with HIV should be informed that the risk of perinatal transmission is estimated to be 15% to 30%, with a recent study showing that the use of Zidovudine during pregnancy and delivery can reduce transmission rates to 8.3% (CDC, 1995c).

Pets can be a source of companionship and affection, but persons with HIV need clear instructions to avoid contact with pet excrement. Whenever possible, persons with HIV should avoid emptying cat litter boxes; if they must empty cat litter, they need to wear gloves and wash their hands afterwards. Persons with dogs should wash their hands immediately after any contact with excrement. Persons with birds or fish should wear gloves to clean cages and tanks. Contact with turtles or reptiles may expose a person to salmonella, so instruct clients to wash their hands thoroughly if they have contact with these pets.

Active injecting drug users should be cautioned about the health hazards of using and sharing contaminated injection equipment, not only because of HIV transmission, but also because of the dangers of hepatitis B, bacterial endocarditis, abscesses, or sepsis. Some states ban the purchase of syringes without a prescription, but you may be able to refer clients to a needle exchange program. Drug users who reuse injection equipment (known as drug *works*) should clean all of their injection equipment with full-strength bleach and rinse afterwards with water (CDC, 1993). Persons who are interested in drug treatment should be referred to either inpatient treatment or 12-step programs such as Narcotics Anonymous (NA).

Referring drug users to needle exchange and teaching them to clean their injection equipment are the principles of the Harm Reduction Model. This strategy was developed to work with active substance users who are not currently receptive to treatment. Harm reduction teaches drug users ways to reduce the harmful health consequences of substance use (Springer, 1991). Harm reduction with other addictive behaviors, such as cigarette smoking, also may be used. For example, if the client smokes two packs a day, encourage him or her to cut down to one and a half packs a day.

Persons with HIV who drink alcohol should be warned that alcohol may react adversely with certain medications, such as didanosine (ddl; Videx). To use harm reduction with an alcohol drinker, advise the person to avoid drinking 2 hours before or after taking medications. If alcohol is a problem for the individual, discuss treatment options or a referral to Alcoholics Anonymous (AA).

If the client is using drugs or alcohol, the nurse must set clear limits regarding acceptable and unacceptable behaviors. Clients should be instructed that they cannot use drugs or alcohol while home care workers are present. Explain that verbal abuse of workers will not be tolerated; clients who exhibit anger or hostility should be offered counseling. It is a good idea to draw up a written contract so the client understands what behaviors may lead to the termination of home care services (Ungvarski & Schmidt, 1995).

Psychosocial Issues

Being diagnosed with AIDS is extremely stressful. It is not uncommon for clients to be anxious, fearful, angry, or depressed. The stress is compounded because of the stigma associated with the disease. Counseling and support groups can be beneficial in alleviating stress and developing healthy coping mechanisms. Try to assess previous coping styles and support systems. For example, did the client find comfort in music, nature, or religion? Relaxation and visualization techniques may be helpful for some individuals. If you are knowledgeable about therapeutic touch, you may wish to use it in your practice. As a person's condition deteriorates, the nurse may need to focus on death and dying issues, comfort measures, and terminal care (see Chapter 22 on Hospice Services).

Friends and family members may be a source of comfort or an additional stress. One of the most difficult issues is disclosing the AIDS diagnosis to significant others. The client may be reluctant to discuss his or her diagnosis because of fears about the response. Mental health professionals, such as psychiatric nurses or social workers, can be helpful in exploring feelings about disclosure; often they will offer to be present when the client decides to disclose. Sexual partners need counseling about HIV testing and referrals for follow-up care if they test positive.

If a client has dependent children, the nurse must assess whether the client is still capable of child care. Family members or friends may be willing and able to assist with the children, but if this is not possible, the client may need a referral to a local social service agency that provides homemakers. It is essential for single parents to plan for future guardianship of their children. Such arrangements can usually be made through the legal department of the local AIDS organization. Legal services also can assist clients to draw up wills.

Follow-Up Health Care

All persons with HIV infection need regular health care follow-up, especially if they are symptomatic. Instruct clients to report any new symptom(s), especially fevers, diarrhea, cough, persistent headaches, severe fatigue, weight loss, skin lesions, or vision changes (NIH, 1993). Women with HIV should report vaginal discharge or severe abdominal pain, which may indicate pelvic inflammatory disease (PID). Instruct women with HIV that they need to have Pap smears at least once a year, and more often if they have ever had an abnormal Pap result. In addition, explain why all clients need to have regular blood work to check the red and white blood cell counts and the functioning of the liver and kidneys.

Whenever possible, clients should be followed by a health care provider or clinic with a high level of knowledge about HIV infection. A recent study found that persons with AIDS who are treated by experienced physicians live longer than clients whose physicians are less knowledgeable about AIDS (Altman, 1996). Unfortunately, many clients' choices of medical follow-up are limited by their insurance. Clients with Medicaid must go to providers who accept Medicaid. If a client is dissatisfied with medical follow-up, direct him or her to call the local AIDS organization. These organizations often have lists of providers who are sensitive to the needs of persons with HIV/AIDS.

DISEASE-SPECIFIC RECOMMENDATIONS

The following are excerpts from United States Public Health Service/Investigational Drug Service Agency *Guidelines for the Prevention of Opportunistic Infections in Persons Infected with Human Immunodeficiency Virus: A Summary;* 1995.

Pneumocystis carinii *Pneumonia (PCP)*

Prevention of Disease

Adults and adolescents with HIV infection (including those who are pregnant) should receive chemoprophylaxis against PCP if they have a CD4+ lymphocyte count of <200, unexplained fever (>100°F) for more than 2 weeks, or a history of oropharyngeal candidiasis.

Trimethoprim-sulfamethoxazole (TMP-SMZ) is the preferred prophylactic agent. TMP-SMZ may offer cross-protection against toxoplasmosis and many bacterial infections. For patients with an adverse reaction that is not life threatening, treatment with TMP-SMZ should be continued if clinically feasible; for those who have discontinued such therapy, its reinstitution should be strongly considered. Whether it is best to reintroduce the drug at the original dose or at a lower and gradually increasing dose or to try a desensitization regimen is unknown.

If TMP-SMZ cannot be tolerated, alternative prophylactic regimens include dapsone, dapsone plus pyrimethamine plus leucovorin, and aerosolized pentamidine administered by the Respirgard II® nebulizer. Regimens including dapsone plus pyrimethamine are also protective against toxoplasmosis but not against most bacterial infections. Because data on their efficacy for PCP prophylaxis are insufficient, the following regimens generally cannot be recommended for this purpose: aerosolized pentamidine administered by other nebulization devices currently available in the United States, intermittently administered parenteral pentamidine, oral pyrimethamine/sulfadoxine, oral clindamycin plus primaquine, oral atovaquone, and intravenous trimetrexate. However, the use of these agents may be considered in unusual situations in which the recommended agents cannot be administered.

Prevention of Recurrence

Adults and adolescents with a history of PCP should receive chemoprophylaxis with the regimens indicated above to prevent recurrence.

Pediatric Notes

Children born to HIV-infected mothers should receive prophylaxis with TMP-SMZ beginning at 4 to 6 weeks of age. Prophylaxis should be discontinued for children who are subsequently found not to be infected with HIV. HIV-infected children and children whose infection status remain unknown should continue to receive prophylaxis for the first year of life.

The need for subsequent prophylaxis should be determined on the basis of age-specific CD4+ lymphocyte thresholds. Children with a history of PCP should receive chemoprophylaxis as indicated to prevent recurrence.

Note Regarding Pregnancy

Chemoprophylaxis for PCP should be administered to pregnant women as to other adults and adolescents, although some providers, because of a general concern about administering drugs during the first trimester of pregnancy, may choose not to initiate such therapy until after the first trimester. Because of the increase in blood plasma volume and the reduced concentrations of drugs during pregnancy, the double-strength (DS) dose of TMP-SMZ (one DS tablet daily) should be used.

Toxoplasmosis Encephalitis

Prevention of Exposure

HIV-infected persons should be tested for immunoglobulin G (IgG) antibody to toxoplasma soon after the diagnosis of HIV infection to detect latent infection with *Toxoplasma gondii.*

All HIV-infected persons, but particularly those who lack IgG antibody to toxoplasma, should be counseled about the various sources of toxoplasmic infection. They should be advised not to eat raw or undercooked meat, particularly undercooked pork, lamb, or venison. Specifically, meat should be cooked to an internal temperature of 150°F; meat cooked until no longer pink inside generally has an internal temperature of 165°F and therefore satisfies this requirement. HIV-infected persons should wash their hands after contact with raw meat and after gardening or other contact with soil; in addition, they should wash fruits and vegetables well before eating them raw. If the patient owns a cat, the litter box should be changed daily, preferably by an HIV-negative, nonpregnant person; alternatively, the patient should wash the hands thoroughly after changing the litter box. Patients should be encouraged to keep their cats inside and not to adopt or handle stray cats. Cats should be fed only canned or dried commercial food or well-cooked table food, not raw or undercooked meats. Patients need not be advised to part with their cats or to have their cats tested for toxoplasmosis.

Prevention of Disease

Toxoplasma-seropositive patients with a CD4+ lymphocyte count of <100 should receive prophylaxis against toxoplasmic encephalitis (TE). The doses of TMP-SMZ recommended for PCP prophylaxis appear to be effective against TE as well. If patients cannot tolerate TMP-SMZ, the regimens including dapsone plus pyrimethamine that are recommended for PCP prophylaxis provide protection against TE. Prophylactic monotherapy with dapsone, pyrimethamine, azithromycin, clarithromycin, or atovaquone cannot be recommended on the basis of current data. Aerosolized pentamidine does not afford protection against TE.

Toxoplasma-seronegative persons who are not taking a PCP prophylactic regimen known to be active against TE should be retested for IgG antibody to toxoplasma when their CD4+ lymphocyte count falls below 100 to determine whether they have seroconverted and are therefore at risk for TE. Patients who have seroconverted should receive prophylaxis for TE as described above.

Prevention of Recurrence

Patients who have had TE should receive life-long suppressive therapy with drugs active against toxoplasma to prevent relapse. The combination of pyrimethamine plus sulfadiazine and leucovorin is highly effective for this purpose. A commonly used regimen for patients who cannot tolerate sulfa drugs is pyrimethamine plus clindamycin; however, only the combination of pyrimethamine plus sulfadiazine appears to provide protection against PCP as well.

Pediatric Note

Current data are insufficient for the formulation of specific guidelines for children. The provider should consider the recommendations for adults; children older than 12 months of age who are seropositive for IgG antibody to toxoplasma, have a CD4+ lymphocyte count of <100, and are not already taking medication effective against toxoplasma may be considered as candidates for chemoprophylaxis. Some providers would consider opting for chemophylaxis for very young children with higher CD4+ lymphocyte consistent with severe immunosuppression and with evidence of toxoplasmic infection.

Notes Regarding Pregnancy

Because of the low incidence of TE during pregnancy and the possible risk associated with pyrimethamine treatment, chemoprophylaxis with pyrimethamine-containing regimens can reasonably be deferred until after pregnancy for women who are seropositive for

IgG antibody to toxoplasma. TMP-SMZ can be administered as described for prophylaxis of PCP. For prophylaxis of recurrent TE, pyrimethamine should be used with caution.

In rare cases, HIV-infected pregnant women with serologic evidence of remote toxoplasmic infection have transmitted toxoplasma to the fetus in utero. Pregnant HIV-infected women who have evidence of primary toxoplasmic infection or active toxoplasmosis (including TE) should be evaluated during pregnancy in consultation with appropriate specialists. Infants born to women with serologic evidence of infections with HIV and toxoplasma should be evaluated for congenital toxoplasmosis.

Cryptosporidiosis

Prevention of Exposure

HIV-infected persons should be educated and counseled about the many ways that *Cryptosporidium* can be transmitted. Modes of transmission include contact with infected adults and diaper-age children, contact with infected animals, consumption of contaminated drinking water, and contact with contaminated water during recreational activities.

HIV-infected persons should avoid contact with human and animal feces. They should be advised to wash their hands after contact with human feces (eg, during diaper changing), after handling of pets, and after gardening or other contact with soil. HIV-infected persons should avoid sexual practices such as oral–anal intercourse that may result in oral exposure to feces.

HIV-infected persons should be advised that newborn and very young pets may pose a small risk of cryptosporidial infection, but they should not be advised to destroy or give away healthy pets. Persons contemplating the acquisition of a new pet should avoid bringing any animal with diarrhea into their households, should avoid purchasing a dog or cat younger than 6 months of age, and should not adopt stray pets. HIV-infected persons who wish to assume the small risk of acquiring a puppy or kitten younger than 6 months of age should request that their veterinarian examine the animal's stool for *Cryptosporidium* before they have contact with the animal.

HIV-infected persons should avoid exposure to calves and lambs and to premises where these animals are raised.

HIV-infected persons should not drink water directly from lakes or rivers. Because water can be accidentally ingested, patients should be advised that swimming in lakes, rivers, or public swimming pools may put them at increased risk for infection.

Several outbreaks of cryptosporidiosis have been linked to municipal water supplies. During outbreaks or in other situations in which a community "boil-water" advisory is issued, boiling of water for 1 minute will eliminate the risk of cryptosporidiosis. Use of submicron personal-use water filters* (ie, home/office

---

*Only filters capable of removing particles 1 μm in diameter and larger should be considered. Sources of bottled water (wells, springs, municipal tap water supplies, rivers, lakes) and methods for its disinfection vary; therefore, all brands should not be presumed to be free of cryptosporidial oocysts. Water from wells and springs is much less likely to be contaminated by oocysts than water from rivers or lakes. Treatment of bottled water by distillation or reverse osmosis ensures oocyst removal. Water passed through an "absolute" 1-μm filter or a filter labeled as meeting NSF standard no. 53 for cyst removal before bottling will provide nearly the same level of protection. Use of "nominal" 1-μm filters by bottlers as the only barrier to cryptosporidia may not result in the removal of >99% of oocysts.

types) or bottled water may reduce the risk. The magnitude of the risk of acquiring cryptosporidiosis from drinking water in a non-outbreak setting is uncertain, and current data are inadequate to recommend that all HIV-infected persons boil or avoid drinking tap water in non-outbreak settings. However, HIV-infected persons who wish to take independent action to reduce the risk of water-borne cryptosporidiosis may choose to take precautions similar to those recommended during outbreaks. Such decisions should be made in conjunction with health care providers. Persons who opt for a personal-use filter or bottled water should be aware of the complexities involved in selecting appropriate products, the lack of enforceable standards for the destruction or removal of oocysts, the cost of the products, and the logistic difficulty of using the products consistently.

Prevention of Disease

No effective chemoprophylactic agents are available for cryptosporidiosis.

Prevention of Recurrence

No drug regimens are known to be effective in preventing recurrence of cryptosporidiosis.

Pediatric Note

No data indicate that formula-based preparation practices for infants should be altered to prevent cryptosporidiosis.

Microsporidiosis

Prevention of Exposure

Other than general attention to handwashing and other personal hygiene measures, no precautions to reduce exposure can be recommended at this time. No chemoprophylactic regimens are known to be effective in preventing microsporidiosis.

Prevention of Recurrence

No chemotherapeutic regimens are known to be effective in preventing the recurrence of microsporidiosis.

Tuberculosis

Prevention of Exposure

HIV-infected persons should be advised that certain activities and occupations may increase the likelihood of exposure to tuberculosis. These include volunteer work or employment in health care facilities, correctional institutions, shelters for the homeless, as well as in other settings identified as high risk by local health authorities. Decisions about whether to continue with activities in these settings should be made in conjunction with the health care provider and should take into account such factors as the patient's specific duties in the workplace, the prevalence of tuberculosis in the community, and the degree to which precautions are taken to prevent the transmission of tuberculosis in the workplace. Whether the patient continues with such activities may affect the frequency with which screening for tuberculosis needs to be conducted.

Prevention of Disease

When HIV infection is first recognized, the patient should be screened by the Mantoux method with intermediate-strength (5-TU) purified protein derivative (PPD). Routine evaluation for anergy is controversial;

some experts recommend anergy testing for persons in settings where there is an increased risk of infection with *Mycobacterium tuberculosis* (ie, in areas where the prevalence of such infection is greater than 10%).

All HIV-infected persons with a positive result in the tuberculin skin test (TST; >5 mm of induration) should undergo chest radiography and clinical evaluation for the exclusion of active tuberculosis. HIV-infected individuals who have symptoms suggestive of tuberculosis should undergo chest radiography and clinical evaluation regardless of their TST status.

All HIV-infected persons with a positive TST result who have no evidence of active tuberculosis and no history of treatment or prophylaxis for tuberculosis should receive 12 months of preventive chemotherapy with isoniazid. Because HIV-infected persons are at risk for peripheral neuropathy, those receiving isoniazid should also receive pyridoxine. The decision to use alternative antimycobacterial agents for chemoprophylaxis should be based on the relative risk of exposure to resistant organisms and may require consultation with public health authorities. The need for direct observation as a means of documenting compliance with chemoprophylaxis should be considered on an individual basis.

HIV-infected individuals who are close contacts of persons with infectious tuberculosis (ie, acid-fast bacilli smear–positive pulmonary disease) should receive preventive therapy—regardless of TST results or prior courses of chemoprophylaxis—after active tuberculosis has been excluded. Such persons should be tested with 5-TU PPD. If the TST is initially negative, the individual should be evaluated again after the discontinuation of contact with the infectious source, and the information should be considered in the course of decisions about whether chemoprophylaxis should continue.

TST-negative, HIV-infected persons from risk groups or geographic areas with a high prevalence of *M tuberculosis* infection (>10%) may be at increased risk of tuberculosis. Some experts recommend preventive therapy for anergic individuals or perhaps for all persons in this category. However, the efficacy of preventive therapy in this group has not been demonstrated, and decisions concerning the use of chemoprophylaxis in these situations must be individualized.

Although the reliability of the TST may diminish as the CD4+ lymphocyte count declines, testing should be repeated at least annually for HIV-infected persons who are TST negative on initial evaluation. In addition to documenting tuberculosis infection, TST conversion in an HIV-infected person should alert health care providers to the possibility of an infectious case in the environment and lead to notification of public health officials for investigation to identify a possible source case.

The administration of bacille Calmette-Guérin (BCG) vaccine to HIV-infected persons is contraindicated because of its potential to cause disseminated disease.

Prevention of Recurrence

Chronic suppressive therapy for a patient who has successfully completed a recommended regimen of treatment for tuberculosis is not necessary.

Pediatric Note

All infants born to HIV-infected mothers should have a TST (5-TU PPD) at 9 to 12 months of age. All children living in households with *M tuberculosis*-infected (TST-positive) persons should be evaluated for tuberculosis; those exposed to a person with active tuberculosis should receive preventive therapy after active tuberculosis has been excluded.

Note Regarding Pregnancy

HIV-infected women who have a positive TST result without evidence of active tuberculosis should receive standard chemoprophylaxis. When possible, chest radiography should be undertaken, and chemoprophylaxis should be initiated after the first trimester to avoid the critical period of major organogenesis. Preventive therapy with isoniazid should be accompanied by treatment with pyridoxine so that peripheral neuropathy does not develop. Alternative regimens (eg, rifampin, rifabutin) should be used with caution during pregnancy.

Disseminated Infection With Mycobacterium avium *Complex*

Prevention of Exposure

Organisms of the *Mycobacterium avium* complex (MAC) are common in environmental sources such as food and water. Current information does not support specific recommendations regarding avoidance of exposure.

Prevention of Disease

Prophylaxis with rifabutin should be considered for HIV-infected adults and adolescents who have a CD4+ lymphocyte count of <75, although some experts would wait until the count is <50. Disseminated MAC disease should be ruled out (by a negative blood culture) before prophylaxis is initiated. Because treatment with rifabutin may result in the development of resistance to rifampin in individuals with active tuberculosis, the latter condition should be excluded before rifabutin prophylaxis is begun. Drug interactions, partial efficacy, and cost are among the other issues that should be considered in decisions about whether to institute prophylaxis for MAC disease. Data on the safety and efficacy of clarithromycin, azithromycin, and combinations of clarithromycin or azithromycin with rifabutin have not yet been reviewed sufficiently to warrant recommendations concerning these regimens.

Although the detection of MAC organisms in the respiratory or gastrointestinal tract may be predictive of the development of disseminated MAC infection, no data are available on the efficacy of prophylaxis with rifabutin or other drugs in patients with MAC organisms at these sites and a negative blood culture. Therefore, routine screening of respiratory or gastrointestinal specimens for MAC cannot be recommended at this time.

Prevention of Recurrence

Patients who are treated for disseminated MAC infection should continue to receive full therapeutic doses for life. The use of a macrolide, usually clarithromycin, is generally recommended in conjunction with at least one other drug, such as ethambutol, clofazimine, ciprofloxacin, or rifabutin.

Pediatric Note

HIV-infected children younger than 12 years of age also develop disseminated MAC infections. Prophylaxis should be considered similar to that recommended for adults and adolescents. For children 6 to 12 years of age, a CD4+ lymphocyte count of <75 is a reasonable threshold for the initiation of chemoprophylaxis. Some adjustment for age is necessary in the interpretation of CD4+ lymphocyte counts of children younger than 6 years of age. No pediatric formulation of rifabutin is currently available, but a dosage of 5 mg/kg has been used in pharmacokinetic studies.

Note Regarding Pregnancy

Information is insufficient for recommendations concerning the use of rifabutin or clarithromycin during pregnancy.

Bacterial Respiratory Infections

Prevention of Exposure

Because *Streptococcus pneumoniae* and *Haemophilus influenzae* are common in the community, there is no effective way to reduce exposure to these bacteria.

Prevention of Disease

As soon as possible after HIV infection is diagnosed, adults should receive a single dose of 23-valent polysaccharide pneumococcal vaccine. This recommendation is especially pertinent in light of the increasing incidence of invasive infections with drug-resistant strains of *S pneumoniae*. Although the administration of protein-polysaccharide conjugate *H influenzae* type b vaccine may be considered, data are insufficient to recommend the use of this vaccine in HIV-infected adults.

TMP-SMZ, administered daily, may be effective in preventing serious bacterial respiratory infections (although not those caused by drug-resistant *S pneumoniae*); this fact should be considered in the selection of an agent for PCP prophylaxis. However, indiscriminate use of this drug (when not indicated for PCP prophylaxis or other specific reasons) may promote the development of resistant organisms.

An absolute neutrophil count that is depressed because of HIV disease or drug therapy may be increased by granulocyte colony-stimulating factor (G-CSF) or granulocyte–macrophage colony-stimulating factor (GM-CSF). However, data are insufficient for recommendations concerning the use of G-CSF or GM-CSF to prevent bacterial infections in HIV-infected patients with neutropenia.

Prevention of Recurrence

Some clinicians may choose to offer antibiotic chemoprophylaxis to HIV-infected patients with recurrent serious bacterial respiratory infections. TMP-SMZ, administered for PCP prophylaxis, is appropriate for drug-sensitive organisms.

Pediatric Notes

Children with HIV infection should receive *H influenzae* type b vaccine in accordance with the guidelines of the Advisory Committee for Immunization Practices and the American Academy of Pediatrics. Children older than 2 years of age should also receive 23-valent polysaccharide pneumococcal vaccine.

To prevent serious bacterial infections in HIV-infected children with documented antibody deficiency, clinicians should use intravenous immunoglobulin (IVIg). The administration of IVIg should be considered also for HIV-infected children with serious bacterial infections, but such treatment may not provide additional benefit to children receiving daily TMP-SMZ.

Note Regarding Pregnancy

Pneumococcal vaccine is not contraindicated during pregnancy.

Candidiasis

Prevention of Exposure

Candida organisms are common on mucosal surfaces and skin. No measures are available to reduce exposure to these fungi.

Prevention of Disease

Although data from a prospective controlled trial indicate that fluconazole can reduce the risk of mucosal (oropharyngeal, esophageal, and vaginal) candidiasis in patients with advanced HIV disease, routine primary prophylaxis is not recommended because of the effectiveness of therapy for acute disease, the low mortality associated with mucosal candidiasis, the potential for resistant *Candida* organisms to develop, the possibility of drug interactions, and the cost of prophylaxis.

Prevention of Recurrence

Many experts do not recommend chronic prophylaxis of recurrent pharyngeal or vulvovaginal candidiasis for the same reasons that they do not recommend primary prophylaxis. However, if recurrences are frequent or severe, intermittent or chronic administration of topical nystatin, topical clotrimazole, or an oral azole (ketoconazole, fluconazole, or itraconazole) may be considered. Other factors that influence choices about such therapy include the impact on the patient's well-being and quality of life, the need for prophylaxis for other fungal infections, cost, toxicities, and drug interactions.

Adults or adolescents with a history of documented esophageal candidiasis, particularly multiple episodes, should be considered candidates for chronic suppressive therapy with fluconazole.

Pediatric Notes

Primary prophylaxis of candidiasis in HIV-infected infants is not indicated. Suppressive therapy with systemic azoles should be considered for infants with severe recurrent mucocutaneous candidiasis and particularly those with esophageal candidiasis.

Cryptococcosis

Prevention of Exposure

Although HIV-infected persons cannot avoid exposure to *Cryptococcus neoformans* completely, avoiding sites that are likely to be heavily contaminated with *C neoformans* (eg, areas heavily contaminated with pigeon droppings) may reduce risk of infection.

Prevention of Disease

Because of the low probability that the results will affect clinical decisions, routine testing of asymptomatic persons for serum cryptococcal antigen is not recommended.

Data from a prospective controlled trial indicate that fluconazole can reduce the frequency of cryptococcal disease among patients with advanced HIV disease; thus, physicians may wish to consider chemoprophylaxis for adult and adolescent patients with a CD4+ lymphocyte count of <50. However, such prophylaxis should not be offered routinely because of the relative infrequency of cryptococcal disease, the possibility of drug interactions, the potential for the development of resistance, and the cost of prophylaxis. The need for prophylaxis or suppressive therapy for other fungal infections (eg, candidiasis) should be considered in the course of decisions about prophylaxis for cryptococcosis.

Prevention of Recurrence

Patients who complete initial therapy for cryptococcosis should receive life-long suppressive treatment with fluconazole.

Pediatric Note

There are no data on which to base specific recommendations for children, but life-long suppressive therapy with fluconazole after an episode of cryptococcosis is appropriate.

Note Regarding Pregnancy

Although treatment with fluconazole is indicated to to prevent the recurrence of cryptococcosis, this drug should be used with caution in pregnant women. At high doses, fluconazole has been associated with both fetal death and increased rates of fetal abnormalities in rats.

Histoplasmosis

Prevention of Exposure

Although HIV-infected persons living in or visiting histoplasmosis-endemic areas cannot completely avoid exposure to *Histoplasma capsulatum,* they should avoid activities known to be associated with increased risk (eg, cleaning chicken coops, disturbing soil beneath bird-roosting sites, and exploring caves).

Prevention of Disease

Routine skin testing with histoplasmin in histoplasmosis-endemic areas is not predictive of this disease and should not be performed. No recommendations can be made regarding chemoprophylaxis for HIV-infected persons in histoplasmosis-endemic areas or for histoplasmin-positive persons in nonendemic areas.

Prevention of Recurrence

Patients who complete initial therapy should receive life-long suppressive treatment with itraconazole.

Pediatric Note

Because primary histoplasmosis can lead to disseminated infection in children, HIV-infected children with histoplasmosis should receive suppressive therapy for life.

Coccidioidomycosis

Prevention of Exposure

Although HIV-infected persons living in or visiting areas in which coccidioidomycosis is endemic cannot completely avoid exposure to *Coccidioides immitis*, they should, when possible, avoid activities associated with increased risk (eg, those involving extensive exposure to disturbed soil as occurs at building excavation sites, on farms, or during dust storms).

Prevention of Disease

Routine skin testing with coccidioidin (Spherulin®) in coccidioidomycosis-endemic areas is not predictive of disease and should not be performed. No recommendation can be made regarding routine chemoprophylaxis for HIV-infected individuals who live in coccidioidomycosis-endemic areas or for skin test–positive persons in nonendemic areas.

Prevention of Recurrence

Patients who complete initial therapy for coccidioidomycosis should receive life-long suppressive treatment. Fluconazole is the preferred agent; alternative drugs include itraconazole, ketoconazole, and amphotericin B.

Pediatric Note

Although no specific data are available on coccidioidomycosis in HIV-infected children, it is reasonable to administer life-long suppressive therapy after an acute episode of the illness.

Cytomegalovirus Disease
Prevention of Exposure

HIV-infected persons who belong to risk groups with relatively low rates of seropositivity for cytomegalovirus (CMV) and who anticipate possible exposure to CMV (eg, through blood transfusion or employment in a child care facility) should be tested for antibody to CMV. These groups include patients who have not had male homosexual contact and those who are not injecting drug users.

HIV-infected adolescents and adults should be advised that CMV is shed in semen, cervical secretions, and saliva and that latex condoms must always be used during sexual contact to reduce the risk of exposure to this virus and to other sexually transmitted pathogens.

HIV-infected adults and adolescents who are child care providers or parents of children in child care facilities should be informed that they—like all children at these facilities—are at increased risk of acquiring CMV infection. Parents and other caretakers of HIV-infected children should be advised of the increased risk to children at these centers. The risk of acquiring CMV infection can be diminished by good hygienic practices such as handwashing.

HIV-exposed infants and HIV-infected children, adolescents, and adults who are seronegative to CMV and require blood transfusion should receive only CMV antibody–negative or leukocyte-reduced cellular blood products in nonemergency situations.

Prevention of Disease

Data on the efficacy and safety of oral ganciclovir have not yet been adequately reviewed; thus, no recommendations concerning this drug can be made. Acyclovir is not effective in preventing CMV disease. Because no chemoprophylactic agent is currently available, the most important method for preventing severe CMV disease is recognition of the early manifestations of the disease. Early recognition of CMV retinitis is most likely when the patient has been educated on this topic and undergoes regular fundus examinations performed by a health care provider. Patients should be made aware of the significance of increased floaters in the eye and should be advised to assess their visual acuity regularly by simple techniques such as reading newsprint.

Prevention of Recurrence

CMV disease is not cured with courses of the currently available antiviral agents ganciclovir and foscarnet. Chronic suppressive or maintenance therapy is indicated. The currently approved regimens include parenteral or oral ganciclovir or parenteral foscarnet. In spite of maintenance therapy, recurrences develop routinely and require reinstitution of high-dose induction therapy.

Pediatric Note

The recommendations for the prevention of CMV disease and of its recurrence apply to children as well as to adolescents and adults. However, oral ganciclovir has not been studied in children.

Herpes Simplex Virus Disease
Prevention of Exposure

HIV-infected persons should use latex condoms during every act of sexual intercourse to reduce the risk of exposure to herpes simplex virus (HSV) and to other sexually transmitted pathogens. They should specifically avoid contact when herpetic lesions (genital or orolabial) are evident.

Prevention of Disease

Prophylaxis of initial episodes of HSV disease is not recommended.

Prevention of Recurrence

Because acute episodes of HSV infection can be treated successfully, chronic therapy with acyclovir is not required after lesions resolve. However, persons with frequent or severe recurrences can be given daily suppressive therapy with oral acyclovir. Intravenous foscarnet can be used for the treatment of infection caused by acyclovir-resistant isolates of HSV, which are routinely resistant to ganciclovir as well.

Pediatric Note

The recommendations for the prevention of initial disease and recurrence apply to children as well as to adolescents and adults.

Note Regarding Pregnancy

The effectiveness of suppressive treatment with acyclovir in reducing the risk of HSV transmission has not been studied. Therefore, no relevant recommendation can be made.

Varicella-Zoster Virus Infection

Prevention of Exposure

HIV-infected children and adults who are susceptible to varicella-zoster virus (VZV)—in other words, those who have no history of chickenpox or are seronegative for VZV—should avoid exposure to persons with chickenpox or shingles.

Prevention of Disease

For the prophylaxis of chickenpox, HIV-infected children and adults who are susceptible to VZV should be given zoster immune globulin within 96 hours after close contact with a patient with chickenpox or shingles. Data are lacking on the effectiveness of acyclovir for preventing chickenpox in HIV-infected children or adults. No preventive measures are currently available for shingles.

Prevention of Recurrence

Recurrence of shingles is unusual, and no drug has been proved to prevent recurrence.

Note Regarding Pregnancy

Zoster immune globulin is not contraindicated during pregnancy and should be given to VZV-susceptible pregnant women after exposure to VZV.

Human Papillomavirus Infection

Prevention of Exposure

HIV-infected persons should use latex condoms during every act of sexual intercourse to reduce the risk of exposure to human papillomavirus (HPV) as well as to other sexually transmitted pathogens.

Prevention of Disease

HPV-Associated Genital Epithelial Cancers in HIV-infected Women. HIV-infected women should have annual cervical Pap smears as part of their initial and routine gynecologic care. In accordance with the recommendations of the Agency for Health Care Policy and Research, a Pap smear should be obtained twice in the first year after diagnosis of HIV infection and, if the results are normal, annually thereafter.

If an HIV-infected woman has a history of abnormal Pap smears, the caregiver may chose to monitor this individual with Pap smears every 6 months.

If the initial or follow-up Pap smear indicates inflammation with reactive squamous cellular changes, further management should be guided by diagnosis of the cause of the inflammation, and another Pap smear should be collected within 3 months. HIV-infected women with Pap smears showing only atypical cells of undetermined significance can be monitored with annual Pap smears.

Controversy exists concerning the management of HIV-infected women with low-grade squamous intraepithelial lesions (SIL) evident on the cervical Pap smear; the natural history of this finding in this population has not yet been well defined. Some experts would collect another Pap smear within 3 months. If subsequent Pap smears again showed low-grade SIL, some of these authorities would refer the patient for colposcopic evaluation and biopsy (if indicated), whereas others would monitor compliant patients with repeat Pap smears at frequent intervals (eg, every 3 to 6 months). Other experts would refer all HIV-infected patients with low-grade SIL for colposcopy.

If a Pap smear indicates high-grade SIL or squamous cell carcinoma, the woman should be referred for colposcopic examination and, if indicated, colposcopically directed biopsy.

HPV-Associated Anal Intraepithelial Neoplasia and Anal Cancer in HIV-Infected Men Who Have Sex With Men. Although the risks for anal intraepithelial neoplasia (AIN) and anal cancer are increased among HIV-infected men who have sex with men, the role of cytologic screening and treatment of AIN in preventing anal cancer in these men is not well defined. Therefore, no recommendations can be made for periodic anal cytologic screening for the detection and treatment of AIN.

Prevention of Recurrence

The risks for recurrence of SIL and cervical cancer after conventional therapy are increased among HIV-infected women. The prevention of illness associated with recurrence depends on careful follow-up of patients after treatment. Patients should be monitored with frequent cytologic screening and, when indicated, with colposcopic examination for recurrent lesions.

Pediatric Note

Newborns have been known to acquire laryngeal HPV from their mothers. No recommendations can be made to prevent such acquisition.

Case Study and Care Planning Exercise

Read the following case study and draw up a care plan for this client:

Angela Cook was diagnosed with AIDS a year ago when she developed PCP. When she was first admitted to your home care agency, she refused to discuss her AIDS diagnosis. She attributed her shortness of breath and cough to cigarette smoking and asthma, and stated that she was fatigued because of the demands of caring for her two children, Mary, age 3, and John, age 10. She agreed to HHA placement 5 days × 4 hours to assist with ADL.

Recently, Angela was hospitalized with fevers, night sweats, weight loss, and diarrhea. Her physician diagnosed MAI and found that her T4 count had dropped to 32. Transfusions were required for MAI-associated anemia. On readmission to home care, her medication regimen includes Bactrim®, Cipro®, clarithromycin, and Epogen® injections three times weekly, plus Proventil Inhaler® as needed.

Angela's recent hospitalization shattered her denial about her diagnosis. She is listless and depressed. Before this hospitalization, she took pride in her appearance; now, she spends all day in her nightgown. She shows little interest in learning to self-inject her Epogen. When you encourage her to eat, she responds: "What for?" She reports occasional diarrhea and intermittent fevers.

On your last visit, Angela confided she was fantasizing about using heroin again, even though she has been drug-free for 5 years and faithfully attended NA. Rose, the HHA, tells you that Angela is no longer capable of caring for her children. Rose says, "I feel sorry for the kids . . . I know it's not my job to cook for them, but I do it anyway." Angela's sister helps out when she can, but she has her own family responsibilities and a full-time job. There are no other dependable family supports.

What are Angela's health problems? Here are examples using nursing diagnosis:

Knowledge deficits: HIV/AIDS, MAI, PCP, medications
Ineffective management of therapeutic regimen
Fatigue
Diarrhea
Altered body temperature: fever
Altered nutrition
Ineffective individual coping
Self-care deficit
High risk for infection transmission
High risk for infection
Altered parent/child attachment
Potential for altered health maintenance: drug use
Risk for caregiver role strain (HHA or sister)

List your nursing interventions:

_____

_____

_____

_____

_____

_____

_____

_____

_____

_____

REFERENCES

Altman, L. K. (1996, February 1). Survival of AIDS patients linked to experience of their doctors. *The New York Times*, p. A12.

Casey, K. M. (1995). Pathophysiology of HIV-1, clinical course and treatment. In J. H. Flaskerud & P. J. Ungvarski (Eds.), *HIV/AIDS: A guide to nursing care* (3rd ed.) (pp. 64–80). Philadelphia: W.B. Saunders.

Centers for Disease Control and Prevention. (1990). Risk for cervical disease in HIV-infected women. *MMWR, 39*(47), 846–849.

Centers for Disease Control and Prevention. (1992). 1993 revised classification system for HIV infection and expanded case definition for AIDS among adults and adolescents. *MMWR, 41*(RR-17), 1–19.

Centers for Disease Control and Prevention. (1993). Use of bleach for disinfection of drug injection equipment. *MMWR, 41,* 418–419.

Centers for Disease Control and Prevention. (1994). Human immunodeficiency virus transmission in household settings: United States. *MMWR, 43*(19), 347, 353–356.

Centers for Disease Control and Prevention. (1995a). USPHA/IDSA guidelines for the prevention of opportunistic infections in persons with immunodeficiency virus: a summary. *MMWR, 44*(RR-8), 5–23.

Centers for Disease Control and Prevention. (1995b). *HIV/AIDS Surveillance Report, 7*(1), 1–34.

Centers for Disease Control and Prevention. (1995c). U.S. public health recommendations for human immunodeficiency virus counseling and voluntary testing for pregnant women. *MMWR, 44*(RR-7), 1–15.

Flaskerud, J. H. (1995). Health promotion and disease prevention. In J. H. Flaskerud & P. J. Ungvarski (Eds.), *HIV/AIDS: A guide to nursing care* (3rd ed.) (pp. 30–63). Philadelphia: W.B. Saunders.

Hoyt, M. J., & Staats, J. A. (1991). Wasting and malnutrition in patients with HIV/AIDS. *Journal of the Association of Nurses in AIDS Care, 2*(3), 16–26.

Hurley, P. M., & Ungvarski, P. J. (1994). Home health care needs of adults living with HIV disease/AIDS in New York City. *Journal of the Association of Nurses in AIDS Care, 5*(2), 33–40.

National Institutes of Health. (1993, April). Infections linked to AIDS: How to help yourself. (NIH publication number 93-3324). Bethesda, MD: U.S. Department of Health and Human Services.

Schmidt, J. (1992). Case management problems and home care. *Journal of the Association of Nurses in AIDS Care, 3*(3), 37–44.

Springer, E. (1991). Effective AIDs prevention with active drug users: The harm reduction model. *Journal of Chemical Dependency Treatment, 4*(2), 141–157.

Ungvarski, P. J., & Schmidt, J. (1995). Community-based and long-term care. In J. H. Flaskerud & P. J. Ungvarski (Eds.), *HIV/AIDS: A guide to nursing care* (3rd ed.) (pp. 339–361). Philadelphia: W.B. Saunders.

Ungvarski, P. J. (1994). Comorbidities of HIV-1/AIDS in adults. *Journal of the Association of Nurses in AIDS Care, 5*(6), 35–44.

18

The Maternal/ Child Visit

Rosalie Rothenberg, RN, EdD,
and Laila N. Sedhom, PhD

**Postpartum Physical
    Assessment**
Newborn Assessment

Conclusions

This chapter focuses on the home visit for the post-partum mother and newborn to help with the transition from hospital to home. Although the nurse usually visits within 24 to 48 hours after discharge, the client may be classified as postpartum any time during the first 6 weeks after delivery. Women are now being discharged as early as 24 hours after delivery. Positive aspects to early discharge include less chance of hospital-source infection, better bonding between baby and family members, and with supports, more rest for the mother at home. There are also disadvantages. The mother's readiness to learn in the hospital during the first 24 hours may be limited because of her physical condition, emotional state, number of phone calls, and family visitors.

The focus of the early postpartum visit is on identification of postdelivery complications, health promotion of the mother and the baby, teaching the mother to care for herself and the baby, and prevention of infections, accidents, and disease. The new mother is usually very receptive to the nurse's teaching and interventions. The nurse may be visiting a first-time mother or one who already has children, a very young or an older mother, a mother who has much or little family support. The needs of each mother and baby are different, and the nurse's care therefore must be individualized. During the home visit, the nurse's attention will be directed to the mother, the new baby, and the family. This chapter provides guidelines for the visit, including physical assessment of both the mother and the baby. Sample forms for the postpartum/newborn home visit are also included. This chapter will guide you in completing the forms.

The early postpartum visit is particularly important because, even after an uncomplicated delivery, mothers may not recognize postpartum complications. Infants may demonstrate health problems that are not evident to hospital professionals during the first day, and the inexperienced mother may have many questions about safely feeding and caring for her new infant. In this chapter, the assessment of both the mother and her newborn infant, identification of most frequently seen problems, teaching the mother self-care and infant care, and strategies of referral and advocacy for the mother and infant are discussed. The nurse's primary role is to help the new mother cope with her new role.

Sometimes you are visiting a mother whose baby remains in the hospital. This is still treated as a postpartum visit, although teaching for her would focus on maternal issues and interaction with a hospitalized infant. Another visit would be made when the baby comes home to address the infant care in the home and special needs of the infant regarding prematurity, post–neonatal intensive care unit (NICU) care, referral for early intervention programs, and other prescribed follow-up care.

In preparation for the visit, read Chapter 10 of this book, "The Initial Visit." The nurse should be familiar with assessment and care of both mothers and infants during the early postpartum period. For this maternal–infant visit, the nurse must read the hospital referral for the physician's orders, pregnancy and birth histories, and any other comments written about the client. The first contact with the mother is by telephone to let her know that a visiting nurse has been ordered for her. Some clients are unaware that their health insurance policy covers this. The nurse should inform the client that both the mother and baby will be seen and ask what is a good time to visit. If the baby is on a schedule, ask when the mother would prefer the visit. If the mother is breast-feeding, try to visit at feeding time so you can observe and teach regarding breast-feeding. The mother should be told to make a list of any concerns, needs, or questions to be discussed at the nurse's visit. Also tell the mother to prepare her insurance cards, any medications that she or the baby is taking, the baby's immunization card, hospital discharge papers, and name of mother's and baby's physicians. Verify her address and apartment number and give her a 2-hour timeframe within which you will visit.

When arriving, first determine where the mother would like to conduct the visit and determine who the mother would like involved in the visit. If the mother does not want any family members involved in the visit, assure privacy for mother and baby. Before beginning the visit, have the mother sign two consents, one for herself and one for the baby. At this time, ask to see the insurance card as the type of insurance will help determine visit frequency.

Begin the visit by taking the history. Postpartum and newborn agency forms should be used for specific guidelines. This helps to focus the visit. Most forms begin with the mother's pregnancy history. Discussing this will let you know if the baby was born premature and any other significant postpartum history. A thorough history will help you to identify significant problems or concerns. Ask the mother about her chief concerns. Her needs may be different from your expectation or perception.

If either the mother or baby is taking medications, ask the mother to tell you the dose, frequency, and route of administration. Assess whether any teaching is needed regarding the medication and its administration. Observe the mother measuring, and if possible, giving the medication.

During the visit, use the physical assessment as an opportunity to teach the mother. Explain what you are doing, what would be signs of problems to report, and how to maintain health in each area. If you demonstrate new skills, provide for return demonstrations and validation of learning. For example, ask the mother how she will take the baby's axillary temperature, let her do that, report the temperature reading, and tell what she will do if it is elevated.

Document *everything* observed, taught, and done at each visit. If it is not written, it was not done! The client's record will be used to justify payment from third-party payors and will indicate the overall quality of care provided by the agency. Thorough documentation of problems will be needed to obtain further services for the client.

Any physical problems should be thoroughly documented and reported to the physician. If you identify family or financial problems, refer to the agency social worker. Approval may be needed for additional home visits or service, depending on the type of insurance the client has.

POSTPARTUM PHYSICAL ASSESSMENT

The *postpartum check,* or physical assessment of the mother during the days after delivery, includes specific areas for the nurse to consider: vital signs, breasts, fundus, lochia, perineum, and episiotomy or Caesarean section incisions. Assessment of these are done to monitor predictable *involution,* or return to the prepregnant physical status, as well as to identify postpartum complications and discomforts.

Individualize

Although the postpartum check includes a consistent set of assessments, it is important to individualize the physical examination. What are this mother's concerns about her physical status? Does her labor and delivery experience indicate special assessment need (eg, perineal tears, Caesarean section delivery)? Does she experience any discomfort now? Is she planning to breast-feed the baby? Is this the first baby? The first pregnancy? Are there other health problems? The physical examination should be used to explain the physical changes after birth of the baby and the best ways for the mother to maintain a healthy state.

Before proceeding with the physical assessment, ask the mother to urinate, because a full bladder may interfere with accurate evaluation of the height of the fundus. This is also the time for the nurse to wash her hands thoroughly. Unsterile gloves should be worn for the examination of the perineum and perineal pad in adherence with universal precautions. Use this opportunity to demonstrate thorough handwashing and to get a return demonstration from the mother. Teach when to wash her hands: before feeding or preparing food, after diapering or handling soiled clothing or materials, before caring for the baby at any time, and before feeding or preparing formula.

The Postpartum Progress Note

See Display 18-1.

Vital Signs

Elevations of temperature, pulse, respirations, and blood pressure may be early indications of infection, inflammation, or other difficulties after delivery of the baby. These may not be elevated until 24 hours or more after discharge from the hospital.

The mother's temperature should be taken orally for at least 2 minutes. Any temperature over 100°F/ 38°C should be considered elevated, and the cause should be investigated. During the rest of the examination, look for other signs of infection or dehydration. Fever also may be related to breast engorgement and body responses to involution. Further care planning regarding the fever would be based on other findings during the assessment. Use this opportunity to evaluate the mother's ability to read the thermometer and her knowledge about taking temperatures of family members and baby. Be sure that the baby's temperature will only be taken by the axillary method, never rectally.

The radial pulse rate should be taken when the mother is at rest. The pulse is likely to be slow for the first day or two after delivery. Elevations over 90 beats per minute may indicate infection, bleeding, anemia, or emotional stress. Respiratory rates also taken at rest show the ability of the body to provide enough oxygen for its needs, and it may be rapid if there is infection, fever, anemia, or respiratory disease. Listen to her lung sounds for clear blowing sounds and absence of rales or rhonchi, indicating respiratory infection.

Lochia

As the lining of the uterus is sloughed off, the vaginal discharge changes from bright red, rubra, with small blood clots and shreds of mucus immediately after delivery, to dark red, serosa, for the first 1 to 3 days; then pale pink for the next 4 to 10 days; and finally alba or scant amounts of pale yellowish-white discharge ending at approximately 20 days. Lochia should be odorless or have a faint menstrual odor. An unpleasant odor may indicate uterine infection and merits immediate action.

The amount of lochia varies with the individual and is estimated by the diameter of the discharge on the perineal pad in 1 hour. *Scant* flow is a spot less than 2 inches in diameter; *small* amount of discharge (less than 25 mL) is indicated by a 4-inch stain; *mod-*

text continued on page 344

DISPLAY 18-1. **Postpartum Progress Note**

Date _____ Patient Name _____ I.D.# _____ D.O.B. _____

Address _____

Pregnancy History: Gravida _____ Para _____ Stillbirths _____

Voluntary Abortions _____ Spontaneous Abortions _____ Date of Delivery _____ Hospital Discharge _____

Delivery—Vaginal _____ C/S _____

Vital Signs: B/P R _____ L _____ P _____ T _____ O/R/A _____ R _____

Lung Sounds Left Lobes _____ Right Lobes _____ Weight _____ Pre-Pregnancy Weight _____

Medications Y _____ N _____ Med, Dose, Frequency, Route _____

Instructions/Teaching Needed _____

Lochia-Rubra _____ Serosa _____ Alba _____

Odor Y _____ N _____ Profuse Y _____ N _____ Light Y _____ N _____ Clots Present Y _____ N _____

Instructions/Teaching Needed _____

Breast: Lactating _____ Non-Lactating _____

Pain Y _____ N _____ Engorged Y _____ N _____ Tender Y _____ N _____ Nipples Cracked Y _____ N _____

Breast Care and Breast Feeding Instruction _____

Abdomen: Bowel Sounds Y _____ N _____ Abdominal Pain Y _____ N _____

Distention Y _____ N _____ Fundus Location _____ Fundus firm Y _____ N _____ Non-Tender Y _____ N _____

Instructions/Teaching Needed _____

Episiotomy/Abdominal Incision-*Specify wound care if indicated* _____

Pain/Tenderness Y _____ N _____ Erythema Y _____ N _____ Ecchymosis Y _____ N _____

Bleeding Y _____ N _____ Edema Y _____ N _____ Drainage Y _____ N _____ Sitz Baths Y _____ N _____

Instructions/Teaching Needed _____

Nausea/Vomiting Y ___ N ___ Adequate Fluid Intake Y ___ N ___
Instructions/Teaching Needed ___

Urinary Status: Number of Times Voided in Past 24 Hours ___ Frequency Y ___ N ___ Retention Y ___ N ___
Burning Y ___ N ___ S/S Urinary Tract Infection Y ___ N ___
Instructions/Teaching Needed ___

Bowel Status: Number of Bowel Movements in Past 24 Hours ___ Constipation Y ___ N ___ Diarrhea Y ___ N ___
Rectal Pain Y ___ N ___ Hemorrhoids Y ___ N ___ Sitz Baths Y ___ N ___
Instruction/Teaching Needed ___

Circulation: Edema Y ___ N ___ Location ___ Measurement L ___ R ___
Leg Cramps Y ___ N ___ Varicose Veins Y ___ N ___
Instructions/Teaching Needed ___

PsychoSocial: Postpartum Blues Y ___ N ___ Insomnia Y ___ N ___ Feeling Overwhelmed Y ___ N ___
MOB Bonding Evident Y ___ N ___ Mother's Concerns ___
FOB Involved Y ___ N ___ Father of Baby Bonding Evident Y ___ N ___ Father's Concern ___
Instructions/Teaching Needed ___

Birth Control: Options Discussed Y ___ N ___ Teaching Needed ___
Resumption of Sexual Relations Discussed Y ___ N ___
Instructions/Teaching Needed ___

Significant Postpartum Findings ___

Need for Further Visits ___

Medical Follow-up ___

Coordination ___

V.N. Signature ___

© With permission. S. Zang

erate discharge of approximately 50 mL is indicated by a spot approximately 6 inches in diameter. Anything more than that would be described as a *large* amount of vaginal discharge/lochia. Excess lochia may be related to lacerations, hematoma, or retained placenta fragments. Increased physical activity may cause the lochia to temporarily increase or return to rubra with a few small clots. The mother may be alarmed by this, and she should be reassured that she is not bleeding. Teach the mother to change her perineal pad at least every 3 or 4 hours, not to touch the inside of the pad, and to wash her hands well after cleaning her perineum. She should call her physician if the lochia has an unpleasant odor or change in character.

Breasts

The breasts and nipples are examined next. Until 24 to 48 hours after delivery, the breasts should be soft to palpation, and colostrum may be expressed from each nipple. By the second to fourth day, the breasts begin to prepare for lactation and become firm, warm, enlarged, heavy, and tender. The blood vessels under the skin of the breasts may then be visible. At first, a small amount of bluish, cloudy milk can be expressed. With time, as breast-feeding becomes established, the milk supply will be regulated by the infant's need and the mother's diet and exercise; the breasts will no longer be engorged. If the mother has begun to breast-feed, inspect her nipples for cracking or irritation and the breasts for reddened or warm areas that might indicate mastitis. Reassure the mother and support her early attempts with breast-feeding. Use this opportunity for teaching breast care and providing reassurance for her progress in establishing breast-feeding.

Observe her technique and assess the rooting and sucking reflexes of the baby. Support the mother to achieve independence and success in her effort to breast-feed. Teach her to alternate the breast she offers to the baby first at each feeding. Explain the technique of breaking suction before removing the baby from the breast. Emphasize the importance of burping between feedings on each breast and at the end of the feeding.

The mother may be concerned about the adequacy of breast milk consumed by the baby. Explain to her that if the baby gains weight and has six or more wet diapers a day, the baby is receiving adequate amounts of milk. Also, the mother can listen for sounds of swallowing while the baby is nursing. Explain to the mother that the breast-fed infant becomes hungry sooner because breast milk is more easily digested than formulas. Refer mother to La Leche League for further support and provide her with pamphlets. Because most medications given to the mother are secreted in the breast milk, make sure that the mother is not taking any medication that may be harmful to the baby.

If the mother is not breast-feeding, engorgement of her breasts should subside in 2 or 3 days. Advise her to wear a support bra and to avoid stimulating her breasts.

If the mother has decided to bottle-feed the baby, support her in this decision. Most mothers will use the formula that was given to them in the hospital. When no formula has been prescribed, the nurse may advise the mother to use Similac, Enfamil, Gerber, Good Start, or SMA formula. Most formulas are interchangeable. If the baby is on a formula with iron, teach mother to only substitute with an iron formula and teach her to monitor baby's bowel status. Formulas are either ready-to-feed, concentrate, or powder form. If the formula is in concentrate form, teach the mother to dilute it by adding one part concentrate to one part water. If the formula is in powder form, teach mother to add one level scoop to each 2 oz. water.

Abdomen

The abdomen should feel soft and nondistended. Record any complaints of abdominal pain or distention; listen for bowel sounds. Muscle tone should return by 6 weeks after delivery, and striae (stretch marks) will fade over time. If client had a Caesarean section, assess the incision for drainage, redness, swelling, or other indications of infection. These should be reported immediately to the physician, and orders for daily dressing changes may be indicated. Teach the mother exercises to strengthen the abdominal muscles, beginning as soon as possible with abdominal breathing and sleeping on the abdomen, and gradually adding pelvic rocking to correct her posture from the tilt of pregnancy. Most strenuous exercises should be delayed until approval by the physician or midwife.

Fundus of the Uterus

The uterus returns to its prepregnant size in the weeks after delivery. This involution is assessed by palpating the height of the fundus of the uterus in relation to the umbilicus and the symphysis pubis. The fundus of the uterus should be felt at the level of the umbilicus on the day of delivery, and approximately

1 cm/1/2 inch lower each day after that. By 8 to 14 days after delivery, the fundus should no longer be able to be felt above the symphysis pubis. In the first days after delivery, a fundus felt higher than expected may indicate a uterus displaced by a full bladder or filled with clots.

The fundus should be palpated with the mother lying flat on a bed or sofa, with her abdomen exposed and privacy provided. The fundus should feel firm as a grapefruit and placed at the midline. A boggy texture, particularly if the fundus is felt higher than expected, may indicate incomplete contraction of the uterine muscles, with an increased possibility of bleeding. Gentle massage of the fundus will help the uterus to become firm and may expel small clots.

Teach the mother to palpate and gently massage the uterus with the palm of her hand. She should notify the physician if bleeding is bright red or clots become excessive. Uterine contractions may continue for up to 48 hours after delivery. Explain this to the mother and follow up with the physician to see if any medication is indicated.

Perineum

Ask the mother to lie on her side, facing away from you. Lift the top buttock to inspect her perineum. A slight amount of swelling and bruised discoloration is expected. The edges of the episiotomy should be together and the same color and degree of swelling as the perineum. Localized swelling or discharge from the incision can indicate infection, and should be reported. Ask the mother if the episiotomy is painful. At the same time, inspect the external rectal area for hemorrhoids or repair of tears from delivery. Pushing during the second stage of labor often distends hemorrhoids, which may be enlarged for several days after delivery. Use this opportunity to teach the mother to wash the perineum with warm soap and water after each voiding, to wipe from front to back, or preferably to pat the area gently. Sitz baths in clean warm water increase circulation to the area and maintain cleanliness. Ice packs or medicated pads may relieve discomfort from the incision or hemorrhoids. Also teach the mother to drink adequate fluids and eat foods with fiber to maintain soft stools. Instruct her to avoid tub bathing, sexual intercourse, or use of tampons until the 6-week checkup by her physician.

Kegel exercises may be started to restore muscle tone to the vagina and perineum, to stimulate circulation to the perineum for healing, and to enhance sexual enjoyment. The mother should be taught to tighten and relax the area around the rectum and vagina for 3 seconds, relax the muscle for 3 seconds, and repeat several times during the day.

Nutrition

Take a brief nutritional history to determine if the mother eats adequate nutrients for postpartum recovery and breast-feeding needs. What are the foods (amounts and types) eaten in the past 24 hours? What does she usually eat? Does she have special dietary needs? If the mother was anemic during pregnancy or had significant blood loss during delivery, teach her about foods high in iron and folic acid. Adolescent mothers need larger amounts of dietary protein and vitamins for growth as well as the usual needs of a new mother. If the mother is breast-feeding, she should be advised that the fat deposited during pregnancy will be used for the increased energy demands of lactation. She should be taught about foods high in calcium and vitamins A and C. It is vital to teach the mother to increase fluids when breast-feeding. If the mother is not breast-feeding, she should be counseled that the weight gained during pregnancy will be lost gradually over the next 2 to 3 months. She may wish to limit foods with empty calories, concentrating on fruits and vegetables, grains, and more nutritious foods. If the family cannot afford foods needed for the postpartum woman, find out if they are eligible for food stamps or WIC (Women, Infants, and Children).

Urinary Status

Large amounts of body fluid are lost in the first week after delivery. The mother may report that she perspires a great deal and urinates frequently for at least 4 or 5 days. Does she have burning on urination or a history of urinary tract infection? She should be encouraged to drink large amounts of liquids and report any pain, burning, or hematuria to the physician after postpartum bleeding has stopped.

Elimination—Bowel Status

Ask the mother if she has had a bowel movement since delivery. A bowel movement is expected by the second or third postpartum day, but may be delayed because of fear of episiotomy or hemorrhoidal pain, dehydration, or weak abdominal muscles after pregnancy. She should be advised to drink adequate amounts of liquids to avoid dehydration. Eating foods with fiber and drinking large amounts of fluids may prevent constipation. If constipated, the mother may need an order for a stool softener, suppository, or mild enema.

Extremities

Inspect the mother's legs for signs of edema, varicose veins, or thrombophlebitis. Assess for edema and any change in size, temperature, color, and pulses. Assess for Homans's sign by dorsiflexing each foot to identify pain in the calf of the leg on stretching. If positive, this may be a sign of thrombophlebitis. If there is edema in the legs, assess both pedal pulses and skin temperature to evaluate circulation and measure the area of edema of both legs. Teach the mother to promote circulation in her legs by walking, avoiding crossing her legs or wearing garters, and elevating her legs at least to the level of her hips if there is edema.

Emotional Response of the Mother

The most usual responses immediately after delivery are fatigue, relief that labor is over, elation and excitement, and feelings of success or failure regarding the labor. During the first 2 or 3 days after delivery, most mothers want to be taken care of and to sleep and rest.

- Mood swings: Many new mothers experience a temporary "let-down" feeling during the first week, crying easily. Possible contributing factors can be fatigue, discomfort, anxiety over her new role, overstimulation, hormonal changes, sleep deprivation, or frustration over inability to console the baby. Teach the mother about "baby blues," or postpartum depression. Encourage the mother to relax with the baby, enjoy the baby, and get to know the baby. Others may offer conflicting advice; reassure her to do things as *she* wishes, taking only advice that fits her lifestyle. The baby will survive the new mother. Help the family to understand and give support.

- Depression: If mood swings persist beyond the first week, are accompanied by lack of interest in the baby, apathy, and *no* crying, this may be more serious. Discuss this with the physician because further evaluation may be needed. The mother may need close monitoring and assistance with infant care and home responsibilities.

Interaction With the Baby

Assess the following: How does the mother hold her baby? Does she talk to the baby, make eye contact? How does she respond to the baby's cries of distress or signs of satiation? Does she discuss the baby or express concerns about the baby? Is the father of the baby available or involved in the baby's care? If either the mother or baby have had birthing problems, attachment may develop slowly.

Who is this baby? The nurse can point out behaviors and characteristics of this baby, characteristics that the infant shares with other family members. Help the mother to recognize her infant's cues/messages. Encourage her to interact with the baby when he or she is alert and not crying. Advise her that babies cry to communicate.

Indications of problems in interaction or potential difficulties include mothers who give evidence of avoidance or withdrawal from the baby, difficulty understanding and responding to the infant's needs, and poor hygiene. A history of no prenatal care, history of social health problems such as child abuse or neglect, drug or alcohol use, psychiatric illness, or poor social support system increase the risk as well. If you find any of these problems, there may be an indication for a social work referral. If you believe that the baby may be at risk, please notify your agency. A referral to Child Welfare Agency (CWA) may be indicated.

Activities of Daily Living

It is important to review with the mother her patterns of eating, sleeping, and usual daily activities. It is also important to find out who is available to shop and prepare food, do laundry, or provide respite during the mother's rest time. If the mother does not have many support systems, teach her about her need to rest when the baby is sleeping. See if she is eligible for a home health aide. If she lives alone or cannot easily manage to shop, ask if there is a grocery store that will deliver food, diapers, or formula.

Home Environment

Assess the home for safety for the infant. Where does the baby sleep? Is there adequate heating, ventilation, and privacy? The home environment can affect the mother's ability to rest and care for the baby. Potential problems may occur if the nurse encounters poverty, crowded housing, or old housing. Once again, a referral to a social worker might be indicated at this time.

Family and Support Systems

Who is in the family? Who lives in this household? What is their relationship with the mother and baby? Who is available to help the mother, to provide a rest for her? Does that person know how to care for the infant? What are the mother's plans for child care if she is returning to work or other activities? Possible supports for the new mother might include family members such as in-laws, siblings who have had babies, parents, friends, a baby nurse, or other hired help in the house. Books, videos, or magazines on infant care and materials sent by insurance companies provide supplemental information. Parenting groups in community health agencies, schools, and churches offer peer support of other new mothers.

Culture and Religion

What expectations do the mother's culture or religion have for new mothers and babies for parenting? While in the hospital, many mothers give no indication of these practices, but in their own homes, these practices are often more important to the mother than the instructions of the health care workers. The mother may have beliefs or practices that others call "old wives tales." These traditions often have a great deal of meaning to a mother and her family. Unless practices are actually dangerous to the mother or baby, the nurse should never try to change them or show disrespect. Try to incorporate these practices into your teaching and planning. If these practices are dangerous, the nurse should negotiate changes with the mother.

Families who are immigrants to this country may not understand the nurse's language or English-language teaching materials. They also may not know resources and processes of the local health care system. Let your agency know. An interpreter from the agency or maybe a family member or friend may be available to help with interviewing.

Sibling Reactions to Baby

It is best to plan ahead for introducing the new baby to siblings. The family should expect to see some jealousy with the mother giving time and attention to the new baby. Young siblings may regress with bed wetting, whining, or a return to the bottle or diaper.

Problems are especially likely at feeding time. Some suggestions for the family are: Let someone else feed the baby occasionally. The mother may give a gift to a sibling from the baby. Allow the sibling to help with care of the baby or a doll substitute. Divert aggressive behavior away from the baby.

Sexuality

This is an appropriate time to discuss the mother's plans for birth control. Caution her that breast-feeding is not a reliable prevention of pregnancy. If she and her partner resume sexual activities before the 6-week postpartum visit, temporary contraception should be used because she may ovulate before her first menstrual period. Until the mother is provided with a newly fitted diaphragm, an intrauterine device (IUD), or a prescription for birth control pills, a well-lubricated condom will provide comfortable and reliable protection from both pregnancy and infection. The mother should be advised NOT to douche until after the 6-week examination, because this can cause infection or air embolus.

NEWBORN ASSESSMENT

A very good physical assessment is needed to assess the baby's successful transition to extrauterine life and health in the first few days of life. In assessing the newborn (Display 18-2), the nurse should bear in mind the following four points:

1. Even though newborns cannot articulate, they speak to us through subtle cues that we can learn to read.

2. When you first see the baby, resist the temptation to disturb the baby. Step back and just observe the baby in a normal resting state.

3. The order of the examination is generally from head to toe, but take advantage of the state of the infant. If the infant is quiet or sleeping, perform a "pre-crying examination," including heart, lungs, femoral pulses, fontanels, and abdomen. More distressing maneuvers should be left to last.

4. Assess the newborn in the presence of the parents. This permits teaching and discussion of parental concerns, and it actively involves the parents in health care of the child. At the same time, parental interactions with the child can be observed.

General Observation

The nurse should assess the environment and the space where the baby will be examined. The area chosen for the infant's examination should be well lit, warm, and free of drafts. Undress the baby and place on a flat surface. Observe the baby in a resting state. The proportions of the newborn's head to the body should be 1:4, with the newborn's body midpoint at the umbilicus. Look at the body symmetry. Is any body part out of place or out of shape? Normal full-term newborns lie in a symmetrical position with the extremities partially flexed, showing good muscle tone, and the legs partially abducted at the hips. The head is slightly flexed and positioned in the midline or turned to one side. Fingers are usually flexed in a tight fist. If one or more extremities are extended, examine the infant further for injury, neurologic deficit, or evidence of gestational immaturity.

text continued on page 358

DISPLAY 18-2. Newborn Progress Note

Date _____ Patient Name _____ I.D.# _____ D.O.B. _____

Address _____

Gestational Age _____ Weeks Reported Apgar _____

Birth Weight _____ Discharge Weight _____ Weight Today _____

Vital Signs:

Axillary Temp. _____ Heart Rate _____ Respiration _____ Color _____ Lung Sounds: Right Lobes _____ Left Lobes _____

Head: Circumference _____ Chest Circumference _____ Length/Height _____

Head: Normocephalic Y _____ N _____ Fontanels Abn. _____ Normal _____ Describe _____

Temperature Taking Taught Y _____ N _____

Instructions/Teaching Needed _____

Medication Ordered Y _____ N _____ Med/Dose/Frequency/Route _____

Teaching Needed _____

Umbilical Cord Y _____ N _____ Drainage Y _____ N _____ Odor Y _____ N _____

Instructions/Teaching Needed _____

Abdomen: Soft Y _____ N _____ Distended Y _____ N _____

G.I.: Stool—Number of Bowel Movements/24 Hours _____ Color of Stool _____ Consistency _____

Urine: Number of Wet Diapers/24 Hours _____ Color of Urine _____

Instructions/Teaching Needed _____

Neuro: Alert Y _____ N _____ Irritable Y _____ N _____ Cry Loud _____ Lusty _____ Shrill _____ Weak _____

Tremors Y _____ N _____ Sleep Pattern _____ Easily Arousable Y _____ N _____

Reflexes Moro Y ____ N ____   Palmer Grasp Y ____ N ____   Stepping Y ____ N ____

Tonic Neck Y ____ N ____   Babinski Y ____ N ____

Instructions/Teaching Needed _____

Skin: Color Pale Y ____ N ____   Icteric Y ____ N ____   Cyanotic Y ____ N ____   Turgor Good ____ Poor ____

Rash Y ____ N ____   Location _____   Treatment _____

Birth Marks Location _____

Instructions/Teaching Needed _____

Nutrition/Hydration: Formula Type _____   Amt./Freq. _____

Breast Feeding/Time at Breast _____   How Often _____

Refusal to Feed Y ____ N ____   Feeding Problems Specify _____

Suck Strong ____ Weak ____   Water Offering Amt./Freq. _____

Instructions/Teaching Needed _____

Circumcision: Site Edema Y ____ N ____   Bleeding Y ____ N ____   Erythema Y ____ N ____

Treatment Ordered _____

Instructions/Teaching Needed _____

Chief Concerns Expressed _____

Parenting Skills Needed _____

Significant Newborn Findings _____

Need for Further Visits _____

Medical Follow-up _____

Coordination _____

V.N. Signature _____

© With permission. S. Zang

The chest should be rounded and not caved in. The abdomen should be rounded too but not too full or enlarged. Study the respiration rate and character. Always count for a full minute. Newborns' breathing is irregular, so a shorter count is inaccurate. Normal rate ranges between 30 and 60 breaths per minute. Report if there are fewer than 20 or more than 60 breaths per minute. Examine the character of the chest movement. Any pulling between the ribs or at the base of the sternum indicates retractions. The newborn's breathing is usually shallow and abdominal. Grunting is not uncommon. In fact, some grunting is normal, but if it continues, it may indicate that the newborn is chilled or in respiratory distress, especially if the grunting is accompanied by flaring nostrils or cyanosis.

Newborns have a periodic breathing pattern because of the immaturity of their respiratory and central nervous systems. It is common for newborns to stop breathing for brief periods. However, pauses lasting 20 seconds or more and accompanied by skin color changes or bradycardia are considered apneic periods and should be reported to the physician.

Do you notice any tremor of the extremities? This is common in newborns but should disappear when you touch the baby. Continuous or pronounced tremor may indicate drug withdrawal, neurologic deficit, or a metabolic problem.

Take an axillary temperature. Never take a rectal temperature on the baby. It should be between 36.5°C and 37.5°C, or 97.6°F to 98.6°F. Teach parents how to take baby's temperature. Have them read it, and teach them how to read it if they are unsure. If the baby has an elevated temperature, it is probably a sign of infection or inflammation. During the rest of the examination, look for other signs of infections.

Next auscultate for heart sounds. Place the stethoscope at the apex of the heart, usually between the fourth or fifth left intercostal space medial to the midclavicular line. Heart rate may vary with crying, activity, sleeping, and feeding. In the normal full-term newborn, heart rate is between 120 and 160 beats per minute while awake, slightly higher while crying, and between 70 and 100 beats per minute while asleep. The apical rate is counted for 1 full minute. Report if the rate is less than 70 beats per minute or greater than 170 beats per minute. Murmurs are common during the neonatal period (first 48 hours of life) as the heart makes its transition from the fetal circulation path. To auscultate for murmurs, place the stethoscope at the left lower sternal border in the third or fourth interspace. If you hear sounds that are not normal, inform the physician.

Next evaluate all peripheral pulses (brachial, radial, femoral, popliteal, and dorsalis pedis) for presence, equality, and strength. Femoral pulses may be difficult to palpate but should be felt along the inguinal ligament midway between the iliac crest and the symphysis pubis.

Auscultate the abdomen for sounds of peristalsis. Their absence may be a sign of intestinal obstruction, especially in the presence of abdominal distention.

Physical Measurements

Length: Place the infant supine with legs extended as much as possible and measure from the crown to the heel of the baby. The normal range is 45 to 55 cm or 18 to 22 in.

Head Circumference: Measure the head at its largest circumference. Place the tape over the most prominent part of the occiput and bring it to just above the eyebrows. The normal range is 32 to 37 cm or 12.5 to 14.5 in.

Chest Circumference: Measure the chest circumference at the nipple line. It is usually approximately 2 cm less than the head circumference.

Weight: Finally, weigh the newborn. Assure parents that this scale is different from the one used in the hospital, and there may be a slight variation in weight. Normal weight for a full-term newborn is 2500 to 4000 g or 5 lbs 8 oz to 8 lbs 19 oz.

Head-to-Toe Examination

Skin Assessment

Skin assessment is part of the overall head-to-toe examination, but because so much important data can be obtained from the baby's skin, it is discussed separately.

Turgor. Assess for proper turgor by gently pulling the skin near the neck or on the lower abdomen to see how quickly it returns to smoothness. Poor turgor is a sign of dehydration, which is very serious for newborns and should be reported.

Newborn skin should feel warm. Cold clammy skin is a sign of heat loss and should be dealt with immediately. Cover the baby to keep warm.

Color. Skin color reflects general health. In assessing skin color, consider the ethnicity of the baby. Caucasian newborns have pinkish-red skin tone. African American newborns have a reddish-brown color. Hispanic newborns have an olive or yellowish skin tone.

Cyanosis. Newborns may exhibit a slight or a transient cyanosis. It is important to distinguish between a mild blueness of the mucosa caused by circulatory changes and central cyanosis caused by circulatory or respiratory insufficiency. A bluish discoloration of hands and feet known as acrocyanosis is a common observation, especially if the newborn is slightly chilled. To make sure this is not a symptom of true cyanosis, rub the sole of the foot vigorously. If pink color returns, the acrocyanosis is caused by heat loss. Take measures to warm the baby and stop the heat loss. Changes in skin color may be the first sign of sepsis or cardiopulmonary or hematologic disorders.

Jaundice or Icterus. Always remember that jaundice can be a serious problem for a newborn. It is always a cue for close following, even though a good percentage of full-term infants develop physiologic jaundice. Physiologic jaundice usually appears on the second or third day. It peaks between second and fourth day, then disappears.

Pathologic jaundice should be suspected if jaundice appears in the first 24 hours or after the third day or if there are reasons to think that the infant might be at risk for pathologic hyperbilirubinemia, for example, from blood incompatibilities, infections, anorexia, dehydration, breast-feeding, etc. Telephone report to the physician and advise the mother to seek immediate medical care if pathologic jaundice is suspected. Teach the mother to monitor the baby's fluid intake.

Jaundice appears first on the head and face, progressing downward to the truck and extremities and finally to the sclera of the eye. To assess for jaundice, press briefly on the bridge of the nose to flush the capillaries. Jaundiced newborns will exhibit a yellow color. In dark-skinned newborns, jaundice is more easily observed in the sclera and buccal mucosa.

Nonpathologic Skin Features

Mongolian spots, a bluish discoloration on the hips or buttocks, is most common in African American and Asian newborns. Assure the mother that these spots will disappear completely without intervention within 2 years.

Telangiectatic nevi, or *stork bites,* are pale pink macular lesions or red spots frequently found on the eyelids, nose, lower occipital bone, and back of the neck, most commonly in babies with light complexions. Explain to the mother that these lesions will become more noticeable during crying and that they usually disappear by the second day.

Erythema toxicum (urticaria neonatorum) is a rash with white vesicles on a red macular base. It usually appears over the trunk and diaper area, but does not appear on the palms of the hands or the soles of the feet. Assure the mother that these lesions clear quickly without intervention.

Milia are small, white, raised spots on the chin, forehead, and bridge of nose. Explain to the mother that these are caused by clogged sebaceous glands and will disappear by themselves during the first 2 weeks of life.

Ecchymoses are bruises from the delivery. Assure parents that these marks will clear up in a matter of 1 or 2 days.

Birthmarks are often a cause of concern for parents. The mother may have guilt feelings and think she is to blame for something she ate or did. Identify birthmarks and correct the mother's misconception about the cause. Assess and document their location, color, size, distribution, and any other characteristics.

Strawberry marks: A raised, clearly delineated, dark red, rough surfaced birthmark that resemble an outside slice of a ripe strawberry. It is commonly found in the head region. Explain to the parents that these marks usually grow for several months and become fixed in size by 8 months, after which they will begin to shrink and then resolve spontaneously. Assure parents that, except in rare cases, these marks are completely gone by the time the child is 7 years old.

Port-wine stains: This is a nonelevated, red-to-purple area of capillaries. It varies in size and shape and commonly appears on the face. Unfortunately, it does not fade with time or disappear; parents need to know that.

Head

Shape. Look for symmetrical, well-formed features. The infant's skull is soft and pliable. The head of the vaginally delivered newborn has probably been molded by the stress of delivery. Explain to parents that this usually corrects itself. For a baby born by Caesarean section, the head is more rounded.

If the head feels spongy and soft, it may be caput succedaneum (edema over the presenting part of the newborn's head), which disappears within 12 hours or few days. It also may be cephalhematoma, which disappears after 2 to 3 weeks or months.

Fontanels. Palpate the anterior and posterior fontanels. They should feel soft and flat while the baby is quiet, and bulging while the baby is coughing or crying. A depressed fontanel is a sign of dehydration. Bulging fontanels while the baby is quiet should be documented and reported to the physician. The anterior fontanel is located between the parietal and frontal bones. It is diamond shaped and open at least as large as the tip of your little finger, approximately 3 to 4 cm long by 2 to 3 cm wide. It closes by 18 months. The posterior fontanel is located between the parietal and occipital bones. It is triangular and 1 to 2 cm wide. It closes between 2 and 4 months.

Eyes

It is somewhat difficult to examine the newborn's eyes because the lids are ordinarily held tightly closed. To encourage the newborn to open his or her eyes, turn off some of the room light or hold the baby upright in your extended arms while supporting the head with your thumbs. Rotate yourself with the baby slowly in one direction. This usually causes the baby to open his or her eyes.

- Eyes should be symmetrical in size and shape. Lids may be edematous and puffy. The iris is usually slate gray, brown, or blue. Explain to parents that eye color becomes permanent at approximately 6 months of age.
- Conjunctiva should be pale pink in color with no discharge. You may note a red, crescent-shaped area in the sclera next to the iris. Explain to the parents that this is of no pathologic significance and will disappear in a week.
- Red conjunctiva with purulent discharge and edema of the lids may appear a few hours after delivery and after instillation of silver nitrate. It disappears without intervention in 1 or 2 days.

Red conjunctiva with purulent exudate or discharge appearing after the second day is abnormal and must be reported. It is probably infectious conjunctivitis and requires treatment.

- Prominent epicanthal folds (mongolian slant) is a normal finding in Asian babies but may suggest Down syndrome in other ethnic groups.
- Pupils are round and should react equally to pen light. Using an ophthalmoscope, assess the red reflex, which indicates an intact lens.
- Eye movements are generally random and uncoordinated. A crossed-eyes appearance is often seen in newborns. Explain to parents that this is caused by weak eye musculature and lack of coordination.

Newborns are nearsighted at birth and will be able to follow and see objects held 8 to 10 inches in front of them. Teach parents that bright-colored or black and white toys are best because newborns respond to such colors.

Ears

Examine ears for shape, position, firmness of cartilage, and hearing. The top of the ear should be in line with the newborn's eyes. Low-set ears are often associated with renal anomalies and chromosomal disorders, and therefore, should be documented and reported to the physician.

To assess the hearing, clap or ring a bell or a rattle near the ear at a distance of about 10 inches. This should elicit a startle or a blink response.

Teach parents that they can use a twisted cotton or a soft washcloth to clean the outer ear, never an applicator. Emphasize the danger of putting anything inside the ear.

Nose

Assess patency of the nasal canals by holding a hand over infant's mouth and one canal and noting the passage of air through the unobstructed opening. The nose should be on the midline of the newborns' face. If the bridge of the nose is flattened, it may indicate chromosomal abnormalities, especially in combination with other facial malformations, and should be reported to the physician.

Passage of thin, white mucus and sneezing is not uncommon, but thick bloody discharge should be reported. Teach parents that the nose usually does not need cleaning. Babies sneeze to clear the nasal passages. Make sure parents understand *not* to use cotton-tipped applicators to clean inside the newborn's nose. Explain that they could injure the delicate tissues of the nose. Only a small twisted piece of cotton moistened with water may be used.

Mouth

Assess lips, mucous membrane, tongue, and hard and soft palate. The mouth should be on the midline of the face. Lips should be pink and dry, with pink and moist mucous membranes. Teach parents that Epstein's pearls, small white spots on the mucous membrane of the mouth, are normal and will disappear in a few weeks. Tongue should be moving freely. To assess for the intactness of the hard and soft palate, sweep the mouth with a gloved finger.

Neck

Assess the neck for symmetry and range of motion. Gently move the head through its full range of motion at the neck: forward bending, backward extension, lateral bending, and rotation to the right and the left. Palpate the clavicles to rule out any evidence of fracture. A fractured clavicle feels like a knot or lump, with decreased movement of the extremity on that side.

Thorax

Moving down to the newborn's thorax, note that the chest should be symmetrical and rounded. The breasts of the newborn in both sexes may be enlarged and engorged with a white liquid. Teach parents not to express, massage, or squeeze the nipples, because this practice may cause a breast abscess. Assure them that this condition lasts only a week or 2 and disappears by itself. Accessory nipples are seen below and medial to the normal nipples and are of no clinical significance.

Abdomen

Before palpating the abdomen, listen for the bowel sounds. Palpation decreases the intensity of the bowel sounds. The abdomen should feel soft and nondistended.

Check the umbilical cord for any redness, drainage, odor, or signs of infection. The cord should be dry, with no oozing or bleeding. An unpleasant odor, drainage, redness, or inflammation may indicate infection and should be reported to the physician. Inform the parents that the umbilical stump will fall off in approximately 10 to 14 days.

Teach the parents to clean around the junction between the cord stump and the skin with alcohol at each diaper change to encourage drying. Explain to parents not to give the baby a tub bath until the cord has separated and the umbilicus has healed. This facilitates drying of the cord. Some cultures prefer to use a cord dressing. Explain to the parents that this is unnecessary and that exposure to air enhances drying.

Urine

The urine of the newborn is clear, straw-colored, and odorless. Newborns urinate frequently. They may urinate 10 to 15 times a day.

Stool

Assess the newborn's stools for color, consistency, and frequency. On the second and probably the third day, the stools are greenish-brown to yellowish-brown. They are called *transitional stools,* and they are less sticky than meconium. Teach the parents that the color and characteristics of stools depend on whether the baby is breast-fed or formula-fed. If the baby is breast-fed, the stools are yellow to golden color with pasty and mushy consistency and distinctive odor. If the baby is formula-fed, the stools are pale yellow to light brown with slightly offensive odor. Stools of formula-fed babies are more formed than those of breast-fed babies. Breast-fed babies may have six or eight stools per day. Formula-fed babies may have four to six stools per day. Teach the parents that the daily number of stools decreases as the baby grows. Teach the parents to report to the physician if the baby passes watery green stools that contain mucus and have a foul odor.

Genitals

Examine the genitals of both males and females. Are they fully developed? Are there any signs of irritation?

Teach parents that female newborns may have enlarged labia and slight vaginal discharge, which may be blood-tinged mucus. Assure parents that the swelling and discharge disappear spontaneously and should not cause any concern.

In male newborns, the scrotum appears relatively large, and the testicles may not have descended at birth, but you should be able to palpate them at the inguinal ring. If the baby is uncircumcised, explain to the parents not to retract the foreskin. If the baby was circumcised before leaving the hospital, assess the site for edema, bleeding, and redness. If there are no specific physician orders for aftercare, teach the parents how to take care of their circumcised baby. In changing the newborn's diaper, teach parents to squeeze water gently over the penis, pat it dry, and loosely put on the diaper. Explain to parents to hold his ankles so he cannot kick against the operative area. Teach the parents that a whitish yellow exudate around the glans is a normal part of the healing process and not indicative of an infection. This exudate will last 2 or 3 days and should not be removed.

Neurologic System

Assessment of the nervous system is performed throughout the physical examination, including the infant's cry, sleeping patterns, and reflexes.

Assess the character of the baby's cry. A full-term newborn's cry is strong. The cry of premature babies is weak and shrill. In the early few weeks, some newborns may cry a total of 2 to 3 hours per day, and others may cry only for 15 to 30 minutes per day. Some newborns may cry for 10 to 15 minutes before they fall asleep. The amount of crying is highly individual. Explain to parents that, in general, newborns do not cry unless they are wet, hungry, ill, or uncomfortable for some reason. Teach parents how to distinguish the newborn's needs from the character of the cry, and assure them that, in time, they will be able to read their child's cues. Emphasize the importance of not feeding the baby every time he or she cries. Newborns may be comforted by swaddling, rocking, and other reassuring activity. Reassure parents that they will not spoil the newborn by picking him or her up and cuddling.

Sometimes the baby is fussy, cries easily and more frequently, and is awake much of the time. This creates a great deal of anxiety on the part of the mother, who may assume that she must be doing something wrong. Assure the mother that this is a normal behavior for this child, and demonstrate how to soothe the baby, for example, rock the baby and walk with the baby, cuddle the baby securely, sing to the baby, play music, and so on.

Reflexes

Moro's Reflex. To assess the Moro's reflex, hold the newborn in a semisitting position and allow his or her head and trunk to fall back slightly. You should observe symmetrical abduction and extension of both arms with the fingers spread. The arms then return to an embracing position and finally relax. Asymmetrical response may suggest injury to the part that lags, and absence of the Moro reflex suggests injury to the brain. Any abnormal findings should be documented and reported to the physician.

Grasp Reflex. To assess the grasp reflex, touch the newborn's palm with a finger. The newborn finger will curl into a grasp tight enough to lift him or her from the surface. Similarly, place a finger against the base of the toes. The newborn toes will curl downward. This reflex disappears by 3 or 4 months. Its persistence suggests damage to the central nervous system.

Stepping. To assess the stepping reflex, hold newborn in an upright position and touch one foot to a flat surface. The newborn will mimic the movement of locomotion. Asymmetrical response may suggest a fracture of the long bone of the leg or injury to the central nervous system and should be reported to the physician.

Tonic Neck Reflex. To assess the tonic neck reflex, turn the newborn's head to one side. You will notice that the newborn's extremities on that side are extended, and the opposite extremities are flexed. This reflex also disappears in a few months. Its persistence is a sign of neurologic injury.

Babinski Reflex. To elicit the Babinski reflex, stroke one foot upward from the heel and across the ball of the foot. You will note that the newborn's toes will hyperextend and fan apart. This reflex disappears by 1 year. Failure to elicit the Babinski reflex is an indication of a deficit in the central nervous system.

CONCLUSIONS

It cannot be emphasized enough that a complete history precedes a good physical assessment of the postpartum mother and the newborn. In summarizing the visit, all findings should be recorded. Physical findings, interactions, teaching, referrals needed, and care given should be addressed. Indicate the mother's ability to learn and interest in learning. What areas were covered in your teaching: temperature taking, formula preparation? What problems were encountered that need further evaluation and care, such as breast-feeding problems, infected episiotomy wound, signs of emotional distress encountered? Make sure forms are signed and dated by the nurse. Report any problem findings to the physician, particularly jaundice or dehydration of the baby. At the end of the visit, make sure that you have addressed and answered the list of concerns, needs, and questions of the mother. Be certain that the mother has follow-up appointments for herself and the baby, or that she knows how to arrange for these. If another home visit or additional services are needed, call the managed care agency for authorization.

Remember, you are the client advocate. If you see any potential problems in the home, and approval for further visits is not given, discuss the problems with your manager, physician, or social worker, because close monitoring of the mother and newborn is vital.

19

Mental Health Services for Home Care Clients

Lawrence Jacobsberg, MD, PHD, Leila Laitman, MD, David Lindy, MD, and Neil Pessin, PhD

In recent years, home care has been a rapidly growing sector of the health care economy. Within this context, mental health home care has become an increasingly important component of essential services offered. This chapter describes the basic approach to making psychiatric home visits in general, as well as specific issues regarding acute home-based care, such as mobile crisis services, and longer-term care, as delivered by psychiatric geriatric home care.

IN THE BEGINNING: SETTING UP THE GOALS OF TREATMENT

Psychiatric home care is not essentially different from psychiatric care as delivered in the traditional settings of office, clinic, or hospital. Careful assessment of the client from a biopsychosocial perspective is, as always, the cornerstone of the treatment plan and subsequent interventions. However, there are several aspects of seeing clients in their home that are of particular concern, and, indeed, are unique to psychiatric home care. They are: the importance of clarity regarding the particular program's mission, the use of the interdisciplinary team, issues of safety, assessment of the home and home system, and methods of engagement.

It is critical to remember that clients typically have multiple psychiatric, medical, family, and socioeconomic problems. Outside the structure of traditional health care settings, this multiplicity of problems can be immediately striking, if not overwhelming, to the home care worker sitting in a client's living room. To triage effectively and allocate appropriate, and usually scarce, resources, each program must be very clear regarding its limits of responsibility and its role in the client's overall treatment.

The intake process begins with a telephone call in which information vital to the particular program is obtained, usually with the aid of a standardized intake form. Such data typically include the client's name, age, address, phone number, insurance information, and native language spoken. Additional information is obtained regarding the source of the referral, household members, and other community agencies involved. Questions are asked about previous mental health treatments, medications, and medical illnesses. An important part of the intake is the "Reason for Seeking Help," in which a detailed inquiry regarding the presenting problem is conducted in an attempt to formulate a specific request or question, which then becomes the focus of the initial home visit.

THE PREVISIT PLAN

Once it is determined that a case is appropriate for a particular program to handle, and it is clear what the goal of the visit is, the team meets to discuss the best approach to the initial visit for this new client. The team relies entirely on the interdisciplinary team model of psychiatric treatment, and teams are typically composed of psychiatric nurses, social workers, and a psychiatrist. This model allows each discipline to make its unique contributions to client care, while also emphasizing collaboration and sharing of tasks as appropriate.

Issues of safety must be addressed at the outset. There is a saying that "all health care is local." This is perhaps particularly true for home care. Programs operating in rural, suburban, and metropolitan areas will each have their own set of local issues to consider. Staff may often make their visits in disadvantaged and potentially dangerous parts of a city. Considerations regarding safety for both staff and clients are critical at the time the team plans its initial visit to a new client. For example, drug-infested areas tend to be safer in the morning. Before the initial visit, obtain as much information as possible about the client's history of violence to self or others, current risk factors for violence, and availability or presence of weapons. Ask about histories of dangerousness regarding other family members or people frequently in the home. Ask family members or referents to be present for home visits if appropriate, and ensure that weapons are removed before the visit. When necessary, the team makes the visit with police escorts. Dangerousness of neighborhoods or buildings where clients live are additional factors to consider.

THE INITIAL VISIT: ONCE YOU ENTER THE HOME

Once goals for the visit and plans for safety are established, a home visit is scheduled. On entering the home, a quick glance from the entrance will give information about the living conditions and the self-sufficiency of the individual. Safety hazards or unsanitary conditions such as exposed wires, cluttered hallways and rooms, presence of vermin or bugs, lack of electricity, and so forth, become obvious. Sometimes you have to forgo your inhibitions about being intrusive so that you can do an adequate job of both safeguarding and treating the client. For example, by looking in the refrigerator or bedroom, a staff member can see if there is fresh food in the house or if sleeping quarters are adequate. With clients prone to denial or distortion, it can be difficult to minimize or exaggerate a problem when observational evidence is available to staff. In addition, evidence of problems with other residents in the home or visitors may be noted, including alcohol bottles, syringes, unsanitary conditions in one room of the residence, etc.

The following could be defined as the assessment of the home system:

- The physical aspects of the home, for example, the nature and condition of the physical space, the adequacy of furnishings and food supplies, the neighborhood or immediate surroundings of the dwelling
- The other significant people in the home, including neighbors, landlords, and professional/paraprofessional staff, or the absence of other people in the home
- Resources in the home, for example, financial, educational, personal, cultural, spiritual, and including access to needed resources in the community, or lack thereof. Although these are ideally aspects of the complete evaluation of any client, the home-based assessment is uniquely positioned to assess these dimensions of a client's life.

The interview itself consists of the usual attempt to outline the current situation and history defined at the time of referral. It also includes a mental status examination. In addition, it includes information gleaned from the assessment of the home. For example, medication regimens for chronically ill clients are often complex. How a client has organized the administration of his or her medication can provide useful ancillary information about cognitive status. A disorganized shoe box filled with new and outdated pill bottles might signal cognitive deficits or drug interactions worsening confusion. Sleep and appetite should be assessed for the disturbances characteristic of depression.

A social assessment takes into account current living situation, pertinent family issues, legal issues, psychiatric family history, employment and income issues, education, and general level of activities of daily living functioning. If substance abuse is suspected, an alcohol and drug screen should be obtained. It is also often important to perform a further assessment of danger in the home, including current evidence of domestic violence, self-mutilation, and extrafamilial violence. Staff should obtain history regarding past and current suicidal or homicidal ideation and acts. "Dangerousness to self" includes neglect of medical condition and lack of appropriate vigor in pursuit of medical treatment, often an example of major depression.

A PARTIALLY WELCOME GUEST

Psychiatric home visits differ from appointments in an office or hospital in that the professional can be felt to be invading the client's home turf. The conventional psychiatric assessment in an office or clinic carries some implicit statement of motivation, in that the client has made the effort to come to the treatment locale. Psychiatric home visits, in contrast, are often initiated by a third party, with the consequent possibility of little client cooperation, or even overt resistance. Clients may not wish to identify themselves as psychiatric, or even as medical clients. To minimize the potentially intrusive quality of the visit, this possibility needs to be acknowledged. Visiting staff need to be polite and careful to behave as guests in the client's home. Tact and acknowledgment of the realities of the situation are the best strategies to maximize client alliance. In addition, other members in the home can be critical resources in engaging or effectively intervening with resistant clients in the home.

Before a visit is initiated, it is important to make appropriate introductions of all parties involved. Staff need to try and walk a thin line between obtaining necessary clinical data at the risk of seeming intrusive while being a guest in the client's home. Staff should give their names and clinical roles during the interview, and names and relationships of those familiar with the client should also be obtained. It is important to be sensitive to issues of confidentiality and determine early on if the client should be interviewed alone or in the presence of others. Sometimes it may even be more appropriate to interview referents rather than the client, if the client is an unreliable historian or too agitated, disorganized, or paranoid to effectively communicate. One very important, but often overlooked, informant is the home health aide or other on-site caregiver, who has valuable and unique data about the client's psychological condition. When sensitive information needs to be communicated, it is preferable that the caretaker do so with both the client and the therapist present. Any risk that the client will react with anger and suspicion is balanced by the possibility of working through the emotional reaction with all parties involved.

TREATMENT PLANNING

The initial home visit is designed to gather the necessary data to formulate an initial diagnostic impression. Ideally, the visit is followed with discussion by the interdisciplinary team so that an appropriate treatment plan can be worked out. Treatment plans are based on the mission of the individual program and must consider possible length of stay within the program, and feasibility and safety of in-home treatment. Critical issues in treatment planning also need to consider available resources in the home and community. The best way to engage reluctant clients and families involves eliciting their views as to what are their most pressing needs, and attempting to help them meet those needs. This usually involves concrete services, including benefits, which means dealing with complicated and sometimes unfriendly bureaucracies.

Some acute crisis situations, however, often require rapid judgments and immediate action. Decisions regarding hospitalization often must be made on the first visit, including arrangements for voluntary or involuntary transport to a psychiatric emergency room. However, hospitalization is only used as the last resort. The nurse must explore every possibility of mobilizing family or community resources to resolve the crisis. Staff also need to be trained to respond to those rare situations in the home that may become unexpectedly dangerous, or, as is usually the case, potentially so.

ACUTE CARE VERSUS CHRONIC CARE

This section demonstrates how these general considerations are applied in two different settings that reflect two basic modes of psychiatric home care: the acute setting, for example, the mobile crisis service, and the more long-term setting, for example, the geriatric service.

As an acute service, mobile crisis visits are geared toward triage, that is, assessment of immediate needs with short-term treatment goals pending appropriate referral. Knowledge of how to help clients negotiate the maze of financial entitlement is invaluable. Psychiatric consultations may be used to institute medications to mobilize clients linked to community-based organizations. Typically, only a few visits are made before linkage within his or her community is accomplished.

Longer-Term Care

Geriatric in-home treatment involves many of the same issues and skills as mobile crisis visits; however, the effort is usually not as concentrated or brief. Cases are not classified as psychiatric crises (though many are), and more physical rather than mental health issues may be involved. Appropriate diagnosis is essential, and treatment is often initiated in the home and then carried out by the client's own physician.

Although geriatric cases may involve diagnoses of psychoses, mood disorders, or substance abuse similar to those of clients seen by the mobile crisis teams, usually the diagnosis of dementia is the primary source of the psychiatric symptoms. A specialized effort needs to be made on geriatric psychiatric home visits to look for dementia, in addition to obtaining the client information previously described.

To make a diagnosis of dementia, the first step is to recognize that some type of memory impairment exists, because this is a prominent early symptom. Dementia symptoms may not be obvious nor be recognized by the client. Often it is the family or care-taker that sees the first signs of a change in function or of psychiatric symptoms such as depression or psychosis. The client also may find ways of compensating for his or her deficits. When health professionals are asked to evaluate these changes, they may be fooled into a misdiagnosis if they rely only on everyday conversation and whether the client is oriented to person, place, and time. Therefore, it is useful to employ a cognitive screening instrument such as the Mini Mental State Examination, which tests the client's ability to register, retain, recall, and recognize information as well as language function, visuomotor skills, and the ability to think abstractly.

A careful history is also essential in determining if dementia is present. Attention should be paid to the onset of symptoms, whether sudden or insidious, and to the nature of the deterioration, whether a steady decline or a stepwise deterioration with a fluctuating course. The client's ability to carry out daily social or occupational functions such as working, shopping, dressing, bathing, handling finances, and other activities of daily living should be investigated.

SPECIAL HANDLING OF DEMENTIA

Once it has been determined that some type of dementia is present, a workup should ensue to make a more exact diagnosis. Prognosis and course of illness can be predicted, making it easier to do psychoeducation and concrete planning with families.

The dementia workup routinely consists of the following tests or procedures:

General physical examination, including vital signs
Neurologic examination to look for focal findings
Blood work, including a complete blood count with
 differential, chemistry screen, thyroid function
 tests, serum vitamin B_{12} and folate levels, and
 serology for syphilis
Urine analysis
Electrocardiogram
Computed tomography scan or magnetic resonance
 imaging of the brain

 In certain cases, a chest radiograph, urine analysis for toxicology, electroencephalogram, lumbar
puncture, arterial blood gas analysis, human immunodeficiency virus infection screening, neuropsycho-
logical testing, or other medical tests would be employed to complete the workup. The need for these
tests would be suggested by findings in the history,
physical examinations, or routine tests. They are not
necessary in every case for screening purposes. In addition, medications and drug levels should be reviewed for side effects that can cause confusion,
memory loss, gait disturbance, or psychiatric symptoms. Drug interactions and the possibility that a
drug is being taken incorrectly or forgotten also
should be considered.

IDEAL WORKUP ONLY IN IDEAL SITUATIONS

Anyone who does home care with elderly clients
quickly discovers that it is often impossible to get the
ideal workup in every client who requires it. Factors
such as client resistance, family resistance, lack of

mobility, lack of facilities or personnel to perform or interpret the workup, and lack of finances or health insurance play a large role in determining what part of the workup gets done. Often, only blood work is feasible, and the diagnosis must rely on best clinical judgment. It is incumbent on professionals in the home care field to try to overcome as many of these barriers as possible by offering information, support, and guidance. In this way adequate diagnoses can be made so that appropriate management can follow.

The dementia workup will, it is hoped, pick up any reversible causes. It is important to note that these same issues often apply with mobile crisis cases, particularly if somatic treatments are indicated. The team must obtain as complete a workup as possible, while recognizing that the optimal inpatient workup is not practical. Often the decision requires a risk–benefit analysis between the risks of treatment and withholding otherwise indicated treatment. It is imperative to use the clinical information gathered during the home visit assessment and to use the team for careful in-home follow-up. Indeed, this kind of careful follow-up is one the great advantages of home-based treatment.

HOME-BASED BEHAVIORAL MANAGEMENT OF DEMENTED CLIENTS

Home-based behavioral management of demented clients can be an important adjunct to the treatment of this catastrophic, irreversible disease. In addition, psychoeducation for caregivers and nonpsychiatric home care staff provided by the geriatric team can also be an invaluable source of support. The first step is to pay close attention to the medical condition of the demented client. When a psychiatric symptom occurs, it should not automatically be assumed to be a natural part of deterioration in dementia. Minor problems such as colds, urinary tract infections, bedsores, and fecal impaction can make big changes in cognitive status or present as psychiatric symptoms. If general health improves, so may the mental state. Thus, minor illnesses should be taken seriously. Hearing and vision deficits should be corrected to the fullest extent possible, which will help in correcting misperceived environmental stimuli.

To help in behavioral management, the client's environment should be kept as constant and structured as possible. If trips are made, even to familiar places, temporary increases in agitation, confusion, or psychiatric symptoms may occur until the client becomes reacclimated to the new environment. These symptoms are to be expected, and it does not mean that the dementia is progressing. Orientating aids such as labels, signs, and calendars help in some situations. Adequate caregiver respite from the burdens of supervision and assistance are necessary as well, because stress in the caregiver can be transmitted to the client, resulting in behavioral problems. Sometimes caregiver shifts are necessary.

When nonpharmacologic interventions fail to provide a safe or tolerable situation, medication to control symptoms should be considered. Medications have side effects even in nondemented clients, but damaged brains are even more sensitive. Medication may be started by the in-home geriatric team or recommended to the client's physician to start and continue.

CONCLUSIONS

Psychiatric home care can provide a unique opportunity to obtain a depth of understanding regarding a client's needs and clinical state. In addition, it allows for treatments that maximize the client's quality of life while minimizing cost to the health care system. This chapter has described the basic approach to the psychiatric home visit in both the acute and the longer-term setting. It should be apparent that this kind of work also provides exciting and gratifying opportunities for the clinicians who venture into the field to deliver these services.

20

High-Tech Home Care

Diane S. Harper, RN, MSN, CANP

Home care infusion nurses must be skilled and knowledgeable in all aspects of infusion therapy, from initiating a peripheral intravenous (IV) to teaching clients and caregivers how to monitor self-infused cancer chemotherapies with central venous access devices. To maintain quality standards, infusion nurses must be certified to care for clients with vascular access devices and meet standards set forth by the State

Department of Health, State Board of Nursing, and Joint Commission on Accreditation of Healthcare Organizations, as well as the accepted intravenous therapy practices as set forth by the Intravenous Nurses Society and the American College of Surgeons.

Nursing support begins simultaneously with the client's discharge planning, regardless of whether this transition is from an inpatient facility or the emergency department. Referral may come from a variety of sources, including acute care facilities, clinics, and physician's offices. Home care coordinators identify appropriate candidates, assuring that services between the referring agency and the home infusion company are coordinated and complete. Coordinators also verify physicians' orders to ensure that pharmacy services and durable medical equipment and supplies needed to provide safe, effective care are in the client's home. The home infusion nurse or home care nurse then becomes responsible for the client's care in his or her place of residence. Collaboration among health care professionals from different health care settings is crucial to achieve positive client outcomes and diminish costly duplication of care.

CLIENT SELECTION FOR HOME INFUSION THERAPY

Client selection is based on the medical diagnosis, medical stability, educability of the client or caregiver, vascular access, and financial resources. Many therapies will be reimbursed by third-party payors only if they are given in the home or on an outpatient basis. The medical diagnosis must be one that can be treated in the home. Medical problems such as osteomyelitis, bacterial endocarditis, cancer, cellulitis, acquired immune deficiency syndrome (AIDS), pneumonia, septic arthritis, and Lyme disease are easily managed in the home care environment. The infusion therapy ordered must be consistent with established medical regimens. If, however, the therapy is experimental, as is the case in some cancer chemotherapies, the protocols to be followed must be readily available in the home or agency.

Each client will have a complete history and physical assessment on the initial visit in the hospital or the home. Determination of suitability for home infusion therapy and client teaching will begin during this assessment.

Ability to perform procedures is another criteria for therapy in the home. Clients must be evaluated to determine if they are able to perform required procedures. If a client cannot perform procedures, then a caregiver can be designated to perform all procedures. For example, Mr. X has sustained a major cerebrovascular accident (CVA) affecting the movement of his extremities, but his wife will perform all procedures to maintain his total parenteral nutrition in the home. A backup system should be in place in the event the wife is unable to provide the care for any reason.

Client or caregiver educability is the third factor in client selection. The client or caregiver must be capable of learning on a cognitive level and have the manual dexterity and visual acuity to perform all procedures. The home infusion and home care nurse serve as facilitator and teacher in this area. Knowledge of different learning styles is a must. Some clients are visual hands-on learners, and some need to read each step carefully to be successful. Collaboration between the nurse and the client/caregiver is essential for safe, effective client administration and outcomes. Essential skills and information that must be taught are:

Mastery of sterile technique
Basic skills of IV therapy and medication administration
Use of equipment
Restricted activities
Medication schedules
Recognition and prevention of side effects
Identification of emergency situations

Fear and anxiety are often barriers to learning in the home care situation. These are normal reactions to what the client/family perceives as complicated, technologically advanced therapies that may be impossible to master. The client and caregiver must have a thorough understanding of the disease process, treatment information, and self-care skills to break down these barriers. The nurse must establish an atmosphere of acceptance and use a combination of teaching strategies to encourage active participation and most importantly to involve the client in the learning process. The following list includes some guidelines for effective client education:

• Divide information into essential and nonessential elements, and teach what is essential first. Emphasis should be placed on what to do, not on what should not be done.
• Do not rely only on verbal or printed information. Combine these and emphasize key points.
• Demonstrate each procedure and then have the client perform the procedure. Repetition in performing skills leads to success.

- Do not suggest alternative procedures until the client has mastered the skill and a routine is established.
- Select an area in the home for teaching that is free from distractions.
- Speak slowly and clearly when giving instructions.
- Incorporate information, schedules, and techniques to fit into the client/caregiver normal, daily routine.

Education should be a part of every nursing encounter with the client/caregiver, and teaching effectiveness must be documented. In home care, the saying "If it wasn't documented, it wasn't done" still holds true. Documentation must be thorough and accurate. Most reimbursement is dependent on the thoroughness and preciseness of nursing documentation. Display 20-1 is an example of a client teaching checklist.

Vascular access, appropriate to the therapy to be administered, is another important criteria in client selection. Short-term antibiotic therapy (5 to 7 days) can be easily managed with a peripheral catheter if the client has suitable venous access. For irritating antibiotics, cancer chemotherapies, and long-term therapies such as total parenteral nutrition (TPN), a central venous access device is preferred. Venous access will include such devices as peripherally inserted central catheters (PICC), central venous access devices (CVAD), and venous access ports (VAP). The type of therapy needed and physician and client preference dictates the decision on which device is used. The perception of body image is a decisive factor for many clients. The client's decision must be supported by

text continued on page 394

DISPLAY 20-1. **Medication Administration/Patient Teaching Checklist**

	Assessment/ Demonstration	Return Demonstration	Performs Independently	Additional Comments
Defines purpose of IV therapy, enteral therapy				
Received emergency phone numbers, disaster plan discussed				
Drug/solution: _____ Dose: _____ Schedule _____				
Drug/solution storage: _____				
Drug/solution side effects: _____				
Aseptic technique: Handwashing, work area				
Aseptic technique: Caps, connections, tubing, dressings				
Access route: Peripheral, port, Hickman/Broviac, Groshong, PICC, midline, IM, sub-Q, enteral, other _____				

Access site inspection: Edema, drainage, erythema, pain, heat, coolness

Flush(s): SASH, _____ cc normal saline, medication, _____ cc normal saline, _____ cc of _____ unit heparin

Infusion device: Intermediate, CADD _____, Sabertech, gravity, advantage, other _____

Infusion type: continuous/intermittent

Environmental: sharps/waste disposal

Patient/caregiver signature: _____   Date: _____

Nurse's signature: _____   Initials: _____   Date: _____

With permission from D. S. Harper, Perspectives in Nursing Care.

the nurse to enable the client to gain control and mastery in using the device.

Financial resources are assessed for home care coverage before acceptance by the home infusion company. Reimbursement is complex and is dependent on the type of insurance the client has. Insurance company approval requires a statement of medical necessity along with the physician's prescription for therapy. Clients may be required to pay a co-payment. Medicare Part B will cover 80% of allowable costs; the remaining 20% is the responsibility of the client. Third-party payors for home infusion therapies include Medicare, Medicaid, commercial insurance, health maintenance organizations (HMOs), preferred provider organizations (PPOs), and managed care companies. HMOs, PPOs, and managed care organizations usually make determinations of eligibility on a case-by-case basis.

The Client/Caregiver Role in Home Infusion Therapy

The client/caregiver role in home care therapy is to maintain responsibility for specific areas of care, including compliance, monitoring, line management, and operating electronic infusion equipment. They are also responsible for knowing client rights and responsibilities. The consent is signed by the client, and a copy is left in the client's home. The client is also asked to sign a consent for treatment and services as well as an assignment of benefits guaranteeing payment to the provider. This ensures that the client/caregiver is well aware of the terms of the agreement.

COMMON THERAPIES ADMINISTERED IN THE HOME

Antibiotic and intravenous drug administration are by far the major therapies provided in the home. Newer technology, especially easy-to-operate infusion pumps, and the development of more potent antibiotics have facilitated the growth of this type of therapy. Intravenous drug administration may include such medications as antiemetics, heparin, interferon, growth hormone, gamma globulin, and cardiovascular and antihypertensive drugs. Initial dosing of any medication should be in a clinically controlled situation, and emergency drugs should be readily available. Protocols for the use of emergency drugs in the home should be established in written policies and procedures.

The nurse must have a broad range of medication knowledge, including administration techniques, side effects, adverse reactions, and incompatibilities. The nurse should at all times carry an up-to-date drug reference book indicating nursing interventions and client teaching information. Also, by law, a pharmacist in the home infusion agency must be available 24 hours a day to answer any questions the client or nurse may have about medication administration.

Incompatible medications are the most frequent cause of peripheral and CVAD failure. Incompatibility may occur when mixing drugs in a syringe or solution container or when delivering multiple IV piggyback drugs through an existing line. The major culprits of incompatibility are pH, light, order of mixing, drug concentration, contact time, and temperature. For example, Dilantin is a very high-pH drug that will crystallize in the presence of a low-pH solution such as

dextrose. This drug can only be mixed and administered with normal saline. If the client has received any
medication or IV fluids containing dextrose, the IV
line must be flushed thoroughly to remove any traces
of dextrose before administering the Dilantin to prevent crystallization and catheter occlusion. See Table
20-1 for some common incompatibilities.

Always remember the five rights of medication
administration: right drug, right client, right dosage,
right time, and right route. This applies to the home
care client as well.

All premixed vials or IV solutions delivered to
the client's home are labeled with the client's name,
name and dosage of medication, and the expiration
date. However, even though the quality controls in
the pharmacy are the same as in any hospital, accidents do happen. Always check the bag or medication
delivery system for your client's information. Do not
give any medication in the home that is not labeled
with the aforementioned information.

The medication is usually premixed, and as
much as 1 week's supply is delivered to the client's
home. This is also true of some IV fluids and TPN
mixtures. You may be directed to maintain the bags
in the refrigerator or freezer, dependent on the stability of the drug. Always take the medication out of the
refrigerator so that it may thaw and come to room
temperature before administering. Cold solutions
cause pain, vasospasm, vasoconstriction, and irritation to the vein. This manifests as very slow infusion
rates, inability to flush, or the client's complaint of
pain.

Hydration therapy has become very popular in
clients with such problems as hyperemesis and before
chemotherapy. The main goal is to maintain fluid bal-

Table 20-1
Common Medication Incompatibilities

Medication	Incompatibility
Acyclovir	Ondansetron
Amikacin	Heparin
Aminophylline	Meperidine, ondansetron, heparin, pencillin G, vancomycin
Amphotericin B	Aminophylline, meperidine, odansetron, potassium, D_5W
Ampicillin	Calcium gluconate, cefazolin, gentamycin, hydralazine, ondansetron, D5.9NSS, erythromycin, heparin, ticarcillin
Ampicillin/ Sulbactam	Aminophylline, ondansetron
Cefazolin	Calcium gluconate, gentamycin
Ceftriaxone	Aminoglycosides, esp. clindamycin
Cimetidine	Aminophylline
Ciprofloxacin	Aminophylline, heparin
Digoxin	Insulin
Erythromycin	Carbamazepine, cyclosporine, digoxin, theophylline, triazolam, warfarin, ergotamine, terfenadine
Furosemide	Hydralazine, meperidine, morphine, ondansetron, quinidine
Gentamycin	Heparin
Heparin	Cefazolin can only be mixed in presence of 0.9 NS morphine sulfate, quinidine, tobramycin
Hydralazine	Aminophylline, streptokianse
Insulin	Aminophylline, diazoxide, sodium bicarbonate
Merperidine	Aminophylline, morphine
Morphine sulfate	Aminophylline, calcium chloride, heparin, sodium bicarbonate, meperidine
Phenytoin	Is not compatible with any other medication and can only be given in the presence of 0.9 normal saline
Tobramycin	Calcium chloride, calcium gluconate, heparin
Vancomycin	Aminophylline, barbiturates, chloramphenicol, chlorothiazide, dexamethasone, heparin, methicillin, sodium bicarbonate, warfarin

ance in the home. Long-term administration of electrolyte solutions is also possible. The nurse in the home therefore must be very familiar with signs and symptoms of electrolyte imbalance (Table 20-2) and anticipate the changes the client will experience.

Signs and symptoms of fluid volume deficit or excess must be constantly assessed in this type of client. Assessment of all body systems is essential to pick up the subtle signs and symptoms of fluid volume changes (Table 20-3). Document and report these findings to the home infusion company, your supervisor, or the physician.

Knowledge of the effects an IV solution has on the fluid compartments of the body is essential to make appropriate patient assessments. *Isotonic* solutions such as 0.9% normal saline, 5% dextrose in water, and lactated Ringer's solution have the same tonicity as serum and plasma and are used to expand plasma volume as they stay within the intravascular space. The 0.9% normal saline is used primarily to provide fluid, sodium, and chloride. The 5% dextrose in water also replaces fluid but does not replace electrolytes. It does, however, provide 170 calories per liter. Lactated Ringer's solution contains all electrolytes but no calories. Patients receiving isotonic solutions should be monitored carefully for a fluid overload and electrolyte imbalance. It is important to remember that 1 liter of isotonic solution expands the vascular volume by 1 liter and that 1 liter of fluid is equal to 1 kg body weight. Home care patients on these fluids should be taught to document daily weights to assess for weight gain and fluid retention/loss. In addition, intake and output are important assessments for the home care nurse when patients are

text continued on page 403

Table 20-2
Assessing Electrolyte Balance

Electrolyte	Principal Functions	Signs and Symptoms of Imbalance
Sodium (Na⁺) Major cation in extra-cellular fluid (ECF) Normal serum level: 135 to 147 mEq/L (135 to 147 mmol/L)	Maintains appropriate ECF osmolarity Influences water distribution (with chloride) Affects concentration, excretion and adsorption of potassium and chloride Helps regulate acid–base balance Aids nerve- and muscle-fiber impulse transmission	*Hyponatremia:* Muscle weakness, decreased skin turgor, headache, tremor, seizures *Hypernatremia:* Thirst, fever, flushed skin, oliguria, and dry, sticky membranes
Potassium (K⁺) Major cation in intra-cellular fluid (ICF) Normal serum level: 3.5 to 5.0 mEq/L (3.5 to 5.0 mmol/L)	Maintains cell electroneutrality Maintains cell osmolarity Assists in conduction of nerve im-pulses Directly affects cardiac muscle contraction Aids nerve- and muscle-fiber impulse transmission	*Hypokalemia:* Decreased GI, skeletal muscle, and cardiac muscle function, decreased reflexes; rapid, weak, irregular pluse; muscle weakness or irritability; decreased blood pressure; nausea and vomiting; paralytic ileus *Hyperkalemia:* Muscle weakness, nausea, diarrhea, oliguria

continued

Table 20-2
Assessing Electrolyte Balance Continued

Electrolyte	Principal Functions	Signs and Symptoms of Imbalance
Calcium (Ca⁺⁺) Major cation in teeth and bones Normal serum level: 4 to 5.5 mEq/L (2 to 2.75 mmol/L)	Enhances bone strength and durability (along with phosphorus) Helps maintain cell-membrane structure, function, and permeability Affects activation, excitation, and contraction of cardiac and skeletal muscles Participates in neurotransmitter release at synapses Helps activate specific steps in blood coagulation Activates serum complement in immune system function	*Hypocalcemia:* Muscle tremor, muscle cramps, tetany, tonic-clonic seizures, paresthesia, bleeding, arrhythmias, hypotension *Hypercalcemia:* Lethargy, headache, muscle flaccidity, nausea, vomiting, anorexia, constipation, polydipsia, hypertension, polyuria
Chloride (Cl⁻) Major anion in ECF Normal serum level: 95 to 105 mEq/L (95 to 105 mmol/L)	Maintains serum osmolarity (along with Na⁺) Combines with major cations to create important compounds such as sodium chloride (NaCl), hydrogen chloride (HCl), potassium chloride (KCl), and calcium chloride (CaCl₂)	*Hypochloremia:* Increased muscle excitability, tetany, decreased respirations *Hyperchloremia:* Stupor, rapid deep breathing, muscle weakness

Phosphorus (P⁻) Major anion in ICF Normal serum level (phosphate level): 2.5 to 5.0 mEq/dL (0.80 to 1.60 mmol/L)	Helps maintains bones and teeth Helps maintain cell integrity Plays major role in acid-base balance (as a urinary buffer) Promotes energy transfer to cells Plays essential role in muscle, red blood cell, and neurologic functions	*Hypophosphatemia:* Paresthesia (circumoral and peripheral), lethargy, speech defects (such as stuttering or stammering) *Hyperphosphatemia:* Renal failure, vague neuro-excitability to tetany, and convulsions, arrthythmias, and muscle twitching with sudden increase in phosphate levels
Magnesium (Mg⁺⁺) Major cation in ICF (closely related to Ca⁺⁺ and P⁻) Normal serum level: 1.3 to 2.1 mEq/L (0.65 to 1.05 mmol/L) with 33% bound to protein and remainder as free cations	Activates intracellular enzymes; active in carbohydrate and protein metabolism Acts on myoneural junction, affecting neuromuscular irritability and contractility of cardiac and skeletal muscles Affects peripheral vasodilation Facilitates Na⁺ and K⁺ movement across all membranes Influences Ca⁺⁺ levels	*Hypomagnesemia:* Dizziness, confusion, convulsions, tremor, leg and foot cramps, arrhythemias, hyperirritability, vasomotor changes, anorexia, nausea *Hypermagnesemia:* drowsiness, lethargy, coma, arrhythmias, hypotension, vague neuromuscular changes (such as tremor), vague GI symptoms (such as nausea), and slow, weak pulse

Table 20-3
Assessing for Fluid Balance

Fluid Deficit	Fluid Excess
Weight loss	Weight gain
Lowered body temperature (if infection is not present)	Elevated blood pressure
Increased or decreased pulse rate	Bounding pulse that is not easily obliterated
Diminished blood pressure, often with postural hypotension	Jugular vein distention
Decreased central venous pressure	Increased respiratory rate
Sunken eyes, dry conjunctiva, decreased tearing	Dyspnea
Poor skin turgor (not a reliable sign in elderly patients)	Moist crackles or rhonchi on auscultation; edema of dependent body parts; sacral edema in patients on bed rest
Lack of moisture in groin and axillae	Good skin turgor
Decreased salivation	Puffy eyelids
Dry, cracked lips	Fuller than normal cheeks
Furrows in tongue	Periorbital edema
Difficulty forming words (patient needs to moisten mouth first)	Hoarseness
Cold limbs (with severe fluid volume deficit)	Slow emptying of hand veins when arm is raised
Indifferent attitude, headache, confusion	
Diminished urine output	
You may also note these laboratory test results: Increased hematocrit Elevated serum electrolytes and BUN Increased serum osmolarity	You may also note these laboratory test results: Decreased hematocrit Decreased serum electrolytes and BUN Decreased serum osmolarity

Abbreviation: BUN, blood urea nitrogen.

unable to participate in their own care. This, too, gives vital information about the patient's ability to use these fluids.

Hypertonic solutions such as 5% dextrose (D_5W) and 0.45% normal saline (½ NS), D_5W and 0.9% normal saline (0.9 NS), and D_5W and lactated Ringer's (LR) solution are used to shift fluid from the cells and tissues into the vascular spaces. This shift of fluid reduces the risk of edema, stabilizes blood pressure, and helps to maintain urine output. You have probably seen these fluids used postoperatively in the hospital to maintain fluid intake. D_5W and ½ NS and D_5W and 0.9 NS supplies 170 calories per liter, sodium and chloride, and fluid volume. D_5W and LR is infused primarily to replace gastric fluid losses. These patients must be watched carefully for circulatory overload and cellular dehydration. These fluids should not be given to patients at risk for diabetic ketoacidosis, because they pull fluid from the cells, thereby causing cellular dehydration. Patients with cardiac and renal impairment cannot handle the extra fluid and are at risk for congestive heart failure and cardiopulmonary fluid overload.

Hypotonic solutions such as 0.33% NS and 0.45% NS are used to shift fluid from the vascular compartments to the cells. Because these fluids can cause such sudden fluid shifts that patients are at great risk for vascular dehydration and cardiovascular collapse, they are not usually ordered in the home care setting.

IV Flow Rates

You will need to calculate IV drug dosages and flow rates in the clients home just as you did in the hospital. Many dosages are based on the client's weight in kilograms. This is easily calculated by dividing the number of pounds by 2.2. Remember, 2.2 lbs = 1 kg. Example: Your order reads to give gentamicin 3 mg/kg/day in divided doses every 8 hours. The client's weight is 110 lbs. 110 ÷ 2.2 = 50; 3 mg × 50 kg = 150 mg/day; 150 mg ÷ 3 daily doses = 50 mg every 8 hours.

Calculating administration rates is also the same as when calculated in the hospital. Typically, you receive an order such as "1000 mL D5.45NS to run over 8 hours."

To calculate: 1000 ÷ 8 = 125 mL/hour. Then set the infusion pump at the correct rate. There are times when you must teach the client to infuse their own medication. This is accomplished effectively by teaching the client to use the drop-per-second method. The nurse calculates the drop factor and then instructs the client in drops per second. For example: 100 mL per hour via a microdrip tubing has the same drop factor as the milliliters per hour. 100 mL per hour = 100 drops per minute. 100 mL per hour via a tubing that delivers 10 drops per minute is calculated: 100 × 10 ÷ 60 = 17 drops per minute. Then divide the drops/ minute by 60 to arrive at how many drops per second: 60 seconds ÷ 17 drops = 1 drop every 4 seconds. Then teach the client to count by saying: drop, 1002, 1003, 1004, drop, 1002, and so forth, and how to adjust the roller clamp to achieve the correct drop factor.

Total parenteral nutrition is another popular therapy. Clients can maintain an active, normal life while receiving the nutrition they need. Clients who receive this therapy may have such problems as malabsorption syndromes, colitis, gastrectomies or colectomies, cancer, CVAs, or failure to thrive. TPN may be a life-long therapy or short-term while the client's bowel heals after resection. Nutrition therapy provides all essential nutrients to maintain lean body mass and nitrogen balance and to promote tissue repair. TPN is mixed to each client's specific metabolic needs. Common components include: 50% dextrose, amino acids, essential electrolytes, minerals, and vitamins. The following is a breakdown of nutrients included in TPN:

Acetate prevents metabolic acidosis and is a precursor of bicarbonate

Amino acids provide nitrogen necessary for protein metabolism and tissue repair

Calcium promotes development of bones and teeth, aids in blood clotting, and plays a role in transmission of nerve impulses as well as contraction and relaxation of muscle

Chloride regulates the acid–base balance and maintains osmotic pressure

$D_{50}W$ provides calories for metabolism

Folic acid is needed for deoxyribonucleic acid formation and promotes growth and development

Lipid emulsions are carriers of fat-soluble vitamins, contribute to the integrity of cell walls, and provide essential fatty acids

Magnesium helps absorb carbohydrates and protein, has a role in calcium metabolism, and aids in muscle, nerve, and cardiac function

Trace elements (zinc, manganese, cobalt) help in wound healing and red blood cell synthesis

Phosphate minimizes the threat of peripheral paresthesia and is involved in the transport of lipids

Potassium is necessary for the anabolism of lean body mass and the normal function of smooth, cardiac, and skeletal muscle contractility

Sodium helps control water distribution and maintain normal fluid balance

Vitamin B complex helps the final absorption of carbohydrates and protein

Vitamin D is essential for bone metabolism and maintenance of serum calcium levels

Vitamin K helps prevent bleeding disorders

TPN is usually administered over 8 to 24 hours through a CVAD such as a Hickman, Broviac, or implanted port. (DO NOT ADMINISTER TPN VIA A PERIPHERAL VEIN.) The infusion is begun slowly (25 to 50 mL/hr) to allow the pancreas to increase endogenous insulin production and decrease the risk of hyperglycemia. Then it is "tapered up" to the ordered hourly rate. At the end of the infusion, the rate is "tapered down" to slow the process of endogenous insulin production. When the therapy is complete or to be discontinued, the client must be weaned from the TPN over 24 to 48 hours.

Intravenous infusion is given administered with a special TPN pump or an electronic infusion device that allows the "taper up" and "taper down" infusion rates. A 0.2- or 1.2-μm filter is usually placed on the IV tubing as close to the access site as possible to trap any particles or large globules. Make sure that the filter's porosity and psi capacity exceeds the psi of the pump used to infuse the solution. This information will be found on the pump and the filter package.

Nursing considerations for the client receiving TPN in the home are varied. The following includes tips on administration and client care monitoring:

• Never immerse TPN in a warm water bath or put in the microwave to speed the warming process before infusion. Heat can interfere with the integrity of the bag and the solution's stability.

- The nurse will, on occasion, add medications to the TPN bag such as heparin, multivitamins, insulin, H_2 antagonists, or steroids. Assure that orders for each additive are in the home. Discuss any concerns you may have with the pharmacist.

- Never shake the bag of TPN. This encourages the formation of fat and air globules in the bag. When adding medications, lay the bag on a clean, hard surface and knead the bag gently to thoroughly to disperse the medication.

- Maintenance of strict aseptic technique in preparing equipment and infusing TPN is essential. This client is at great risk of catheter-related sepsis and infection because of the high glucose content of the fluid.

- Change the IV tubing and filter every 24 hours, and do not allow the solution to hang for more than 24 hours.

- Assess the client for signs and symptoms of electrolyte and fluid imbalance at each visit. (See Tables 20-2 and 20-3 for assessment of electrolyte and fluid balance.)

- Assess daily or weekly weights. A weight gain of greater than 2 pounds per week can be a sign of fluid volume excess.

- Question the client about vomiting, diarrhea, or increased ostomy or fistula drainage, which may indicate fluid volume deficit.

- Ensure that laboratory monitoring is performed in accordance with the physician's orders. Laboratory testing is usually ordered biweekly, bimonthly, or monthly, depending on length of therapy, the client's clinical condition, and response to TPN therapy.

• Glucose monitoring in the home is a must. Fingerstick glucose may be assessed by the client or nurse once per day or as ordered by the physician. The client should be taught urine glucose monitoring by the double-voiding method.

• A daily or weekly client log should be maintained, indicating weight, temperature, glucose and urine monitoring, and any symptoms associated with changes in the client's condition.

Complications of TPN therapy are many (Table 20-4). The most common are metabolic complications associated with the TPN administration, such as hyper/hypoglycemia. The second most common complication is infusion related, such as too-rapid infusion and extravasation. Other complications deal with catheter-related and mechanical complications.

Pain management may be ordered for postsurgical clients, the client with chronic pain, or the cancer client. Continuous or intermittent self-administration of analgesics allows clients to remain with their families and maintain a degree of comfort previously only given in the hospital. Pain medication in the home is delivered most frequently by continuous IV infusion through patient-controlled analgesia (PCA), portable pumps, and by intrathecal and subcutaneous routes. In clients with pain that is difficult to control, IV pain management may supplemented with oral pain medications by combining drugs such as MS Contin® and IV Dilaudid®. In home care, the nurse plays the key role in successful pain management by constant client assessment and noninvasive therapies such as distraction, relaxation, guided imagery, and self-hypnosis taught by the nurse.

Client monitoring and documentation should contain the following:

- The client's pain rating using a scale of 0 to 10 (0 = no pain; 10 = most severe pain)
- Description of the pain in the client's own words
- Onset, location, intensity, and duration of pain
- Any associated activity
- Medications used for pain relief in addition to the prescribed drugs
- Any behavioral component that increases or decreases pain
- Presence of any side effects that are bothersome to the client, such as nausea, vomiting, orthostatic hypotension, urinary retention, and pruritus

Medications used most frequently for intravenous pain relief are morphine sulfate, meperidine hydrochloride (Demerol®), and hydromorphone hydrochloride (Dilaudid®). The nurse must be diligent in assessing side effects and adverse reactions. The possible side effects and management of IV, subcutaneous, and intraspinal narcotic analgesics are:

- Respiratory depression: decrease dosage of drug. Assure that Narcan® is available to reverse depressants effects.
- Nausea/vomiting: antiemetics such as prochlorperazine (Compazine®) may be helpful. This usually resolves over time.
- Constipation: encourage activity, a diet high in bulk-forming food, and daily use of a stool softener or peristaltic agent.

Table 20-4
Common TPN Complications

Complications	Signs and Symptoms	Interventions
Metabolic complications		
Hyperglycemia	Fatigue, restlessness, confusion, anxiety, weakness, and (in severe cases) delirium or coma; poluria, dehydration, elevated blood and urine glucose levels	Start insulin therapy or adjust TPN rate
Hypoglycemia	Sweating, shaking, irritability when infusion stopped	Infuse dextrose 10%
Hyperosmolar non-ketotic syndrome	Confusion, lethargy seizures, coma, hyperglycemia, dehydration, glycosuria	Stop dextrose Give insulin and 0.45% sodium cloride to rehydrate
Hypokalemia	Muscle weakness, paralysis, Paresthesia, arrhythmias	Increase potassium supplementation
Hypomagnesemia	Tingling around mouth, paresthesia in fingers, mental changes, hyperreflexia	Increase magnesium supplementation
Hypophosphatemia	Irritability, weakness, paresthesia, coma, respiratory arrest	Increase phosphate supplementation

Hypocalcemia		Increase calcium supplementation
Metabolic acidosis	Polyuria, dehydration, elevated blood and urine glucose levels Increased serum chloride level Decreased serum bicarbonate level	Use of acetate or lactate salts of sodium or hydrogen
Hepatic dysfunction	Increased serum transaminase, lactate dehydrogenase, and bilirubin levels	Use special hepatic formulations Decrease carbohydrate and add IV lipids

Infusion-related complications

Too rapid an infusion	Nausea, headache, lethargy	Assess the infusion rate Assess the infusion pump Stop IV infusion
Extravasation	Swelling of tissue around the insertion site; pain	Assess patient for cardiopulmonary abnormalities. Chest x-ray may be performed
Phlebitis	Pain, tenderness, reddness, and warmth	Apply gentle heat to the insertion site Elevate the insertion site, if possible

- Sedation: decrease dosage of drug while other causes are ruled out.
- Urinary retention: change the type of narcotic. Demerol is the most frequent cause. Intermittent catheterization or administration of bethanechol (Urecholine®) may be necessary.
- Pruritus: caused by the interaction of narcotic with the dorsal horn, not by the release of histamine. This is best treated with narcotic antagonist such as Narcan or Nubain, not diphenhydramine (Benadryl®).
- Postural hypotension*: teach client to avoid arising too quickly from bed or chair.
- Numbness*: change dosage or type of analgesia.

Patient-controlled analgesia (PCA) allows the client to self-administer an IV analgesic and maintain therapeutic levels to allow pain control without sedation. The physician's order and documentation at each visit must include:

- Loading dose, given IV push at start of therapy
- Lock-out interval, during which the device cannot be activated, no matter how many times the client pushes the button
- The amount of medication the client will receive on an hourly basis
- The amount of drug the client will receive when the bolus button is pushed
- The maximum amount of drug the client can receive in a specified period
- Any problems with the delivery device
- Client or caregiver knowledge of operating or troubleshooting the device

---

*Not a side effect of intraspinal narcotics.

Intraspinal is a term used to denote both epidural and intrathecal administration of medications and is most often delivered to clients with intractable pain. These methods allow for smaller doses of analgesics than does the IV or subcutaneous routes. The rational for this method of drug administration is that the drug is delivered directly to the receptors in the brain and spinal cord.

Intrathecal catheters are placed in the space between epidural space and the dura mater surrounding the spinal cord, which contains the cerebrospinal fluid. In intrathecal administration, anesthetic agents such as Marcaine may be added to the ordered narcotic to produce a sympathetic blocking effect. Sympathetic blocking decreases activation of sympathetic pathways, thereby reducing epinephrine release, which in turn decreases the workload of the heart, the client experiences less anxiety, and the end result is lowered vital signs and a more comfortable client.

Intrathecal narcotic administration requires 10 times less medication than does the epidural route. Certain antineoplastic agents and antibiotics also may be delivered intrathecally. The major disadvantages to the use of intrathecal catheters is the potential for infection, spinal fluid leak, and the control of side effects of medication, which can be life threatening.

Epidural catheters are placed in the epidural space, which surrounds the spinal cord and dura matter. This space is not separated until air or medication is injected between them. Multiple studies have shown that, postoperatively, epidural pain management is far superior to systemic administration for abdominal, pelvic, thoracic, or spinal surgery, and obstetrics. Strict sterile technique must be used in caring for both types of catheters, because infection is a major disadvantage to their use. Intrathecal and epidural catheters require special handling and care.

- These catheters are not sutured in place. They are laid along the spinal column and over the shoulder, then taped in place to provide stability and protection. Care must be taken not to pull on the catheter dressing.
- Preservative-free medications must be used.
- It is the recommendation of the Intravenous Nurse's Society Standards of Practice (1990) that medications be infused using an electronic infusion device.
- Both catheters must be clearly labeled to prevent accidental infusion of other medications or fluids.
- Narcotic antagonist such as Narcan or an agonist/antagonist such as Nubain are the preferred antidotes to narcotic side effects.

ADMINISTRATION OF MEDICATION WITH AN INTRASPINAL CATHETER

1. Assemble equipment; wash hands
2. Inspect insertion site for signs of infection or drainage
3. Verify that a preservative-free narcotic is mixed in normal saline.
4. Assess client baseline data and vital signs

5. Use sterile gloves and scrub the injection cap with povidone-iodine for 2 full minutes. Wipe the excess iodine with a sterile 2 × 2 gauze pad.

6. Enter the injection cap using an empty 3-mL syringe. Aspirate gently; less than 1 mL clear or slightly bloody fluid should return. Discard the syringe.

7. Rescrub the injection cap with iodine solution and wipe the excess with a sterile 2 × 2.

8. Begin infusion with pump or inject intermittent dose at a rate of approximately 5 mL/min.

9. Assess catheter injection cap for tightness, and tighten as needed.

10. Document the procedure.

11. Assess client frequently, measuring vital signs every 15 minutes × 2, then every 4 hours. Assess level of consciousness every hour for 24 hours, then every 4 hours. (The family should be taught how to assess level of consciousness for continuous monitoring if the client does not have 24-hour nursing care.)

DRESSING CHANGE MANAGEMENT OF INTRASPINAL CATHETERS

1. Wash hands for at least 1 full minute using an antimicrobial soap. This is a sterile procedure.

2. Remove the old dressing. Use a cotton ball dipped in normal saline to assist in removing the dressing.

3. Wet cotton-tipped applicators in povidone-iodine solution and clean in a circular pattern from

the catheter insertion site outwards. Allow to dry. If there are any crusted areas, use a cotton-tipped applicator soaked in hydrogen peroxide before using the povidone-iodine solution. *Never use alcohol to clean an intraspinal catheter insertion site.* This may cause migration of alcohol into the intraspinal spaces and cause neural damage.

4. Apply new transparent dressing.
5. Remove the tape holding the catheter up the spinal column and shoulder, clean the skin using normal saline, allow to dry, and retape.

Cancer chemotherapy has become a widely used treatment modality in the home. Clients no longer have to travel long distances. This is especially important for clients who cannot drive or who are in pain. They can remain in the comfort of their home in a favorite recliner, bed, or couch. It has also been shown that clients who stay at home have fewer incidents of side effects such as nausea and vomiting associated with motion and travel. The biggest obstacle to home chemotherapy is the lack of Medicare reimbursement. Medicare does not cover the drugs involved, and this is by far the largest group of clients who need chemotherapy. Most commercial insurances and some Medicaid programs, however, do cover these expenses.

Chemotherapeutic agents may be administered orally, topically, parenterally, or by direct perfusion into a body organ or cavity. Intravenous administration is the most common route and may be delivered by IV push, Y-site injection, IV piggyback, or IV continuous infusion using a bag or pump cassette. Many clients may be hydrated and medicated before administration of antineoplastic agents to decrease possible side effects and fluid volume imbalances.

NURSING RESPONSIBILITIES IN ADMINISTRATION OF NEOPLASTIC AGENTS

- Knowledge of the cell cycle and malignant cell growth
- Knowledge of the drug class, side effects, adverse reactions, and methods and rates of administration
- Being able to distinguish palliative from curative therapy
- Knowledge of drug properties: vesicant or non-vesicant
- Understanding of the vascular system
- Client education as to the physical and psychological drug side effects
- Knowledge of OSHA standards for disposal of cytotoxic agents
- Awareness of personal risks and safety factors in cytotoxic administration

Every client should have a complete history and physical assessment before administration of any chemotherapeutic agent to evaluate and assess side effects and adverse reactions to the medication (Table 20-5). Serum blood studies are usually performed 1 week before and 1 week after administration to assess fluid and electrolyte balance, blood counts, platelet counts, and liver and kidney function. If low red blood cell (RBC), white blood cell (WBC), or

Table 20-5
Considerations in Administration of Neoplastic Agents

Antineoplastic Agent	Key Points in Administration	Side Effects
Alkylating agents Mustargen Cytoxan TSPA Ifosfamide Vesicant	Cell-cycle nonspecific Keep patient well hydrated Monitor BUN, creatinine Monitor IV Site	Leukopenia, thrombocytopenia, nausea, vomiting anorexia, alopecia, stomatitis, headache, vomiting, weakness, metallic taste, nail and skin hyperpigmentation, nasal stuffiness
Antimetabolites 5-FU Mexate Cytosar-U Cytarabine	Cell-cycle specific in S phase Assess pain in chest or stomach, diarrhea, or black stools Monitor BUN, creatinine Protect from light Leucovorin given with high doses to minimize side effects	Dermatitis, hyperpigmentation, leukopenia, alopecia, nausea, vomiting, anorexia, diarrhea, pharyngitis, headache
Antitumor antibiotics Doxorubicin	Cell-cycle nonspecific	Hypersensitivity reactions, fever, chills, pruritic

Drug	Nursing considerations	Side effects
Bleomycin Mitomycin-C Dactinomycin Mithramycin Vesicant	Administer antipyretics as needed Assess stomach pain, black stools Asculate lungs daily	erythema, alopecia, stomatitis, nausea, vomiting, diarrhea, leukopenia, thrombocytopenia, urine color changes
Steroids Diethystilbestrol Betamethasone	Cell-cycle nonspecific Give emotional support for side effects	Side effects are gender related
Plant alkaloids Vinblastine Vincristine Etoposide Vesicant	Cell-cycle specific in M phase Assess jaw pain, numbness, tingling, and loss of deep tendon reflexes	Leukopenia, alopecia, nausea, vomiting, anorexia, constipation, abdominal pain, headache, depression, hyperbilirubinemia, pheripheral neuropathies, transient hypotension with rapid administration, bronchospasm
Nitrosoureas Dacarbazine Cisplatin Streptozocin	Cell-cycle nonspecific Can cross blood–brain barrier Assess BUN, creatinine, liver function	Leukopenia, thrombocytopenia, nausea, anorexia, diarrhea, nephrotoxicity, glucose intolerance, alopecia, facial flushing

platelet counts are identified before preadministration, the dose may be delayed until these have improved.

A very common side effect of most cancer chemotherapies is a syndrome called *nadir*. During this period, the client is at very high risk for infection from low WBC counts, anemia from low RBC counts, and bleeding from low platelet counts. Each drug has a specific timeframe in which nadir occurs. This can be anywhere from 3 days to 14 days post-chemotherapy administration. The nurse must be aware of this time and instruct the client to take his or her temperature every day and report to the physician any elevation, as well as chills, fatigue, or unusual bleeding.

Knowledge of personal safety factors in antineoplastic agent administration is a must to protect yourself from exposure. Personal protective gear is usually included in the box delivered to the client's home by the pharmacy:

A moisture-repellent gown, gloves, mask, and goggles or eyewear is recommended.

Work surfaces should be covered with a plastic-backed, absorbent pad.

You should not eat, drink, smoke, or apply makeup in the area where chemotherapy is being administered.

Gloves should be talc-free, disposable, and of thick latex.

Gloves should be disposed of immediately after use.

Wash hands before and after removing gloves.

Syringes, tubings, and all connections should have a Luer-lok device.

When disconnecting syringes or connections, cover
with a gauze pad wrapped around the site to prevent droplet leakage.

Dispose of all contained articles, including the IV delivery system, into the special chemo/biohazard
container provided by the pharmacy.

Venous sampling is performed for thousands of
clients at home. Blood samples to monitor antibiotic
levels (peaks and troughs), WBC counts for oncology
clients, and serum chemistries for the client receiving
TPN are easily drawn from CVADs or through peripheral venipuncture. Blood samples should always
be drawn from the arm without an IV whenever possible, because laboratory values may be altered by IV
fluids. Care must be taken for the safe handling of
laboratory samples and to ensure proper disposal of
medical wastes.

Blood and component therapy is a fast-growing
area of home infusion therapy. The most frequently
used products are normal serum albumin, immune
globulin, cryoprecipitate, factor VIII concentrate,
platelets, and blood administration. Very strict criteria for client selection has been set forth by State Departments of Health, the American Association of
Blood Banks, and the Food and Drug Administration
in the delivery of blood products in the home. The
client will have pretransfusion testing just as if the he
or she were in the hospital. Policies and procedures
are developed and must be strictly adhered to in
administration and in the event of transfusion reactions or delayed effects of blood component administration.

THE HOME CARE NURSE'S RESPONSIBILITY IN INFUSION THERAPY

Client assessment is the most crucial factor in safe, effective delivery of home infusion therapy. A review of systems relevant to the client's problem should be made at each visit to assess changes in client condition. Complete vital signs and a focused physical assessment also should be performed and correlated with any available laboratory data. Assess the vascular access device and medication delivery systems as well as the client's knowledge of these. Discuss with the client and caregiver any new developments in the client's condition or visits to physicians and the outcomes of these visits. This is the perfect time to elicit questions and educate clients regarding their knowledge of the disease process, progression of therapy, medication administration, and equipment to achieve a more positive client outcome. Then document your assessment in the nurse's notes or a client visit form. Copies of notes and client visit forms should be in the client's home for review and comparison by all nurses involved in the client's care. Assessment and documentation should include:

- Complete client assessment
- Vascular access device and medication delivery system
  - Patency
  - Ability to flush
  - Any problems
- Any changes in client condition
- Venous sampling
- Client's knowledge and tolerance of therapy

- Client teaching and a reflection of understanding
- Any client problems, corrective actions, and the name of the agency and person who was notified of the problem.

Care and maintenance of vascular access devices is another important responsibility in high-tech home care. All nurses involved in the client's care should be knowledgeable about the different types of devices, their advantages and disadvantages, and basic care issues. Your State Board of Nursing and Department of Health have issued regulations delineating who can manipulate venous access devices. These state boards of regulation also state that nurses must be certified by a state or nationally recognized association in peripheral and central IV therapy to perform this care in the home, so that quality standards are maintained.

Peripheral venous cannulation may be instituted for short-term IV therapy such as intermittent administration of antibiotics. Peripheral cannulation in the home should only be performed by nurses experienced in peripheral IV sticks, because the inexperienced nurse will inevitably meet the difficult-to-access client on their first or second visit. Multiple unsuccessful attempts will be viewed by the client as poor nursing care, an inexperienced nurse, or inability to maintain access in the home, which increases the clients's anxiety and will interfere with successful therapy outcomes. The rule of thumb in home care is: for two unsuccessful sticks, notify the agency and request a second nurse to attempt access.

Selection of the appropriate vein (Table 20-6) and venipuncture device is an important factor. In home infusion therapy, the digital and metacarpal veins are not routinely selected (unless the client has

Table 20-6
Selecting Peripheral Venipuncture Sites

Site	Advantages	Disadvantages
Digital veins		
Run along lateral and dorsal portions of fingers	May be used for short-term therapy May be used when other means are not available	Fingers must be splinted with a tongue blade, decreasing ability to use hand Uncomfortable for patient Infiltration occurs easily Can not be used in veins in dorsum of hand already used Only 27- or 25-gauge catheters can be used
Metacarpal veins		
On dorsum of hand, formed by union of digital veins between knuckles	Easily accessible Lie flat on back of hand In adult or large child, bones of hand act as splint 25- or 23-gauge catheters can be used for intermittent infusion	Wrist movement decreased unless a short catheter is used Insertion more painful because more nerve endings in hands Site becomes phlebitic more easily

Accessory cephalic
Runs along radial bone as a continuation of metacarpal veins of thumb

Large vein excellent for venipuncture
Readily accepts large-gauge needles
Doesn't impair mobility
Doesn't require an armboard in older child or adult

Sometimes difficult to position catheter flush with skin
Usually uncomfortable. Venipuncture device at bend of wrist, so movement causes discomfort

Cephalic vein
Runs along radial side of forearm and upper arm

Large vein excellent for venipuncture
Readily accepts large gauge
Doesn't impair mobility

Proximity to elbow may decrease joint movement
Vein tends to roll during insertion

Median antebrachial vein
Arises from palm and runs along ulnar side of forearm

Vein holds winged needle well
A last resort when no other means are available

Many nerve endings in area may cause painful venipuncture
Infiltration occurs easily in this area

Basiliac vein
Runs along ulnar side of forearm and upper arm

Will take a large-gauge needle
Straight strong vein suitable for large-gauge venipuncture devices

Uncomfortable position for patient during insertion
Penetration of dermal layer of skin where nerve endings are located causes pain
Vein tends to roll during insertion

continued

Table 20-6
Selecting Peripheral Venipuncture Sites Continued

Site	Advantages	Disadvantages
Antecubital Vein		
Located in antecubital fossa (median, cephalic, located on radial side: median basilic, on ulnar side; median cubital rises in front of elbow joint)	Large veins facilitate drawing blood Often visible or palpable in children when other veins won't dialate May be used when in an emergency or as a last resort	Difficult to splint elbow area with armboard Median cephalic vein crosses in front of brachial artery Veins may be small and scarred if blood has been drawn frequently from this site

Note. Venipuncture sites located in the forearm offer the most advantages. This chart includes some of the major benefits and drawbacks of several common sites as well as the nursing considerations in their use.

no other access sites), because the client must be able to use his or her hands to perform self-administration and participate in their activities of daily living. Over-the-needle catheters are the devices of choice; the smallest device possible should be used to permit efficient infusion of fluids, which allows for client comfort and mobility.

Considerations in size selection include:

- Size and condition of the vein
- The viscosity of the fluid to be infused
- The client's age
- The expected length of therapy
- Gauge of catheter
  - 16 gauge: major surgery or trauma
  - 18 gauge: blood and blood products, administration of viscous medications
  - 20 gauge: most applications
  - 22 gauge: most applications, especially children and the elderly
  - 24 gauge: pediatric clients and neonates, subcutaneous continuous infusions

Site selection should be made based on the following points:

- Use the nondominant arm when possible.
- Never select a vein in an edematous or impaired arm; avoid areas of flexion.
- Consider accessibility; but the most prominent, accessible vein is not always the best choice because of sclerosis or previous multiple use.
- Perform all subsequent venipunctures proximal to a previously used or injured vein.

Peripheral venous access devices are routinely changed every 3 days. If the client is to have 14 days of antibiotics, this means four to five sticks during the course of therapy. Preservation of venous access is essential, especially in a child or in the elderly (Table 20-7).

Procedure for Venipuncture

1. Wash hands and gather all equipment. Select site and appropriate-sized catheter.
2. Prepare all equipment, prime tubings, pumps, and medication administration devices.
3. Rewash hands and put on gloves.
4. Place tourniquet 2 to 3 inches above selected site.
5. Clean site selected with alcohol, using a circular motion from inside to outside at least 2 inches around, three times. Then perform same procedure using povidone-iodine solution.
6. Anchor skin and vein with thumb below selected site to minimize movement of skin and vein rolling.
7. Insert the needle of choice, bevel up, at a 30- to 45-degree angle using the direct or indirect method:

    Direct method: Insert directly over the vein. All layers of the vein are penetrated with one motion.

    Indirect method: Cannula insertion alongside the vein; cannula gently inserted distal to the point where the needle will enter vein; parallel alignment maintained and cannula advanced through subcutaneous tissue; vein then relocated and angle of cannula decreased and vein entered.
8. When the needle enters the vein, you will get a steady backflow of blood into the flashback chamber. Cautiously, move the cannula up the

Table 20-7
Tips for Successful Venous Access

Patient Type	Problem	Intervention
Obese patient	Unable to palpate or see vein	Create a visual image of the venous anatomy; select a catheter long enough to reach the patient's veins (1 1/2 to 2 inches); warm packs may be applied; use multiple-tourniquet method (one tourniquet 2 to 3 inches above and one 2 to 3 inches below for 2 minutes).
Edematous patient	Fluid in extremity	Displace fluid using digital pressure; elevate extremity for 10 to 15 minutes before applying tourniquet. Cannulate quickly because fluid will return to site.
Elderly patient	Fragile skin and veins; Veins roll when stick attempted	Use minimal tourniquet pressure or no tourniquet; high pressure in veins will cause collapse on insertion of needle. Use smallest catheter; use direct entry; decrease angle of entry by 15 degrees. Anchor vein with thumb during insertion.
Dehydrated	Poor venous filling	Leave tourniquet on to promote vein distention. Use warm packs. Wipe skin with alcohol and tap with finger to make vein more prominent.
Infants	Unable to palpate or see veins	Warm soaks or transillumination of veins. Use smaller tourniquet with minimal pressure. Extremity must be stabilized. Use 24- or 26-gauge catheters. May not see flashback of blood in chamber.

lumen, threading it into the vein. Hold the
catheter hub with the thumb and middle finger,
and use the index finger to advance the catheter.
9. Release the tourniquet.
10. Remove the stylet from the catheter.
11. Place a primed extension tubing or adapter on
the catheter.
12. Anchor as per agency policy.
13. Cover the transparent semipermeable dressing.
Do not cover the insertion site with tape or an-
choring material.
14. Label dressing with date, size of catheter, and
your initials.
15. Dispose of all contaminated articles in the proper
waste disposal bag.
16. Wash hands.
17. Document the following in the client's chart or
on the client visit form:
a. Date and time of venipuncture
b. Number of attempts required
c. Site location
d. Catheter gauge and length
e. Presence of any complications and action
taken to correct the problem
f. Client/caregiver teaching and a reflection of
understanding

CVADs and VAPs are commonly used for long-
term therapies. These include midline and PICC,
Hickman/Broviac, and Groshong catheters, all of
which may be single-lumen, double-lumen, or triple-
lumen. Midline and PICC catheters are designed for
shorter-term use of weeks to months, and Hickman/
Broviac/Groshong catheters may be in place for several years with proper care and maintenance. The sin-

gle most important factor in caring for these catheters is patency. Patency (lack of obstruction) is maintained by proper flushing before, between, and after medication administration. Other factors contributing to catheter patency are IV flow rates maintained at less than osmotic pressure, periodic flushing of unused lumens or unused catheters, and medication and fluid incompatibilities that cause precipitates to form inside the catheter.

VAPs are implanted under the client's skin and may be single- or double-lumen. These are long-term (months to years) catheters and must be maintained with flushing even when they are unused for long periods. VAPs are accessed using noncoring needles so that the integrity of the membrane is not broken. Do not try to access these ports without experience.

The home care nurse may be responsible for maintenance of the catheter, which includes dressing changes and flushing. Each agency must have a written protocol describing how to perform the dressing change, how often it should be changed, and flushing guidelines. A general guideline for dressing changes is PICC and midline catheters, twice per week; Hickman/Broviac/Groshongs, once per week; VAPs, once per week and any time the integrity of the dressing is breached. Follow the guidelines exactly, and report any signs of infection or infiltration to the home infusion company and your supervisor immediately. During the dressing change, the extension set and the infusion cap will be changed also.

General flushing guidelines are as follows: PICC and midline catheters: 3 mL NS and 3 mL heparin 10 U/mL; Hickman/Broviac's: 5 mL NS and 5 mL heparin 10 U/mL; Groshong catheters: 5 mL NS. Never instill heparin into a Groshong catheter.

Obtaining blood samples from a CVAD is a common practice, especially when the patient has poor venous access. When the patient has a multilumen catheter, access a used port to obtain the sample. If the patient has a single-lumen device or all lumens are in use, turn off IV fluids for 1 full minute to ensure a pure blood sample. Then follow the directions below:

1. Gather equipment and wash your hands. This is a sterile procedure.
2. Equipment
   1 Vacuum tube holder
   1 Multiple-sample needle: 22-gauge × 1 inch
   Appropriate number and type of vacuum tubes
   Prefill and air-purge two syringes with 0.9% sodium chloride, 10 mL
   1 Empty 10-mL syringe with 22-gauge needles attached
   1 Prefilled, air-purged syringe with appropriate heparin dose
   4 Povidone-iodine swabs
   1 Alcohol swab
   Tape and sterile gauze pads
3. Put on gloves.
4. Cleanse rubber end of injection cap with povidone-iodine for 30 seconds. Allow to dry by placing on sterile gauze pad.
5. Prepare vacuum tube holder and needle. Insert tube into vacuum tube holder, but do not insert tube into needle, because the vacuum will be lost.
6. Pick up and hold catheter hub using a sterile gauze pad. Do not touch the end of the injection cap. Insert the needle of one of the syringes of NS

in the center of the injection cap and flush to remove heparin or other solutions that were infusing.

7. Insert one empty 10-mL syringe into the injection cap and withdraw 10 mL blood, then discard this syringe.

8. Recleanse the injection cap with povidone-iodine for 30 seconds and allow to dry.

9. Insert needle of vacuum tube into the center of the injection cap. Fully insert vacuum tube into needle and allow tube to fill with blood, then remove tube. Repeat, inserting tubes into needle until all required tubes are filled.

10. Be sure to gently rotate any blood tubes containing anticoagulants, such as complete blood count or prothrombin time/partial thromboplastin time tubes.

11. Recleanse the injection cap with povidone-iodine for 30 seconds and allow to dry.

12. Insert needle of second prefilled NS syringe into injection cap to cleanse blood from tubing and flush.

13. Recleanse the injection cap with povidone-iodine for 30 seconds and allow to dry.

14. Insert needle of prefilled, air-purged heparin syringe into the injection cap and gently flush. Before the syringe is completely empty (approximately 9 mL), clamp the tubing. Apply pressure on the plunger while withdrawing needle and syringe.

   Observe the injection cap. If all blood has not been flushed thoroughly, change the injection cap.

15. Remove clamp and tape catheter on chest wall or reconnect the ordered infusion.

16. Discard all wasted syringes in the appropriate hazardous waste disposal container.
17. Label all vacuum tubes with the appropriate information and place in a biohazard bag usually provided by the laboratory.
18. Remove gloves and wash hands.

Use of CVADs and VAPs present some common problems that will face any nurse caring for clients with long-term catheters. The two most common problems are the inability to flush or withdraw blood from the catheter. Tables 20-8 and 20-9 cover some of the most common problems and how to manage them. Your home care agency will have specific guidelines on when to call the infusion company and when to try to manage the problem yourself. Always check with your supervisor if you are in doubt.

Documentation of care CVADs and VAPs should include

- Date and time of dressing change
- Appearance of insertion site
- Size and type of needle used to access a VAP
- Blood return present
- Ease of flushing and what was used to flush
- Name of nurse performing dressing change

MANAGING SUPPLIES AND DURABLE MEDICAL EQUIPMENT

Managing supplies and durable medical equipment is a team effort in high-tech home care nursing. At each nursing visit, the client's supplies should be assessed and the home infusion agency notified of any items in short supply. Supplies should be correlated to the number of days of medication or fluids to be infused. Does the client have enough medication to get through the weekend and Monday morning? For example: You must know the agency's policy on IV tubing changes. If the tubing is to be changed every 24 hours on a continuous infusion and the client has 4 days of therapy to complete, there should be four tubings as well as four prn adapters to access the Medlok. All nurses caring for the client should assess supplies to maintain uninterrupted services and continuity of care for the client. The pharmacy compiles a list of supplies and equipment and knows approximately when deliveries should be made. However, sometimes problems occur; maybe the client used two tubings on one day instead of one. This would mean the client is short one tubing.

Basic items to assess at each visit should include:

IV tubing, extension tubings
PRN adapters
Gauze sponges and protective pads for preparing solutions
Peripheral access devices
IV start kits or dressing change kits
Adequate amounts of medication bags, IV fluids, or IV additives
Gloves
Hazardous waste disposal units (these should be changed when 3/4 full)
Alcohol or povidone-iodine preparations

Durable medical equipment also should be checked at each visit to ensure proper working order. Ask the client/caregiver if they have encountered any problems with the infusion device or PCA. Assure that there are sufficient numbers of batteries in the

text continued on page 440

Table 20-8
Common CVAD Problems

Problem	Possible Cause	Nursing Interventions
Unable to infuse fluids Unable to withdraw blood	Closed clamps Catheter kinks Thrombus formation Catheter movement against vessel wall with negative pressure	Assess clamps and all tubing Change patient's position Raise the arm on the same side as the catheter Turn patient from side to side Instruct patient to cough, sit up, or take several deep breaths Perform valsalva maneuver Remove dressing and assess catheter Try to flush with 10 mL normal saline Attempt to aspirate the clot with gentle quick pulls on the barrel of the syringe; if blood returns, discard, and flush with 10 mL normal saline If unable to withdraw blood, notify home infusion company and doctor
Leakage of fluid at insertion site	Catheter displacement Subcutaneous tract leaking lymph fluid Tear in catheter	Assess for signs of distress in patient Assess dressing and observe site for redness Notify home infusion company and doctor

Problem	Causes	Interventions
Disconnected catheter	Tubing not secured to catheter Excessive patient movement	Clamp catheter Attach sterile syringe to end of catheter hub Replace extension set with new sterile setup. *Do not re-connect contaminated tubing* Clean catheter hub with alcohol and povidone-iodine. *Do not soak the hub* Replace with sterile IV tubing or Medlok device to the extension set
Catheter obstruction	Improper flushing Flow rate too slow Incompatible solutions causing precipitate formation Catheter tip against vessel wall Thrombus formation	Flush with normal saline and heparin or restart infusion Turn patient side to side and check for flow Attempt to aspirate the catheter. Do not force clot into the catheter Notify the home infusion company and the physician Possibly, infuse thrombolytic or neutralizing agents Possibly remove catheter Document all interventions

Table 20-9
Common VAP Problems

Possible Causes	Nursing Interventions
Unable to withdraw blood or flush	
Closed clamp or kinked tubing	Check clamp and infusion tubing
Catheter tip lodged against vessel wall	Teach patient to change position
	Reposition patient
	Raise the arm on the same side as the cathether
	Turn patient from side to side
	Instruct patient to cough, sit up, or take several deep breaths
	Flush with 10 mL normal saline
	D/C current access to VAP and reaccess with a new needle
Needle not advanced far enough into septum; needle placed incorrectly	Reaccess device with a new needle
	Educate patient in the proper placement of needle and to push down firmly on the needle and verify correct position by aspirating for blood

Clot formation

Assess patency by attempting to flush catheter with 10 mL normal saline

Notify home infusion company and request urokinase instillation

Assess patient knowledge of flush procedures and instruct patient to recognize symptoms of clot formation

Notify home infusion company and doctor immediately

Catheter, migration, port rotation, catheter kinked

Instruct patient to notify home infusion company and doctor if any difficulty in flushing or administration of infusion

Unable to palpate VAP

Deeply implanted port

Palpate area of port scar

Use deep palpation technique

Nofity home infusion company for nursing assessment visit

Reaccess VAP using 1 1/2" or 2" noncoring needle

home if the client is using a PCA. Check electronic infusion device cords for fraying, and make sure the devices are plugged in when not in use to maintain their internal batteries.

Hospital beds should be assessed in each position for ease of movement, along with side rails for client safety.

The nurse caring for the client should notify the agency immediately for any unsafe situations and to order any needed supplies. Any supply shortages or equipment problems should be noted on the Client Progress Note. Document the name of the person you spoke to at the agency about the problem. You also must ensure that the client/caregiver knows how to call the agency for any problems encountered with any equipment or supply shortages.

DOCUMENTATION IN HIGH-TECH HOME CARE THERAPY

Documentation is the principal means of communication between all of the health care team members in high-tech home care. Client care records are used by insurers to justify client supplies and equipment costs as well as the medical need for home care therapies and nursing services. Review organizations will analyze your documentation to evaluate client care. The courts will examine what you have documented to justify malpractice. Incident reports should be completed for any unexpected client outcome or event to receive immediate attention by the agency. Incident reports are also used to track client problems, provide statistics on the incidence of client problems, and to protect the nurse in cases of litigation. All client documentation should be in the hands of the agency within 24 to 48 hours of the visit.

Nursing plans of care are written to communicate expected client outcomes. These should be updated with any change in the client's condition, addition of new diagnoses, or client problems. Some common nursing diagnoses used in high-tech home care nursing are:

Infection
Fluid Volume Deficit/Excess
Acute/Chronic Pain
Altered Nutrition: Less Than Body Requirements
Knowledge Deficit
Altered Health Maintenance
Impaired Home Maintenance Management
Anxiety/Fear

Client/caregiver education is provided at every encounter and documented on the Client Progress Note. Along with the areas of documentation already discussed in this chapter, the following should be documented at each visit:

Appearance of the infusion catheter site
Observation of catheter patency
IV therapy management
   Date and time of tubing changes; list all accessory
      tubings
   Date, time, and contents of IV fluids and medica-
      tions
   IV flow rate and any rate changes
   Electronic equipment used to regulate flow
   Time medication or fluid infusion begun and com-
      pleted

Presence of any complications and actions taken to resolve the problem

Time and date IV therapy is discontinued and whether the catheter is intact when removed

Client/caregiver ability to perform all procedures

Client/caregiver compliance with regimen

Client weight and vital signs, including temperature and blood or urine glucose levels (if indicated)

Provision of all client and caregiver education

QUALITY ASSURANCE IN HIGH-TECH HOME CARE

Quality assurance and *risk management* programs are mandated by the Joint Commission on Accreditation of Healthcare Organizations (JCAHO) and State Health Departments. The purpose of these programs are to identify and monitor important aspects of care, identify and correct problems as they occur, and document optimal client outcomes. All agencies must be able to provide documentation of client visits, a plan of care, adequate policies, procedures, protocols, and statistics on the incidence of complications during therapy. This is accomplished by periodic chart reviews within the home infusion agency. Because JCAHO and State Health Departments make unannounced spot visits to agencies, it is essential that your documentation be thorough and precise at the time of the client visit. You will be asked to participate in continuing education programs or documentation seminars to maintain high levels of accuracy and completeness.

21

Skin and Wound Care

Maritza Cunningham, RN, BSN, and Patricia Lang, RN

STATEMENT OF NEED

As a hospital-based nurse who has entered the field of home care, you will be caring for many clients with wounds. Caring for wounds in the home is a skilled nursing service that ranges from the simple to the complex.

Patients are being discharged from acute care settings at an earlier stage in their recovery. Nurses are encountering clients with fresh postoperative wounds that require early assessment, care, and teaching. Pressure ulcers and other types of wounds continue to provide extreme challenges to home health care nurses.

The services your patient will receive are directly related to your ability to assess wounds, choose the proper plan of care, and document your findings. During your orientation, your learning goals for wound care should be to:

- Recognize the family dynamics and their impact on wound healing
- Increase your knowledge of the wound healing process
- Know the principles of risk assessment and prevention
- Enhance your skills in wound assessment and documentation
- Develop your knowledge of wound management principles

ANATOMY AND PHYSIOLOGY

When presented with an open wound, it is critical to have an understanding of which layers of skin have been affected. The skin consists of the epidermis, dermis, and subcutaneous tissue. Each layer contains structures that allow for wound repair.

Epidermis is the outermost layer of the skin. It regenerates every 4 to 6 weeks. The epidermis is avascular and thin. It contains melanin, which gives skin its color. Skin has a pH balance of 4.5 to 5.5. This is commonly referred to as the protective acid mantel. Clients at home need to be taught to avoid substances that will disrupt the pH of the skin, such as harsh soap and contact with urine or stool.

Dermis is highly vascular. It has a network of capillaries that provide oxygen and nutrients to tissue. It has nerve endings that allow for response to stimulation. Sebaceous glands and hair follicles contribute to the lubrication of skin and maintenance of pH balance. Dermis houses fibroblast cells, which are responsible for the formation of collagen. Collagen gives skin its strength. Elastin is formed in the dermis and is what gives skin its recoil.

Subcutaneous tissue is composed of adipose (fat) tissue, muscle, and connective tissue. Blood vessels and nerves are also present. This layer protects, insulates, and cushions the body.

When you admit a patient to home care, a thorough skin inspection should be done. During the skin assessment, you can teach the patient and family of the many functions of skin. Skin protects us from organisms in the environment. Skin encases tissues and organs in place.

Thermoregulation is an important function of skin. We shiver when we are cold, and this helps warm us. We perspire when we are hot, and this help cool us. Skin is a sensitive organ that initiates a response to heat, cold, pressure, pain, and pleasure. When skin is exposed to sunlight, vitamin D synthesis takes place. This facilitates the metabolism of calcium. Elimination of electrolytes, water, and waste takes place in part through skin.

CLASSIFICATION OF WOUNDS

The purpose of classifying wounds is to have a common language when layers of tissue damage are being described. The Agency for Health Care Policy and Research (AHCPR) has set forth guidelines and language as to how to classify a wound. There are two accepted systems of classification. One is the wound thickness classification, which is used to describe all wounds except pressure ulcers. Pressure ulcers are described by stages.

Wound Thickness Classification

Wounds caused by trauma, surgery, vascular impairment, and cancer are classified by their thickness. Partial-thickness wounds involve the epidermis and part of the dermis. They may present as a blister, skin tear, or abrasion. These wounds usually heal promptly.

Full-thickness wounds involve the epidermis, dermis, and subcutaneous tissue. Damage may extend further to muscle, tendon, and bone. Healing is slow because of extensive tissue loss.

Pressure Ulcer Classifications

Wounds that are caused by pressure and shearing are staged. The staging system identifies how many layers of tissue damage have occurred. A pressure ulcer develops when an area of soft tissue is compressed between a bone and a hard surface. This deprives tissue of blood, oxygen, and nutrients, resulting in ischemia, which leads to tissue destruction.

A pressure ulcer is the correct term for what used to be called a bed sore or decubitus ulcer. They are a cause of great human suffering and expense. Pressure ulcers are classified by stages, each stage indicating the extent of tissue damage.

Stage I pressure ulcers present as nonblanchable erythema (persistent redness) on intact skin, the
heralding sign of tissue damage. When assessing
darkly pigmented skin, look for a heightened intensity of the skin tone or discoloration. Feel for
heat and edema.

Stage II pressure ulcers present skin loss that involves
the epidermis and part of the dermis. The ulcer is
superficial and presents clinically as an abrasion,
blister, or shallow crater.

Stage III pressure ulcer refers to skin loss that involves
damage to the epidermis, dermis, and subcutaneous tissue and may extend to, but not through,
underlying fascia. The ulcer may present as a
deep crater with or without undermining of adja-
cent tissue. The patient's body build will determine the depth of the wound (cachectic versus
obese).

Stage IV pressure ulcers represent extensive destruction that involves the epidermis, dermis, subcutaneous tissue, muscle, bone, or supporting
structures such as tendon and joint capsules.

SOURCES OF SKIN BREAKDOWN

Shearing forces are often present in conjunction with
pressure. This occurs when the head of the bed is elevated higher than 30 degrees. Gravity causes the body
to slide down in bed. The tissues attached to the bone
are pulled in a downward direction while surface tissue is trapped in place. The tissues are torn away
from each other, and blood vessels are stretched and
obstructed. Shearing forces may account for a high

number of wounds that are superficially small with intact skin, but may cause more extensive damage to the inner layers of tissue. This can be avoided by keeping the head of the bed at 30 degrees or lower. When moving the client up in bed, a draw sheet should be used to lift the client off the bed surface. Consider ordering a Hoyer lift or trapeze for clients who have only one caregiver. Remember, have the caregiver demonstrate and explain all procedures to you. Teaching is a skilled nursing service that is reimbursable. Furthermore, the documentation needs to reflect that prevention of skin breakdown was taught.

Friction is created by two surfaces moving across one another. Friction works in combination with shear when the client is dragged up in bed. Ulcers resulting from friction appear superficial as an abrasion, but in combination with other factors can often deteriorate into a pressure ulcer. Patients with spastic conditions or clients who wear braces or appliances that rub against the skin are at risk for developing friction ulcers.

Teach the family and caregivers to keep the sheets free of wrinkles and debris such as crumbs and other objects. Pad appliances and have the client wear long cotton socks to insulate the skin from direct trauma.

WOUND HEALING PHASES

All wounds follow the same healing phases: inflammatory phase and maturation phase. The rate of healing is determined by many health factors related to the specific patient, and of course the severity of the wound.

The *inflammatory phase* starts when the tissue is first injured. The tissue responds with a localized area of edema, erythema, and pain. The body then mobilizes its line of defense. Platelets form fibrin clots to control bleeding.

Neutrophils and macrophages move in to engulf bacteria and foreign matter. Antihistamines are mobilized to reduce swelling. Finally, growth factors are released to begin wound repair. In a healthy patient, this process may take 4 to 6 days.

When you examine the injured area, you will note heat, edema, pain, and erythema. This is a normal localized response.

The *proliferative phase* is also called the granulation phase. In a healthy patient, it may take 4 to 24 days. Granulation tissue appears beefy red and granular. It is made of newly formed capillaries (angiogenesis), collagen, and fibroblasts and will fill in the base of the wound. Epithelial cells begin to appear at the margin of the wound and continue to migrate toward the center of the wound until the wound is resurfaced and closed. Epithelial tissue is thin, velvety, and silvery in appearance.

The *maturation phase* in a healthy patient may take 3 months to 2 years. During this phase, the newly formed tissue further remodels itself and strengthens the scar tissue through continued production of collagen. This improves tensile strength to 70% of the original strength. Tensile strength is the ability of the skin to withstand traumatic assault. Scar tissue is more likely to break down under pressure, friction, shear, or trauma than is skin that has never been injured.

An exciting challenge that nurses have is to favorably impact the rate at which a wound moves through these phases. The type of wound healing is just one consideration to the length of time it will take to heal the wound.

TYPES OF HEALING

There are only three ways that a wound will heal: primary closure, secondary closure, and tertiary closure.

Primary Closure

Wound healing by primary closure refers to surgical wounds. There has been minimal tissue loss. The wound margins are approximated and held in place by sutures, staples, or butterflies. Healing will occur rapidly.

Secondary Closure

In this case, wound margins are not pinned together. This is an open wound. The wound may involve the epidermis, dermis, subcutaneous tissue, and possibly fascia. These wounds heal by the formation of granulation tissue in the wound bed. As the wound bed fills in, the depth is reduced. Epithelial tissue develops at the wound margins, and size is reduced. This is often a slow process.

Third Intention Closure/Delayed Primary Closure

In this situation, the wound has been left open with the intention of a surgical closure at a later time.

Often the presence of infection prevents immediate surgical closure.

DELAYED HEALING

Unfortunately, the question most often asked about a wound is, "How long will it take to heal?" You will be asked this by the client, caregiver, Medicare, Medicaid, insurance company, or health maintenance organization (HMO). Even your supervisor and quality assurance will ask.

There is no simple or sure answer to the question. Each client must be assessed as an individual. Many factors affect healing rates, and it is up to you to identify and correct them. Factors that may delay healing include age, weight, history of chronic diseases, immunosuppressants, medications, infection, necrosis, and wound-cleansing solutions.

Age

Clients older than age 65 years heal at a slower rate. The older the client, the more prone the client is to chronic disease that changes the tissue's ability to heal.

Weight

The obese client will heal slowly because adipose tissue lacks ample capillary perfusion.

The cachectic client is often undernourished, dehydrated, and has poor circulation. There is no cushion between their bony prominences and the bed surface. Healing will be slow, if it occurs at all.

Diabetes

Blood glucose fluctuations and insulin slow the rate of granulation and collagen tissue formation. Neuropathy further reduces the client's ability to feel pain, which is essential to avoid trauma and recognize infection. Blood sugar needs to be controlled, and skin needs to be protected from injury.

Cardiopulmonary

Oxygenated blood pumped to every cell of the body is what keeps the tissues healthy. When there are changes in the volume and quality of blood delivered, the healing process slows down.

Chronic Diseases

Chronic diseases such as diabetes, cancer, or renal disease may have a negative impact on wound healing. It is important to document the presence of chronic disease and to be aware of its physiologic effect on your client.

Immunosuppression

Nursing interventions and wound care need to be based on sensitivity to the client's physical and psychological needs. Clients with a diagnosis of cancer, acquired immune deficiency syndrome (AIDS), or renal failure are severely immunosuppressed. Their ability to heal is severely altered. These clients are actively experiencing some level of hormonal and metabolic changes that damage cells and tissue.

Nutritional intake is crucial. Suggest high-calorie, protein-rich foods and give examples of them unless there are dietary restrictions.

The wound care treatment will vary. At times your intention will be to heal, and at other times to control skin breakdown, infection, and pain.

Medications

Steroids decrease the production of fibroblast cells, which are essential in the production of collagen. The effect of steroids on wound tissue results in weak tissue that lacks tensile strength. Vitamin A is often ordered to decrease the damaging effect of steroids on healing tissue. Clients that require insulin also produce a weak collagen and heal very slowly. Those on chemotherapy and immunosuppressants have macrophage cells damaged, making them more prone to infection because these cells are no longer available to kill bacteria and remove debris. The inflammatory process is suppressed, and the healing phases are delayed.

Infection

When a client is referred to home care with an active wound, there must be a regular assessment for infection at the wound site. All chronic wounds are contaminated, but this does not mean that they are infected. If the bacterial load becomes too great, clinical signs of infection will appear. The site becomes painful. There is erythema (redness) extending well beyond the wound margins into the surrounding tissue (periwound). The area feels hot. There is induration, which means the area has become firm, hard, and swollen because of fluid collection at the site. The exudate (drainage) increases and is probably prevalent with a pungent odor. There might be fever. A temperature elevation of 101°F or higher requires that the physician be informed immediately.

The physician may order wound cultures and certainly will order systemic antibiotics, either oral or intravenous. Irrigation is helpful in removing purulent drainage and slough from the wound.

The volume of normal saline used in small wounds should be 300 mL; a large wound should receive 500 mL. To deliver the saline with enough force to dislodge slough and debris, a 35-mL syringe with a 19-gauge needle should be used as per AHCPR guidelines.

Because wound healing ceases during an infection, there should be no delay in initiating treatment. Make sure you record all your observations and communications with the physician.

Necrosis

Necrotic tissue is dead tissue. When present in the wound bed, it impedes healing. Necrotic tissue increases the potential for infection. It must be removed.

When the wound bed has necrotic tissue, it is not possible to determine how many layers of tissue have been damaged. The wound cannot be staged.

Necrotic tissue presents as eschar or fibrin slough:

Eschar is hard, dry, black, leathery, tough dead tissue.
Fibrin slough is soft, wet, slippery, yellow, white, or gray dead tissue. Fibrin is stringy and securely attached to the wound bed.

You must document the type and characteristics of the necrotic tissue. This will serve as supportive evidence for the need of skilled nursing visits and related wound care treatments.

Debridement is the removal of necrotic tissue. There are four methods used to accomplish this. They are mechanical, chemical, autolytic, and surgical.

Mechanical debridement is a traditional and conservative method of debridement. An example is wet to dry gauze dressing changes. It *must* be understood that it is a form of nonselective debridement. The technique consists of an application of damp gauze into the wound bed. It is allowed to dry and later pulled off, bringing along fibrin slough and granulation tissue. Black eschar does not respond to this type of debridement. This procedure is painful. It is best to wet the gauze with saline before removal.

Chemical debridement consists of application of enzymes capable of digesting fibrin slough or eschar. It is a prescription item ordered by the physician. There are several products on the market. You must read the enclosed literature for application instructions. In a week or 2, the wound should be much cleaner. Remember, discontinue use when the wound bed is free of necrosis.

Autolytic debridement is accomplished by maintaining moisture on the wound bed. This allows the wound to use its own enzymes to lyse fibrin slough and eschar tissue. Several types of dressings are designed to support autolytic debridement. They are transparent films, hydrogels, and hydrocolloids. Autolytic debridement is gentle to granulation tissue and is often preferred by home care nurses.

Surgical debridement is the removal of necrotic tissue with a sharp instrument. Areas of fibrin slough and eschar are mediums for bacterial infection and do best when removed promptly by surgical debridement. The procedure is performed by a physician in the hospital, clinic, and occasionally in the home. It is quick, nonselective, and often painful.

Solutions

Some solutions are compatible with healing, and others are toxic. The physician will order the solution for wound cleansing and irrigation, and it should appear on the physician's order.

The AHCPR recommends the use of *normal saline* for wound cleansing and irrigation. Normal saline is physiologic and not harmful to cells.

Traditionally, disinfecting solutions such as hydrogen peroxide, povidone-iodine, acetic acid, and Dakin's solution have been used. The AHCPR recommends that these solutions not be used.

If any of these are prescribed, contact the physician and suggest a change to normal saline. Otherwise, use the following guidelines:

Hydrogen peroxide: If used, it must be diluted to at least ¼ strength and followed by an irrigation of normal saline. Never use for packing.
Acetic acid: This is not recommended. It is ordered as a 0.5% dilution to treat gram-negative and grampositive organisms. Follow with a normal saline irrigation.
Dakin's solution: This is not recommended. It is usually ordered as 0.25/0.5 strength for its germicidal, debriding, and odor-controlling properties. Follow with a normal saline irrigation.
Povidone-iodine: This is not recommended. It is a broad-spectrum antiseptic. If used, dilute to a

0.01% strength. Follow with a normal saline irrigation.

Soap and water: If used, instruct the client to rinse soap residue with water and follow with a normal saline irrigation.

LEG ULCERS

Venous Stasis Ulcer

Some of the most persistent, slow-healing wounds are leg ulcers. These are caused by distended varicose veins. They are usually located by the inner ankle (medial malleolus). The surrounding skin is discolored with a darker tone (hyperpigmentation). Pain is not severe. Pedal pulses are usually palpable unless obscured by tissue edema. These wounds are often large, shallow, and have irregular margins. The wound bed will be granular, red, and wet.

The most important aspect of treatment is promoting venous return. This is done through the application of a sustained compression bandages. Several new products on the market serve this purpose. The traditional method of treatment is application of an Unna's boot and compression bandage. Topical treatment alone has minimal impact. Ask a certified wound/ostomy specialist which product is appropriate for your client. Instruct the client to elevate the lower limbs as often as possible. Instruct in weight reduction, limiting smoking.

Arterial Leg Ulcers

It is important to differentiate an arterial from a venous ulcer. Venous ulcer treatment can do great harm to an arterial ulcer.

The arteries are occluded and blood, oxygen, and nutrients do not perfuse the tissues. These ulcers are located on the toes, feet, and lower legs. The skin appears waxy and hairless with no pigment changes. Toenails thicken and develop ridges. Pain is usually present and increases when the leg is elevated, while walking, and at night. Pedal pulses are usually absent. Feet become red when in a dependent position. Edema is limited to the wound area. These ulcers are usually small, deep, dry, and may be necrotic. There is high risk for infection and gangrene. An eschar on an arterial leg ulcer must *not* be removed, because the underlying tissue is likely to become necrotic also.

The most satisfactory treatment is revascularization through surgical intervention. If the client is not a surgical candidate, a conservative treatment plan should be developed.

Pain can be reduced by using moist wound dressings that will not stick to the wound bed. An additional benefit is the provision of moisture to the wound bed for enhanced healing. Although pain heightens with exercise, an exercise plan is essential to preserve the remaining circulation. A physical therapist may be needed to teach a home exercise program.

Diabetic Ulcers

Diabetic ulcers are caused by a combination of arterial insufficiency and neuropathy. They are commonly found on the toes and plantar surface of the foot. The skin is thick and callous (hyperkeratotic). Pain is usually absent because of neuropathy. Presence of a pulse is not necessarily indicative of good circulation. These wounds are small, deep, and dry, with thick callous margins. There is high risk for infection and gangrene.

Control of blood glucose levels is essential for wound healing. Treatment is the same as for an arterial ulcer. The client should have an evaluation for orthotic shoes. Instruct the client to follow guidelines for diabetic foot care.

RISK FACTORS FOR SKIN BREAKDOWN

As we discussed, skin breakdown occurs when the forces of pressure, shear, and friction are present. Other factors such as age, weight, and chronic diseases also may cause delayed healing. Additional factors for skin breakdown are moisture, immobility, and poor nutrition.

Moisture

Moisture contributes to the risk of skin breakdown because moisture macerates skin. This means skin becomes soft, white, waterlogged, and weakened. The pH of the skin is altered.

The most common cause is urine. Many homebound clients suffer from urinary incontinence.

During assessment, inquire about the status of urinary and bowel control. If incontinence is present, instruct the caregiver to cleanse the perineal area immediately after each episode. Mild soap should be used and rinsed well with clear water. The area should be dried thoroughly. A skin barrier should be applied. Barriers seal the skin, protecting it from urine. Barriers are available as ointments, sprays, or film wipes.

The client's bed must also be kept dry. Linens may require frequent changing. A protective draw-sheet or disposable under pad will be helpful. Explore other methods of containing urine. The preferred choice will be to restore continence. Implement a toileting schedule.

If toileting is unsuccessful, use of a urinal, bedpan, or commode may alleviate the problem. A male client may benefit from using an external catheter. Diapering is used as a last resort. Instruct the caregiver to change the client frequently, as soon as there is moisture. If a wound is present and is contaminated by urine, consider recommending temporary use of an indwelling catheter.

Other fluids that can macerate and excoriate skin are perspiration that is trapped in skin folds, for example, under breasts. If wound exudate accumulates and pools on the periwound skin, maceration and skin breakdown can occur.

Immobility

Assess the client's mobility as it relates to issues of skin integrity, safety, and the capability of the caregiver. Assess and document if the client is bed bound, paraplegic, quadriplegic, or hemiplegic. The inability to move independently or respond to painful stimuli places these clients at high risk of tissue ischemia and pressure ulcers. The weak or debilitated client with slow movement or balance deficit is likely to be immobile for prolonged periods.

Have the client demonstrate the level of activity he or she can accomplish. Can the client ambulate, transfer from bed to chair, or turn from side to side in bed? Identify the potential for an injury or an accident. Make the client and caregiver aware of any deficits. Consider the inclusion of a therapist in the plan of care.

If the caregivers assist with activity, assess their willingness and ability to help the client. Often the caregiver has good intentions but is not familiar with body mechanics. Have the caregiver demonstrate a position change or a linen change. Take the opportunity to guide and teach appropriate techniques.

For a family member caring for a client with mobility deficits, it is labor intensive and energy draining. You can offer emotional support and positive feedback for the prevention of skin breakdown. Encourage the caregiver to seek additional resources for help in the home. Often family and friends are willing participants and can reduce the burden of care significantly. If there is no such support, the services of a home health aide are justified.

It is important that the caregiver understands the principles of pressure ulcer development. Demonstrate to the caregiver how to turn the client and inspect all bony prominences for skin integrity.

The immobile client will require an every-2-hour turning schedule. When turning the client to the side, avoid placing full body weight on the iliac crest and trochanter. Place the client laterally at a 30-degree angle. Use of pillows and rolled towels will help support proper positioning and provide comfort to the client. Emphasize that heels should not be in contact with the bed surface because heels are at greatest risk for breakdown.

There are many pressure-reducing and pressure-relieving mattresses and beds available to the homebound client. Pressure-reducing mattresses include 4-inch-thick foam, alternating air, static air, or gel and water overlays. Pressure relief may be accomplished with use of low-air-loss or air-fluidized surfaces. Refer to AHCPR guidelines:

> *US Dept. of Health and Human Services*
> *Agency for Health Care Policy and Research*
> *Executive Office Building, Suite 501*
> *2101 East Jefferson Street*
> *Rockville, MD 20852*

The chairbound client's areas of greatest risk are the ischium, coccyx, and sacrum. Clients need to be taught not to sit in one position for prolonged periods. They need to shift positions or raise themselves off the seat at least every half-hour to relieve pressure. Obtaining a specialty cushion that redistributes weight and decreases pressure over bony prominences is a basic necessity for the wheelchair-bound client. Use of a foam donut is contraindicated because they are a source of pressure. If redness appears at the area, it should not be massaged until it disappears, because this will cause further tissue damage. The client should keep weight off the area.

The client with partial mobility will need to be encouraged to gradually increase the level of activity. Have the client walk with you around the room. Stop, look at a picture, move on to the hall, listen to the stories. This is a good time for conversation and getting to know the client as a person. If the client remains weak and has poor balance, consider a referral to physical therapy.

Communicate to the physician the deficits in mobility and sensory perception. You may recommend additional services and equipment such as occupational therapy, a home health aide, a trapeze, a Hoyer lift, a wheelchair, a walker, or a cane.

Nutrition

The client's nutritional status has a profound effect on wound healing outcomes. Deficiencies may result in skin breakdown or delayed healing. You will need to assess the client's nutritional status. Is the client obese? Obesity does not always correlate to a good nutritional status. Obese clients may often take in too many calories with foods that have poor nutritional value.

Do the dentures fit properly? If not, suggest that they be repaired. Does the client have sores in the mouth? Recommend salt water rinse before and after meals. Is there difficulty with digestion? Perhaps the client would benefit from digestive enzymes. Does the client state that he or she has lost his or her appetite? Look in the refrigerator. Do you see foods with nutritional value? Can the client afford three meals a day? You may need to arrange for assistance from a religious organization, food pantry, food stamps, or a charitable organization. Who prepares the meals?

Ask the caregiver to list the foods eaten daily, and how much: baked 1/2 potato, 1/2 cup spinach, 3/4 fish fillet.

Protein, minerals, carbohydrates, and vitamins are available in the basic food groups. Discussed next are the most important ones for wound healing.

Vitamin A helps prevent cellular destruction or injury, and is involved in collagen synthesis. Vitamin A is necessary for good vision, growth, strong immunity, and reproduction. Sources are fish, liver, and leafy, dark green, yellow, or orange vegetables such as sweet potatoes, carrots, spinach, squash, turnips, and cantaloupe.

Vitamin D supports bone formation, cell metabolism, and immunity. Sources are fish such as herring, salmon, and tuna, and dairy products such as milk and cheese.

Vitamin E helps protect cellular function, enhances collagen synthesis, and may increase sexual potency. Sources are seed/vegetable oils, wheat germ, soybeans, grains, and nuts.

Vitamin K aids blood clotting. Sources are green leafy vegetables such as spinach, turnip greens, lettuce, broccoli, cabbage, liver, and bacon.

Vitamin C is an antioxidant that aids in collagen/connective tissue/cartilage formation. Sources are fresh citrus fruits and green and yellow vegetables. A supplement of vitamin C 500 mg twice per day is recommended for wound healing.

Vitamin B complex, thiamine, riboflavin, niacin, B_6, and B_{12}, support many functions of cell production, such as energy and protein metabolism for antibody and white blood cell production. Sources are meat, fish, shellfish, and grains.

Zinc assists in cell proliferation. Sources are oysters, wheat germ, meat, fish, and dairy products.

Protein assists in wound repair. Sources are meat, fish, grains, and nuts.

Carbohydrates are required for energy. Sources are grains, cereal, pasta, and rice.

You should discuss food preferences with your client. Determine at what times of day he or she likes to eat. Perhaps small, frequent meals will increase the client's intake. Encourage the caregiver to socialize with the client at mealtime.

If the client is not able to eat enough to support nutritional needs, suggest a food supplement. Should the client lose weight, become weak, and wound healing is delayed, discuss with the physician the need for an albumin and lymphocyte count. Some laboratories will go to the client's home to draw the blood, or you may need to send the client to the clinic or physician's office.

Normal serum albumin ratios are 3.5 to 5.0 g/dL. A level of 3.0 g/dL indicates mild deficiency, and 2.5 g/dL or less indicates severe deficiency, which will delay or halt healing. Serum albumin less than 3.5 g/dL and a total lymphocyte count less than 1,500 cells/mm^3 indicates significant malnutrition. If the client has recently lost 15% body weight, the nutritional status is compromised.

If your agency has a nutritionist available, request a consult. The nutritionist may recommend a more aggressive regimen, which may include a G tube. Discuss the recommendations with the physician for orders.

WOUND ASSESSMENT AND DOCUMENTATION

The AHCPR, which was formed by clinical experts in the area of wound care, have set forth guidelines that include the description of wound characteristics. The terminology used in this section follows the AHCPR guidelines. The wound record needs to be accurate and reflect the ongoing changes in the wound.

The assessment is carried out each time the wound is examined and cared for. The documentation of all key elements is done on admission, at least once a week and more often if there are changes.

Location

Name the location of the wound by its anatomic location, such as sacrum or scapula. As a home care nurse, your assessment should include the whole skin, starting at the head and ending at the toes. Your goal is to discover any areas of actual or potential skin breakdown not identified in the original referral. Clearly state the number of wounds and type of skin impairment found and whether they were acquired in the hospital or the home.

Wound Classification

Determine how many layers of skin have been broken, and label according to the cause of injury (see section on Wound Classification).

Staging System

Only used to identify pressure ulcers.

    Stage I   Stage II   Stage III   Stage IV

Thickness Systems

All other causes of tissue breakdown are either:

Partial-Thickness Wound (PTW): blisters, skin tears, abrasions

Full-Thickness Wound (FTW): surgical sites, leg ulcers, cancer lesions, burns

Size

The unit of measurement is the centimeter. To properly measure a wound, you will need a linear instrument (a ruler) and cotton swab (Q-tip®). You will also need to *imagine a clock* superimposed on the wound, where 12 o'clock is the direction of the head, 6 o'clock the feet, and 3 o'clock and 9 o'clock are the sides. The clock will help to better locate and identify key elements in the wounds.

Length

To determine the length, you will measure the largest open area from the head-to-toe plane. Use an imaginary clock; the head is 12, the toe is 6. The longest part of the wound may be 11 to 5. This is also head to toe and is the area you should measure.

Width

To determine the width, you will measure the widest open area. Use your imaginary clock; side to side is 9 to 3. The widest part of the wound may be 8 to 4. This is also side to side and is the section you should measure.

Depth

To measure depth, hold a sterile cotton-tipped applicator in a vertical position and insert into the deepest area of the wound. Grasp the applicator at the point that corresponds to the wound margin, and measure from the tip of the applicator to your fingertips.

Wound Margin/Edges

This is the edge where intact skin ends and the open wound begins. Margins in a healthy wound are *attached* to the wound base; there is no space between the margin and the wound tissue. Complex wounds have margins that are rolled under or detached from underlying tissue. These conditions may indicate the presence of undermining and tunneling. A related condition but undetectable by wound margin is the sinus tract.

Undermining

Tissue under the wound margin is no longer attached to the wound bed because there has been tissue loss. Even though the superficial skin is intact, the wound appears smaller than the actual size.

Explore the wound margin with a sterile Q-tip®. Slide into the underlying space and move along the margin like the hands of a clock. Note the depth and extent of undermining along the wound margin. Using your imaginary clock, document as such: 3 cm ranging from 1 o'clock to 4 o'clock.

Problem. Extensive tissue loss will require additional time for wound closure to occur.

Nursing Care. Cleanse undermined area by irrigation of normal saline. Lightly pack the area to fill dead space and absorb exudate.

Caregiver. Inform the caregiver and the client that the ulcer is larger than it appears to be, so that they can adjust their expectations.

Tunneling

Tunneling is a pathway that extends in one direction under the margin of the skin. A sterile Q-tip® can be introduced into the tunnel in one direction only. The open area is not visible.

Problem. Tunnels often accumulate exudate and become a vessel for bacterial collection. An abscess can develop.

Nursing Care. Irrigate well with normal saline and pack lightly to fill dead space and absorb exudate. Document the extent of the tunnel and width using centimeters.

Caregiver. Observe client for fever, pain, or redness in the affected area. If these symptoms develop, the caregiver should notify the home care nurse. If the temperature is higher than 101°F, the physician should be notified.

Sinus Tract

The sinus tract is a small, narrow channel that involves a cavity longer than the visible opening, perhaps the size of a pinhead, and cannot be explored with a sterile Q-tip®.

Problem. A sinus tract will delay the healing rate. A sinus often produces large amounts of exudate. Development of an abscess is possible. A sinus tract may reach the bone and be an indication of osteomyelitis.

Nursing Care. Document amount of drainage and location of sinus in the wound. Irrigate wound with normal saline to remove exudate and reduce bacterial load. Assess site for potential abscess formation. Inform physician of your findings. There may be a need for further diagnostic studies, such as radiography or bone scan.

Caregiver. Instruct caregiver to report fever or increased pain (same as tunneling).

Characteristics of Wound Bed Tissue

Granulation

Granulation tissue is beefy, red, or pink. Revascularization of capillaries is taking place.

Problem. Granulation tissue is delicate, and newly formed capillaries are fragile.

Nursing Care. This tissue needs to be protected and nurtured because it is the foundation on which wound healing takes place. Irrigate gently, and protect from trauma and contamination. Apply a dressing that will provide moisture to the wound bed. Maintain the client's nutritional status.

Document the percentage of granular tissue present and its color. Example: "Granular tissue unevenly distributed on 40% of wound bed. Color ranging from pink to beefy red."

Epithelial Tissue

Epithelial tissue first appears at the wound margins and is evidence of wound closure taking place. Its appearance is pinkish and silvery.

Problem. Epithelial tissue is fragile and can be adversely affected by excessive moisture or trauma. It can take up to 2 years for this tissue to recover strength.

Nursing Care. Irrigate gently, and protect from trauma. Use an absorbent dressing that will spare epithelial tissue from maceration. Continue to encourage sound nutritional intake.

Document percentage of epithelial tissue present, pattern of distribution, and color. Example: "Epithelial tissue is pink, silvery, and shiny. Evident along wound margin, covering 25% of wound bed."

Caregiver. Inform caregiver that healing will proceed rapidly, and soon there will be no need for skilled nursing service. The healed wound will not require dressings, but the area should be protected from trauma.

Necrotic Tissue

Necrotic tissue is dead tissue. The presence of necrotic tissue halts wound healing. An ulcer cannot be staged nor can depth be determined because the necrosis covers the layers of tissue. There are two types of necrotic tissue.

Fibrin slough is soft, slippery, and can be yellow, gray, tan, or white.
Eschar is black, leathery, hard, and dry.

Problem. As tissue decays, bacteria will proliferate, increasing risk for infection. The wound remains in the inflammatory phase, so expect an increase in exudate.

Nursing Care. Identify and remove the cause of the necrosis, for example, pressure and diminished circulation. Notify the physician and jointly plan a method of debridement—sharp, autolytic, chemical, or mechanical. Irrigate wound bed with a large volume of saline. The type of wound dressing used should support the method of debridement.

Documentation should include a description of the type of necrotic tissue and the percentage of wound bed covered. Example: "Fibrin slough—yellow, thick, covering and attached to 75% of the wound bed."

Exudate

Exudate, also called drainage, is any fluid produced by the wound. It is rich in cells that benefit the wound healing process.

Serous is watery and clear.
Serous sanguinous includes both serous drainage and
    blood.
Purulent drainage contains leukocytes, bacteria, and
    debris.

Problem. Excess wound exudate will macerate the periwound area and can disrupt the dressing placement. Purulent exudate will house bacteria over the wound bed.

Nursing Care. It is important to remove all exudate and debris. Irrigate the wound with normal saline. Contain exudate with an absorbent dressing to prevent maceration of the periwound and ensure that the dressing stays intact.

Document the amount, color, and effect of exudate on periwound skin. Example: "Large amount serosanguinous exudate—wets 6 layers of 4×4 gauze, macerating the periwound."

Caregiver. Have caregiver demonstrate how to change or reinforce the dressing to prevent maceration.

Periwound Skin

Periwound skin is the skin surrounding the open wound. The condition of the periwound helps determine the risk for further breakdown. Describe the periwound in the following terms:

Maceration is softened or waterlogged skin as a result of exposure to moisture.

Erythema is a generalized redness. The term is only descriptive. The possible cause of redness must be stated: pressure, friction, shear, or sign of infection.

Induration is a term used to describe firm, hardened tissue. This is an indication of tissue trauma or infection.

Problem. The periwound skin is compromised under each of these conditions. Signs of erythema or induration may signify infection or continued pressure to the tissue.

Nursing Care. Assess for clinical signs of infection. Relieve pressure from the affected area.

  Document the extent of maceration or reddening of the area. State this in centimeters. Identify the absence or presence of clinical signs of infection (include vital signs). State your activities to relieve the condition. Example: "Firm, hard, reddened, and macerated area measuring 3 cm around periwound.

Client admits to no position change for past 4 hours (source of pressure). Client turned to side at 30-degree angle to relieve pressure. Client and caregiver agree to adhere to the turning schedule."

Caregiver. Re-emphasize the principles of pressure relief, skin inspection, and potential consequences.

By using the above wound care language, you will be able to communicate in an objective, accurate, and consistent manner. After assessing the wound, you will be able to recommend a treatment plan based on the wound characteristics.

WOUND CARE PRODUCTS AND TREATMENTS

In this past decade, great advances have been made in wound healing. It has been discovered and proves that moist wounds heal 30% to 35% faster than dry wounds. This fact has altered methods of managing wounds. We no longer leave wounds open to air, shine a heat lamp on them, or treat them with dry, sterile dressings. We have learned to take advantage of the positive effects of wound exudate through use of contemporary wound dressings that retain moisture on the wound bed.

Now that you are in home care, there is a wide selection of contemporary dressings. This could be overwhelming, because there are thousands of brands, sizes, and types of dressings on the market.

Rather than learn and understand each dressing, it is wise to group dressings into categories. Then associate the functions of each category with your client's wound characteristics.

Some wounds can be treated with a primary dressing only. This dressing contacts the wound bed. Other wounds may require a primary and secondary dressing. This is used to cover and retain the primary dressing.

Gauze is considered a traditional dressing. The product will offer numerous functions, depending on how it is used as a primary dressing.

Wet to dry gauze is used for removal of fibrin slough. The gauze is moistened with saline, fluffed, and placed on the wound bed to dry. When the gauze is removed, mechanical debridement takes place; slough and granular tissue adhere to the interstices of the gauze. This is a nonselective debridement.

Wet to moist gauze is used to keep the wound bed moist. The gauze is dampened with normal saline, fluffed, and placed on the wound bed. Removal of the gauze in a moist state spares some disruption of granular tissue.

Another function of wet to moist gauze is to obliterate dead space such as undermining, tunneling, and space in deep wounds. Wet to dry dressing changes are not recommended for granular wounds. This treatment is ineffective for the removal of black eschar.

Calcium alginate's primary function is to absorb exudate. When the dressing comes in contact with wound fluid, it transforms into a gel. This dressing is effective in preventing maceration. Calcium alginates will fill dead space and maintain moisture over the wound bed. Calcium alginates can be used and are effective in supporting the proliferation of granular tissues. This moisture retention facilitates autolytic debridement and is indicated for use as a primary dressing for heavily exuding wounds or wounds with fibrin slough. A secondary dressing such as transparent film, hydrocolloid, or foam is necessary. This can remain in place for up to 4 days. Contraindications are wounds with small amounts of exudate or black eschar. Calcium alginate is made of natural fibers derived from seaweed.

Hydrocolloid dressings maintain a moist wound environment by absorbing and retaining wound fluid, which will promote autolytic debridement. This dressing is occlusive, meaning there is no vapor or oxygen exchange over the wound bed. A securely sealed hydrocolloid provides a barrier from contaminants such as feces or urine.

A hydrocolloid could be used as a primary dressing to granular or sloughing wounds with little depth. A deep wound can be filled with a hydrocolloid paste or a calcium alginate and covered with hydrocolloid as a secondary dressing. This may remain in place 3 to 5 days.

Hydrocolloid is contraindicated in infected wounds, or wounds with excessive amounts of thick slough and debris. It needs to be used with caution on the immunosuppressed client. Hydrocolloids comprise colloids, elastomers, and adhesives.

Hydrogel's primary function is to maintain moisture on the wound bed. This facilitates the proliferation of granulation and epithelial tissue. Hydrogels are soothing and do not adhere to the wound bed. Hydrogels are compatible with topical ointments such as antibiotics. Autolytic debridement of eschar and slough is enhanced with a hydrogel. It is often used as a space filler and may be used in combination with gauze to lightly pack undermining and tunneling.

The hydrogel is always used as a primary dressing, whether it is a hydrogel wafer or the viscous gel. There is a requirement for a secondary dressing to retain the gel in place. This could be a transparent film, foam wafer, hydrocolloid wafer, or an absorbent pad. Gels can be left in place for up to 3 days. Hydrogels are contraindicated for heavily exudating wounds. Avoid gel contact with periwound skin. Hydrogels comprise water or glycerin in a polymer formulation.

Transparent film traps wound exudate to hydrate necrotic tissue and promote autolytic debridement. It provides a barrier from feces and urine, but allows fluid vapor to pass into the environment. This dressing is adhesive and nonabsorbent.

Transparent film can be used as a primary dressing on partial thickness or stage I and II wounds. Visualization of the wound bed is possible without removal of the dressing. The dressing may remain in place up to 3 days. As a secondary dressing, film is used to retain a viscous hydrogel, calcium alginate, foam, or moist gauze. Films are not to be used as a primary dressing in a moderate to heavily draining wound. Films comprise adhesives, elastomers, and copolymers.

Foam dressings are highly absorbent, nonadhesive wafers. They maintain moisture on the wound bed and assist with autolytic debridement without damaging granulation tissue. Because foams are thick, they insulate and protect the wound.

Foams are used as a primary dressing on moderate to heavily draining wounds. Foam can be used as a secondary dressing over hydrogel or calcium alginate. This dressing can remain in place up to 5 days, depending on the amount of exudate. Foam should not be used on dry eschar, or on wounds with small amounts of exudate. Foam is a hydrophilic polyurethane wafer.

See Tables 21-1 and 21-2 for wound care products and treatments.

text continued on page 483

Table 21-1
Wound Care Products and Treatments

Dressing	Function	Indications/Benefit	Practical Consideration
Wet to dry gauze	Nonselective mechanical debridement Absorb exudate Fill dead space	Presence of fibrin slough Does not spare granulation tissue Moderate to heavy drainage Deep or large wound Tunneling or undermining	Must be done daily, increases cost of service Dry cells repair and migrate more slowly than moist ones Gauze packing strips are good tunnels
Wet to moist	Provide moisture to wound bed Minimal absorption Fills dead space	Granulating wound Small to moderate drainage Deep or large wound Tunneling or undermining	Wound will appear larger as necrosis is removed
Hydrocolloid (colloids, elastomers, and adhesive)	Autolytic debridement Maintains exudate on wound bed Spares granulation tissue Occludes the wound Provides barrier to contaminants Moderate absorption Self-adhesive	Necrotic wounds Enhances cell migration Granulating wounds Use in presence of incontinence on noninfected wounds Slight to moderate drainage Avoids skin damage due to tape	Lifted edges will offer pathway for contamination Excessive drainage will lift dressing out of place Do not remove prematurely—tugging may damage peri-wound skin Apply liquid barrier film Can leave in place up to 5 days

Dressing	Function	Indications	Application
Foam (hydrophilic polyurethane wafer)	Can be used as secondary dressing with filler as primary Highly absorbent Protects granulation tissue Maintains a moist wound bed Supports autolytic debridement Protects wound base from trauma To fill space	Undermined or tunneled wound Moderate to high exudating wounds Granulating wounds Enhances cell migration Use full-thickness wounds Stages II, III, IV	If foam becomes saturated with exudate, change so as to prevent maceration Soft-conforming Secure with tape, nets, or montgomery straps Do not use on eschar Up to 5 days
Hydrogel (water or glycerin, polymer formulation)	Provide moisture toward bed Soothing Nonadherent Minimal to nonabsorptive Compatible with topical antibiotics Autolytic debridement of eschar and slough	Granulating wounds Epithelial wounds Small to moderate exudate Partial-/full-thickness wounds Necrotic wounds Stages II, III, IV	Not for large exudate Secondary dressing foam–hydrocolloid ABD pad Avoid periwound contact Up to 3 days

continued

Table 21-1
Wound Care Products and Treatments Continued

Dressing	Function	Indications/Benefit	Practical Consideration
Calcium Alginate (derived from seaweed, natural fiber)	Highly absorbent Forms gel over wound bed Nonadherent Fills dead space Autolytic debridement	Moderate to high exudating wounds Spares granulation tissue Maintains a moist wound bed Protects granulation tissue Stages II to IV PTW FTW	Prevent maceration May dehydrate a slightly exuding wound
Transparent Films (elostomers, copolymers)	Autolytic debridement Collects wound fluid Hydrates the wound bed Permeable to vapors Provides a barrier to contaminants	Use on fibrin slough Debridement of slough Debridement of eschar Facilitates granulation Epithelialization Protect from soiling, urine, stool Primary dressing on stages I, II PTW Secondary dressing to secure clacium alginate, gauze, hydrogel, or foam Stages III, IV FTW	Effective in softening eschar Excessive exudate will cause maceration Able to visualize wound bed Up to 3 days

Table 21-2
Wound Healing Progression

Initial Assessment	2 to 3 Weeks Later	4 to 6 Weeks Later	6 to 8 Weeks Later
Size: 4 × 6 × 0.5 cm	3 × 5 × 1 cm	1 × 4 × 5 cm	0.5 × 1.5 × < 0.1 cm
Undermine: 3 cm 1 to 5 o'clock	2 cm 1 to 5 o'clock	0	0
Tunnel: 4 cm 11 o'clock	3.5 cm 11 o'clock	1 cm	0
Slough: 60% yellow, thin, loose	0	0	0
Granulation: 40%	100%	100%	100%
Epithelium: 0	1 cm	2 to 3 cm	2.5 to 5.5 cm
Exudate: Moderate, serous sanquinous	Moderate to large, yellow and thick	Slight to moderate, serous	Slight serous
Periwound: Macerated	Clear	Clear	Clear
Treatment: Irrigate with normal saline	Continue same treatment	Discontinue irrigation	Prepare for discharge
Remove slough			Continue treatment to closure
Cleanse and hydrate wound bed			Instruct client that area is fragile and should be protected
Stimulate circulation			Continue use of seat cushion

continued

Table 21-2
Wound Healing Progression   Continued

Initial Assessment	2 to 3 Weeks Later	4 to 6 Weeks Later	6 to 8 Weeks Later
Primary dressing: Calcium alginate	Calcium alginate	Calcium alginate	
Autolytic debridement	No longer need autolytic debridement	Dead space filled with granulation	
Highly absorbent	Continue need for absorption	Exudate diminished	
Fills dead space	Fill dead space		
Secondary dressing: Hydrocolloid wafer	Same	Continue hydrocolloid	
Provides barrier to contaminants		Provide moisture to wound bed	
Self-adhesive and long wear time		Absorb exudate	
Liquid barrier film to periwound		Provide barrier to contaminants	
Safeguards skin from denuding on removal		Continue irrigation	
Frequency: Three times/week		Cleanse and hydrate Stimulate circulation	

Reimbursement

Caring for wounds is costly. All payors—Medicare, Medicaid, Blue Cross, HMOs, managed care companies—are seeking to institute cost containment measures. As a nurse, it is your vivid, objective, factual, accurate, and consistent documentation that will make the insurance industry responsive to clients' needs by reimbursing for services needed.

Thorough documentation of the wound is the best protection for the client and your home care agency. There are many formats of documentation: narrative, focus charting, computerized, S.O.A.P. (Subjective, Objective, Assessment, and Plan), and so forth. Regardless of the format used, the key elements of wound assessment must be included. The record and all its documentation becomes a permanent legal document accessible to many for different purposes—research, litigation, and reimbursement. Let your contribution in the area of wound care stand on its own as thorough, accurate, complete, and objective.

Case Study

You have just received your first referral as a home care nurse. The information from the hospital states that Mr. J is 76 years old. He has a sacral pressure ulcer. He was admitted with a hypoglycemic episode; glucose is now stabilized at a range of 130 to 150. He is able to self-inject 12 units NPH insulin in the morning. Mr. J is 6'1" and weighs 150 pounds. Wound care orders are to clean wound with H_2O_2 and cover with wet to dry gauze using normal saline. You call Mr. J and

484 o UNIT 3 Clinical Challenges

make arrangements to see him early in the morning, before the insulin is administered.

When you arrive, Mrs. J, who is 72 years old, opens the door and states, "I am so glad you're here . . . the hospital told me you would help with the sore." Mrs. J escorts you to the kitchen. Mr. J is sitting in a foam donut cushion (not recommended) and is demanding his breakfast. Mrs. J states that she has been handling Mr. J's insulin for quite some time because he tends to be forgetful (mental status). You observe Mrs. J test the blood glucose and administer the insulin. Mrs. J demonstrates competency in these procedures.

Mr. J enjoys a breakfast of one hard boiled egg, one piece toast and jelly, and coffee with milk. Mrs. J states that Mr. J used to have a better appetite. She agrees to record the foods he eats over the next 3 days (nutritional assessment).

You note that Mrs. J assists Mr. J from the chair. She states, "That hospitalization seems to have weakened my husband" (mobility impairment). As you walk down the hall with them, you continue to observe for other problems.

Mr. J begins to hurry. Mrs. J asks, "Do you need the bottle?" (incontinence). Mrs. J states that her husband has accidents because he cannot get to the toilet fast enough.

As you prepare Mr. J for a thorough skin assessment, Mrs. J says that she is overwhelmed and exhausted. "Now that he is weak, I have to bathe him, run for the bottle, wash extra laundry. I need a little help until he's back on his feet" (activities of daily living deficiency). When you inquire of family members, their only daughter lives 120 miles away and visits once a month (support systems).

Mrs. J is looking forward to her husband's recovery so they can travel to their daughter's home and visit with their grandchild (attitude).

You invite Mrs. J to participate in the implementation of infection control principles, such as handwashing and waste disposal. Mrs. J is willing to learn skin inspection and pressure relief principles, but cannot bring herself to touch the dressing. The following display shows Mr. J.'s wound assessment and documentation:

Mr. J's Wound Assessment and Documentation
Location: sacrum   *Stage:* III
Size: length 4 cm; width 6 cm; depth .5 cm
Margins: smooth even
Undermining: 3 cm 1 to 5 o'clock
Tunneling: 4 cm 11 o'clock   *Sinus tract:* none
Granulation: 40% pink to red   *Epithelialization:* none
Fibrin Slough: 60% yellow, thin, and loose
Exudate: moderate serous sanquinous saturates dressing
Periwound: macerated, white soft skin
Erythema: none   *Induation:* none

You call the doctor with your findings and recommendations:

Nutrition:	Multivitamin qd
	Vitamin C 500 mg bid
Mobility:	Physical therapy
	Home exercise program

continued

ADL:	Home health aide 5 x wk, 4 hr/day for personal care
Equipment:	Specialty seat cushion
Wound Treatment:	D/C H_2O_2
	Irrigate wound with normal saline
	Use 35-cc syringe with 19-g needle to promote mechanical debridement and circulation
	Primary dressing: calcium alginate for absorption, autolytic debridement, and fill dead space
	Secondary dressing: hydrocolloid wafer barrier to contamination—less frequent changes

Periwound protection: Liquid skin barrier application per dressing change

Skilled nursing visits: Reduce to three times a week (tiw).

The physician approves of your plan and agrees to sign orders (Health Care Financing Administration [HCFA] 485). You inform Mr. and Mrs. J of the new care plan. They are pleased and eager to participate.

22

Hospice Services for Home Care Clients

Eileen M. Hanley, RN, BSN, MBA

This chapter discusses the philosophy of hospice care and how hospice services are organized in the United States. Additionally, the chapter discusses the services provided through hospice programs and the clients best suited for hospice services. Included also is discussion of the needs of the terminally ill client at home and the role of the hospice nurse.

PHILOSOPHY

The term *hospice* originated in the Middle Ages and was used to describe places where travelers could find respite and rest from their journeys. The relationship to a journey is important to the modern interpretation of the word *hospice* as well. Those who work in the hospice field believe that their role is to assist the dying throughout this journey and to support them and their loved ones during this process. This is a process that begins with the acknowledgment that perhaps a change in the goal of treatment should be considered. This process requires a redefining of the purpose of treatment from one of curative treatment to one that emphasizes comfort and symptom control and support for these objectives.

The philosophy behind hospice care is that of offering comfort to those who are dying. Based on a belief that death is experienced on many levels and in many different ways, hospice promotes an interdisciplinary approach to care of the terminally ill. Although most people think of the physical symptoms that clients may experience, such as pain or respiratory distress, when they think of the focus of care for the terminally ill, for many it is the psychological and spiritual suffering that may be of greater concern. The hospice philosophy also believes that support is necessary for the family and loved ones of the person who is dying; therefore, the "client" of the hospice program is the client *and* family.

Contrary to popular belief, a person selecting hospice care is not "giving up." A common fallacy regarding hospice services is that programs will require that clients discontinue all treatments and medications. This creates an anxiety that clients will be left in pain or discomfort. Hospice programs take an aggressive approach to maximizing the quality of life for those who are dying. A common maxim of hospice care is that although hospice cannot add days to the client's life, it can add life to their days. Hospice is a program that offers the opportunity for more to be done for the client and caregivers than any other program can offer when the goal of treatment is comfort and not cure.

This is particularly important for nurses to understand, because one of the greatest frustrations nurses have in caring for the terminally ill is that they feel they have no hope to offer the client. Nurses have a lot to offer dying clients, but it requires that we think differently about the purpose of our work.

Another aspect of the hospice philosophy is that of caregiver support. Although it is not a federal regulation that there is an informal caregiver involved, some programs do require this. The purpose of the caregiver is to render custodial services and to support the client in the event that he or she can no longer participate in the care and to assist the client with decision making about their care.

Hospice care recognizes the significant role caregivers play in the care of their loved ones. Family members are often anxious about their ability to care for their dying loved one, but they want to fulfill the wishes of the dying person to remain at home. The reality is that these caregivers, with the support of the hospice program, are often able to maintain the person at home and are very pleased that they were able to accommodate their loved ones' wishes. Some hospice programs have developed supportive care for those clients who may have no caregivers involved.

Client autonomy is another major characteristic of the hospice philosophy. The ability of the client/family to direct the care begins with the choice to enter into a hospice program and continues throughout the time spent on the program. An informed consent is required for admission into hospice care. The content of the consent may vary depending on the program, but at a minimum, it requires that the client is aware that the hospice program will not take any means to prolong life or hasten death.

A hospice program cannot require a do-not-resuscitate (DNR) order as a point of admission. Many programs will encourage clients and families to discuss their feelings about advance directives. Because of the need for informed consent, it is of utmost importance for the home care nurse to accurately describe the benefits of the hospice program and be able to answer the questions about hospice services.

The client/family participates in the development of the plan of care by deciding which services they will take advantage of and how they wish the care to be rendered. For example, although there are many different disciplines and supports available, the client may not wish to avail himself or herself of all of these benefits. This is acceptable and not a reason to discontinue service of the program.

HOSPICE MODEL OF CARE

Hospice services in the United States are organized under the auspices of the Health Care Financing Administration in the form of Medicare certification. Certified hospice programs are organized and regulated as a separate entity from home care, although most services are provided in the home care setting.

Hospice programs have different standards and regulations, which are not interchangeable with those of Certified Home Health Agencies (CHHA). Although hospice started as a voluntary grassroots movement in this country, the federal government formalized the Hospice Medicare benefit in 1985. Since that time, only programs that are certified by Medicare can use the term *hospice* to define their services for the terminally ill. Other health care entities may provide care to the terminally ill and promote similar services as certified programs. These are often referred to as *palliative care programs*.

Hospice care as defined by Medicare is an interdisciplinary model of care that offers palliative care or alleviation of symptoms and support over a continuum of sites and over time. Hospice is unique because, although most services are provided in the client's home, the hospice is also responsible for care in the inpatient setting. Hospice care also can be provided in skilled nursing facilities. The purpose of the hospice service is to insure that clients and their families have access to expert pain and symptom control and spiritual and psychological support services.

Below are the core services that make up the **hospice interdisciplinary team:**

Team coordinator
Registered nurse
Physician
Social worker
Pastoral care counselor
Volunteer
Home health aide
Bereavement counselor

Other professionals that may be used intermittently include:

Occupational therapist
Music therapist
Nutritionist
Physical therapist
Recreational therapist

One of the greatest benefits of hospice services to the client and family is that most hospice insurance plans include reimbursement for medications, durable medical equipment, and supplies related to the terminal illness. This benefit can be an enormous cost saver for the client and family, because medications can be very expensive, and most other insurances do not cover prescriptions nor many of the supplies needed.

Some unique features of certified hospice programs follow.

Inpatient Services

Certified hospice programs are also responsible for providing inpatient care for short-term acute medical needs related to the terminal illness and for respite for family caregivers. Hospice programs administered by a home care agency or administered as an independent free-standing program may contract with a local hospital or develop a free-standing unit for inpatient services.

In hospital-based programs, the hospice will usually have a designated unit within the hospital for this service. Inpatient care is used for short-term stays during periods of crisis or medical management. It also may be used for respite purposes when the family caregiver needs a rest from the stresses of managing the client at home.

Typical reasons for using the inpatient unit include: symptom management, such as transfusion or acute and intractable pain, or care for a client who is actively dying and the family can no longer manage the client at home. When the client is in the inpatient unit, members of the hospice team will continue to visit and supervise the client's care, ensuring that the hospice plan of care is being followed. Hospice inpatient care will provide medical treatments and other treatments only as necessary. Routine diagnostic tests are typically not ordered unless necessary to treat the client palliatively. Every effort is made to make the client's stay as comfortable and homelike as possible.

Bereavement Services

One of the most unique aspects of certified hospice programs is the inclusion of bereavement services for the caregivers for a year after the death of the client. In most home care programs, services are immediately discontinued when the client dies. Because there is no reimbursement mechanism for counseling services to family and caregivers after the death of the client, the nurse is unable to offer the family support services. This often leads to feelings of frustration and abandonment in the home care nurse. However, in hospice, bereavement services are made available in some form to the immediate support system of that client.

Volunteer Services

The hospice movement began as a volunteer movement when concerned individuals began programs to care for the dying in a more humane and compassion-

ate way. When the federal government showed interest in formalizing the model, the founders of hospice
in the United States ensured that the volunteer component remained an essential part of the program.
Today, the use of volunteers is mandated for certified
hospice programs. Volunteers serve a variety of functions in hospice programs. They provide professional
visits, consultation, pastoral care, or bereavement
counseling. Some may function as respite workers,
friendly visitors, or telephone reassurance. Others
may help the program in administrative ways, such as
office operations and fund raising.

Volunteers are critical members of the interdisciplinary team. Their documentation of their encounters with clients and family is considered part of the
medical record. It is not unusual for the volunteer to
be the team member that perhaps has the most mean-
ingful relationship with the client and family. In addition, the volunteer may be the one person who can
have the greatest impact on the family and enhance
the care rendered by other members of the team.

Reimbursement

Under the Medicare hospice benefit, there are four
levels of care, each associated with a daily or per diem
rate. The hospice program is based on the type of reimbursement whereby hospice programs must manage the care needs of the client within a limited reimbursement rate. In hospice, the program must
manage all of the care needs of the client within one
of the four rates associated with the level of care.

The four levels of reimbursement include a routine home care day, a continuous care day, inpatient

general, and inpatient respite. Each of these rates is determined on a regional basis. The model of hospice reimbursement could be said to be a precursor of what managed care companies are trying to do with capitated models of reimbursement.

WHAT ARE THE NEEDS OF THE TERMINALLY ILL?

Physical Needs

Most often when we think of the dying, we think of their pain. Although it is true that pain is certainly one of the more common symptoms of those dying of cancer and other diseases, it is not the only physical symptom that accompanies the advanced stages of illness. Often the client manifests other physical signs, such as nausea and vomiting, severe constipation, respiratory distress, or insomnia. There may be psychological or neurological symptoms such as depression, confusion, anxiety, and agitation. In other words, the terminally ill can manifest an infinite variety of symptoms, all of which require aggressive management to try to add quality to their days.

Aggressive management means frequent assessment of response to treatment and adjustment of dosages and regimens. In hospice, it is not unusual for clients to be monitored every few hours for their response to a particular drug regimen so that the prescription can be quickly modified to relieve pain. This assessment is often handled by frequent phone calls during the day to ascertain whether the medication is effective. This aggressive management also means that a variety of methods are used to alleviate symptoms. Hospice programs have vast experience in finding the right combinations of medications that can best meet the increasing and changing needs of the terminally ill client. As a nurse caring for the dying client with pain, you will have to consistently assess the client's response to the medications and communicate with the physician for necessary changes in dosages or medications. Although most programs may have protocols in place, it will always be the attending physician who will direct the pain management and other care rendered. The nurses may use the protocols to discuss pain management with the attending physician.

A Special Word About Pain Assessment

Although not every client will manifest signs of pain, it is important to try to quantify as objectively as possible the client's level of pain, the interventions used, and the response to the interventions. Most hospice programs will use some tool that helps the nurse measure the client's level of pain. These are usually client self-assessments that use a scale of 0 to 10, with 0 being the absence of pain and 10 being the worst pain the client has ever had. Some scales can use faces or colors to help the client describe the pain. These tools should be used together with the staff's clinical observation of the client, so that there can be some comparison and basis for intervention in cases in which there appear to be discrepancies between the stated levels of pain and the observed levels of pain. Clients may understate or overstate their pain for a variety of reasons. It is also not uncommon for family members to interpret the client's pain and medicate them or withhold medication based on their belief of what is best for the client. In such situations, the nurse's assessment and observational skills are critical to adequate symptom control.

There can be many reasons for inconsistencies; however, the important thing is for the hospice team to be aware of any problems and patterns in assessing pain. Using a tool is helpful in minimizing discrepancies that may occur when different team members are making the visits. A consistent and documented assessment of pain will enable the hospice program to monitor the effectiveness of interventions.

Most hospice programs will use specific protocols, depending on the specific type of pain and other symptoms that may be accompanying the pain. These protocols are usually based on the preferences of the medical director of the hospice program. It is safe to say that most hospice programs take a low-tech approach to pain to achieve adequate comfort levels. Programs use intravenous drips or client-controlled analgesia pumps if that is an effective means.

Although the reliance on medications is primarily for the alleviation of symptoms, the use of other means such as massage, therapeutic touch, prayer, music, or meditation is encouraged as well. Before the more emotional or spiritual needs of the client can be met, they must be made physically comfortable. The client may be in need of other forms of nursing care, for instance, those associated with wound management or infusion therapies.

Psychological/Spiritual Needs

Clients may be pain free but continue to suffer terribly because they have a psychic or spiritual pain that may only be relieved by the intervention of counseling. This is why an interdisciplinary approach is so important in the care of the dying.

A thorough assessment of the client and family's psychosocial and spiritual needs should be made by a qualified pastoral or psychological counselor. This assessment should be discussed with the attending physician and other members of the interdisciplinary team to identify the best means of addressing the problem.

THE ROLE OF THE HOME CARE NURSE

As a home care nurse, you may be the first person to consider that hospice may be an appropriate program for your clients. Many professionals feel uncomfortable bringing the subject of hospice up with their clients. They think that they are telling clients that there is no longer any hope. This is not true. When clients are at the point of deciding on whether to continue curative treatment, they are most in need of knowledgeable advice and someone who can offer them hope for comfort.

Clients who have decided they no longer want to aggressively treat their disease may still want aggressive treatment of their symptoms. They are afraid that they will be in pain and discomfort, and they are anxious about what the next months will be like. They are also afraid of being abandoned by friends and family. Most importantly, they want to make the time they have remaining as good as it can be. They want to be comfortable enough to be able to spend time with their children and friends. They want to know that their life has had meaning, and that they will be missed.

It is the nurse's responsibility to inform clients/ families of what their choices are. If the hospice program can offer services and benefits that a client cannot obtain from regular home care service, it would be less than adequate nursing care to withhold that information from the client. Many home care nurses believe that they provide hospice care because they care for people who are dying.

There is more to hospice care than the services of the nurse and a home health aide. There is also more to care of the dying than meeting their physiologic needs. Care of the dying offers nurses the opportunity to practice in a holistic manner, responding to the psychological and spiritual needs of the client as well as to their physical needs. This is best done using an interdisciplinary approach. It can become very overwhelming for the nurse to attempt to meet all the needs of the client/family without additional support. It would be inappropriate to begin discussions of hospice care with a client or family that has not been given a limited prognosis or who are not ready for this discussion. You may want to approach the subject if the client:

Does not want any more hospital admissions

Is not receiving adequate pain or symptom management

Is concerned about the need to care for unfinished business

May be seeking out opportunities to discuss spiritual issues

Wants to stop aggressive curative treatment

Is incurring overwhelming costs for medications and
supplies

or if

The caregiver is feeling increasing difficulty in managing the client

The nurse is having increasing difficulty in finding
resources to help with the management of the
client's needs or is finding that it is impossible to
coordinate all the resources needed

The nurse believes the type of support needed cannot
be offered

When the above issues are detected, it may indicate that there may be a shift in focus in the client's
expectations and goals of care. This may change your
relationship with the client. Suddenly, because the
client and family are beginning to accept the in-
evitability of the client's death, your role as the nurse
coordinating the care will change. It is important for
you to be able to remain objective while supporting
the client, family, and their needs. This can be very
difficult for the nurse in home care for the following
reasons:

You may be in conflict with the client's wishes about
ceasing curative care.

Certified home care programs do not support long-
term care unless there is a skilled need (hospice
does not require this).

Most home care programs do not have access to the
other disciplines that are most needed by the terminally ill, such as psychological and spiritual
counseling.

Productivity expectations of most home care nurses
do not allow for long extended visits that may be
occasionally necessary with the terminally ill.
You may believe that you do not have the expertise to
meet the needs of the client or the support you
think necessary to enable you to do this type of
work.
You may feel conflicted about the decision to transfer
the client to a hospice program resulting in discharging the client from your care.

The nurse may be in the position of teaching the
physician about hospice services. Hospice programs
encourage clients to retain their attending physicians.
The role of the hospice medical director and team
physicians is that of consultation to the attending
physicians when requested and to ensure that the
client is an appropriate hospice client.

Although anyone can make a referral to a hospice
program, including the client and family, eventually it
is necessary to speak with the physician regarding the
client's eligibility. Hospice programs must confirm
the prognosis with the client's physician. If the home
care nurse finds resistance from the physician regarding the need for hospice services yet the client does
have a life expectancy of 6 months or less and is seeking a palliative course of treatment, it is appropriate
to leave literature for the client/family and inform
them of their options. Hospice programs can call
physicians and usually help to minimize their concerns.

Should the client and family decide that a hospice program is not what they want, then you must
help them find other resources to supplement nursing
services. It will be important for the nurse to find

other ways to help support the client/family needs while maintaining the ability to handle the stresses of caring for the client.

The client will need the nurse to help facilitate access to social work counseling to help with end-of-life care issues such as guardianship issues, funeral planning, or family counseling, as well as anticipatory grief work. The client also may need access to a lawyer and religious support. Additionally, you will most likely have frequent conversations with the attending physician to manage the increasingly complex symptoms that often accompany the more advanced stages of illness.

HOSPICE PROCEDURES

Admission Criteria

- Physician is willing to certify that the client has a prognosis of 6 months or less
- Client is seeking a palliative course of treatment
- Client or their health care proxy is willing to sign an informed consent, which acknowledges that the hospice program will not take any measures that will prolong life or hasten death
- Willingness of client to participate in the plan of care
- Clients with any terminal illness (including the terminal phases of chronic illness such as acquired immune deficiency syndrome, amyotrophic lateral sclerosis)

Certain criteria will differ among programs, such as:

Care to children
Infusion services
Palliative chemotherapy or radiation
Nursing home care
Day care
Need for caregiver living with the client

If you have questions about the particular admission criteria of your local hospice program, information about the hospice program in your community can be obtained from the National Hospice Organization (1-800-658-8898). Each state has a hospice organization that can also serve as a resource for professionals as well as families. Encourage family members to call different hospice programs in the community to see which they think will best meet their needs.

Not every community will have a choice of programs, but if so, there may be subtle differences among the programs that may be important to the client/family. For instance, some hospice programs may be run by religious affiliations. The client may be concerned about which hospital is used for in-client care or the type of volunteer and bereavement services offered. You as the nurse could call the hospice programs and ask for material that can be given to the client/family for review.

Referral Procedures

Once you have identified the hospice program that you would like the client to consider, the hospice program will need to know the following information:

Client demographics such as the name, significant other contact information, address

Diagnosis and prognosis

Physician data

Insurance

The client's care needs, for example, wound care, infusions, medications, or any other treatments

Once received, the hospice program will use this information to contact the physician regarding his or her willingness to participate in the plan of care and their willingness to certify the 6-month prognosis of the client

The hospice program will also want to confirm with the insurance company that the client has a hospice benefit or that the insurance company is willing to reimburse for this service

The hospice program will also want to confirm with the client and family their interest in the hospice program and their willingness to accept the hospice program

Assessment

The first visit by the hospice nurse is an evaluation visit, where the nurse explains the program in greater detail and answers any questions about the program for the client and family. The team member making the first visit should also speak with the intake staff who took the referral to determine the level of knowledge and anxiety of the client and family. It is also helpful to ensure that the primary caregiver will be present for the first visit. Another suggestion is to ask the family to gather all medications and important papers such as health care proxy or DNR forms or communications from the physicians and have them available for the nurse to review at the time of the visit. It may be useful to try to interview the client and family separately as well as jointly. This helps the nurse get a truly accurate picture of what is happening. Sometimes clients and families will try to protect one another from the truth and need and want some privacy. It is also beneficial to see how they communicate with one another. In certain cases, it has been found helpful to have the nurse and social worker make a joint visit. This is most helpful in circumstances in which there may be some discrepancy between the concerns of the family or caregiver and the client or perhaps hesitation on the part of the client to accept hospice or situations in which there may be other social or family concerns. Clients must sign an informed consent if he or she wants to come onto the program. At that visit, the hospice nurse does a thorough assessment of the clinical and psychological needs of the client/family. The following information is what should be covered in the interview:

Medical surgical history

Prescription and nonprescription medications currently being taken

Other treatments used for symptom control

Response to medications and treatments

Is the client self-administering medications, or is the family responsible for this?

Feelings about future hospitalizations (are they willing to be admitted to hospice inpatient unit or prefer another facility, or do they not want hospitalization at all?)

Goals for treatment (palliative or curative)

Knowledge about diagnosis and prognosis (nurse will have to be sensitive when broaching this subject with client and family members, who may not be aware of true prognosis and diagnosis)

What services do they wish from the hospice program?

What are the needs of the caregiver?

What is the family constellation, and what are the concerns of the family and client toward each other?

Are they interested in spiritual or volunteer services?

Are there any other community resources involved in the care of the client (eg, Meals on Wheels; telephone reassurance; religious affiliations)?

Wishes about advanced directives

Clients' and caregivers' emotional state and concerns

Caregivers' willingness and ability to participate in care

Once the nurse has elicited this information, he or she should begin to explain the benefits and policies of the hospice program. This would include the covered services; the financial responsibility if any of the client and family; what they can expect of the hospice team; what the expectations of the caregivers might be; what hospitals the hospice program uses for in-hospital care. The nurse should review the informed consent with the client or caregiver and answer any questions they might have.

If the nurse believes that the client may be eligible for the hospice program and the client and family are interested in accepting the hospice program, the nurse should follow agency policies. The nurse should confer with the other members of the interdisciplinary team to determine the eligibility of the client for acceptance into the program. It is important to attempt this conference during the home visit so that the client's care needs can be addressed immediately by the hospice program.

Additionally, during this time, the client and family often wish to think about whether this is the right program for them. Remember, client autonomy is a major belief of the hospice philosophy, and therefore it is always the client/family choice to come on or come off a hospice program.

If the client is on another type of home care program and the client/family does decide to enroll in the hospice program, the nurse will be required to discharge the client. Recently, some home care agency–based hospice programs have been experimenting with models that would allow the clients to maintain their relationship with their home care nurse and home health aide. Some hospice programs will offer support services to home care clients who do not want to sever their relationship with their nurses in the home care agency, so they will offer social work or pastoral care support. Other programs may offer hospice training for home care staff so that the nurse will meet the regulatory standards of the hospice program. The nurse could then be a member of the interdisciplinary team for that client only. You may want to check with your agency to see if any accommodations have been made to help bridge the gap between home care and hospice services.

The most important thing for the home care nurse to remember is to remain objective and help the client assess which program will best meet the client and family needs. Remember that hospice services can be most effective for all members of the family when a referral is made early enough for the client and family to take advantage of all of the services that the program has to offer.

Many times referrals are made only when the client is actively dying. When referrals are made so late, it usually means that the client has spent significant time in pain and discomfort, and the family has received little support. The interdisciplinary team can be most effective when they have several months to help the client. That is not to say that making a referral in the last few weeks or days of life is inappropriate. It is more appropriate to make the referral as early as possible, but it is never futile to make the referral. When clients are referred in the last few days of life, the hospice program offers crisis management rather than their more traditional care. For those families who are spending their last days and hours together, that is what is most needed at that point.

The nurse who is conducting the visit will set up the preliminary plan of care to address the immediate needs of the client and caregiver. This usually includes, at a minimum, getting medical equipment and supplies in the home, obtaining orders for pain medications and ensuring the delivery of the same, and arranging for personal care attendants. The nurse may need to consider the need for other services such as physical therapy, occupational therapy, or nutritional service. It must be remembered that these services should be considered not for restorative but for palliative purposes. Most frequently these services are used in short-term consultative basis.

On subsequent visits, the nursing staff and other team members will want to document and track the progression of the client's illness and response to interventions. It is important that all disciplines document accurately and thoroughly their findings of the client's status, the progression of disease, the interventions, and response to the same. Visit frequency is dependent on the needs of the client and the number of disciplines who are involved in the care of the client and family.

The interdisciplinary teams usually meet weekly to discuss the care needs of all of the clients. It is at this time that the team members discuss their individual findings and how their findings result in alterations or modifications to the plan of care. New goals may be developed, and unmet goals for comfort may need to be modified. It may be that new services will be put in place, such as volunteers or social work, when the client or family may have refused these services in the past. The team meeting ensures that all team members are familiar with every aspect of the client and caregivers needs so that when they need to cover for a vacationing staff member or if they are working on call they will be familiar with the case.

THE HOSPICE NURSE

Hospice nursing is an extremely satisfying career, professionally as well as personally. Job satisfaction tends to be very high, and the professionalism of hospice nurses serves as a model for the whole profession. It takes a very dedicated and skilled professional to meet the demands of this specialty, but with those demands come many rewards. It is critically important that the nurse working in hospice be emotionally mature enough to handle the demands of the role. Oftentimes the staff members that are most effective in doing this work are those who have experienced personal loss and have come to terms with their own beliefs about death and dying. It is important that team members' own beliefs not be imposed on their clients. If the staff have not worked out their own issues with death, it will be difficult for them to be effective in helping others to cope at this difficult time.

Hospice nurses spend their time visiting clients in their home and visiting the in-hospital units if their client is admitted to the facility. They are responsible for coordinating the physical aspects of care and for maintaining ongoing communication with the attending physicians about changes in the client's status and the need to modify medication regimens to achieve adequate symptom control.

Nurses who choose to work in a hospice setting will be an integral part of an interdisciplinary team approach. Managers recruit nurses who have a solid generalist background in medicine, oncology, or other acute care fields and who have excellent clinical assessment skills. It is preferable to have several years of experience before seeking a position in hospice care. It is also preferable that the nurse has some experience in home care because so much of the client's care is rendered in the home setting.

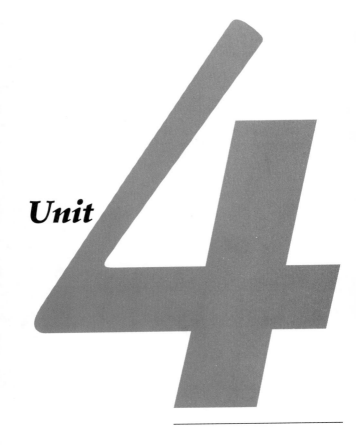

Unit

4

PROFESSIONAL ISSUES

23

Client Teaching and Learning

Patrice Kenneally Nicholas, RN, DNSc, ANP

This chapter discusses the process of teaching and learning in the home care setting. It involves all members of the health care team, the client, the family, or significant others. With decreased hospital length of stay and greater client acuity at discharge, client and family education in the home care setting is essential. The clients that we care for in the home often have chronic illnesses requiring long-term management. If the client has been hospitalized, he or she is frequently discharged earlier with more teaching needs. Teaching priorities must focus on assessing the client as a learner, planning and implementing the teaching, intervening when different types of learning problems exist, and evaluating the client's success in learning.

TEACHING AND LEARNING: WHAT ARE THEY?

In planning to teach clients in the home, it is necessary to consider their current diagnosis, medical history, current medications, level of orientation, and family supports. But first, we need to determine the roles of the teacher and the learner.

At the initial visit, the nurse meets the client, and at times the client's family or significant other. One of the most important aspects of the visit is determining what the nurse thinks the client needs to be taught and what the learner, the client, thinks he or she needs to learn. The nurse needs to evaluate the client by doing a full physical and mental assessment to see how involved the client is capable of being in the plan of care. The nurse also needs to evaluate how involved the client's spouse or family can be or how involved they want to be. If the nurse assesses that there is no one who is able to learn a procedure or technique, the nurse needs to visit until all skilled nursing needs are met. Teaching should still include the client and family member in every aspect of the plan of care.

Readiness to learn is a complex process involving the client's current knowledge, motivation for learning, anxiety level, and acceptance or denial of illness. An issue impacting on home care is what happens when you want to teach someone who does not want to learn. This is discussed later in the chapter, along with other approaches for teaching clients with disabilities or impairments that impact on learning.

The environment is another factor essential for successful teaching. The client needs to be involved in deciding the best place for teaching. A bright place with a clean surface and a table to allow for hands-on demonstration of material is helpful. Particular skills, such as wound care, insulin administration, and medication teaching, all require an environment that offers a comfortable place for the client and nurse to work together.

COLLABORATION BETWEEN NURSE AND CLIENT

If the process of collaboration works well for the client and nurse at the first visit, then it may be likely that teaching and learning can be achieved. It is helpful to include family members if they are committed to the client's health status, while acknowledging that sometimes the family's schedules or work are barriers to their involvement. Using written materials is a way of communicating with committed family members who cannot be present during the home visit. The first home visit enables the nurse to perform a family assessment while beginning to coordinate client education. Evaluating family dynamics, the availability of home and community resources, and teaching needs among family members is critical to the success of teaching in the home.

In some teaching situations, linking clients with similar diagnoses can support client education. The social support and education that occurs with two clients in a similar situation can facilitate the learning. Maintaining confidentiality is, of course, most important, but the client's awareness of other clients who are successfully dealing with a similar health problem may be helpful. This approach has been successfully used in teaching with older diabetics learning insulin administration. For the client beginning to learn the technique of drawing up and administering the insulin, meeting with another client who has accomplished insulin administration can facilitate the process. Although the nurse's role is pivotal, the experienced client often has tips for both medication and dietary management. Because hospitalized clients may receive teaching before discharge, coordination with the discharge planner may be helpful. The nurse should ask several important questions to assess the client's baseline knowledge and readiness to learn: What was he or she taught in the hospital or clinic? What does the client know about his or her illness? Does the client know his or her current medications? Is there specific diet teaching that has been done, or is needed? What is the client's understanding of the illness and teaching needs?

Clients who are referred for home care teaching from ambulatory settings by primary care providers will need coordination with the physician, nurse, and home health aide. The teaching plan and documentation will facilitate the continuity of care with all of the client's providers.

Collaborating in teaching in the home care setting may require working closely with other home care services, including intravenous (IV) therapy services, nutritional services, and other professional associations (eg, acquired immune deficiency syndrome [AIDS] support groups, American Diabetes Association, American Lung Association). Teaching in the home is optimal when all of the possible resources are brought together.

GOAL SETTING IN CLIENT EDUCATION

After the first visit, the nurse, client, and any involved family members should have agreed on a learning goal with specific achievable and measurable steps (behavioral objectives) for future home visits. If the client, nurse, and family are not in agreement, additional discussion by the nurse may be needed to clarify expectations and focus on the goal. Negotiation with all involved (nurse, client, family) may be necessary to achieve the goal. For example, the diabetic client who previously was managed on oral hypoglycemic agents and is now highly anxious about changing to insulin may need additional educational support to convey the knowledge about diabetes, its chronicity, and the need for the client to change to insulin from oral hypoglycemics.

The leap from oral agents to insulin administration can be a great adjustment for clients, requiring the support of all available resources. Asking the client what impact the change from oral medications to insulin injections will have is a good starting point. When we instruct the client, we must assess how motivated the client is to learn.

If there are any potential learning problems, such as visual or hearing impairment, cultural issues, anxiety, denial, or confusion, the nurse must plan the teaching to accommodate these problems. Following are examples of potential learning problems and suggestions for management. Acknowledging the learning problem will help the nurse and client to address the specific strategies that will help meet the learning goal.

The Client With Visual Impairment

For oral medications, a prefilled pill box can be used, which the nurse or family member prepares weekly. Teaching the client with a visual impairment requires auditory-oriented materials and verbal instructions. Also, using tapes with specific instructions can be helpful to reinforce the teaching. Using charts or graphs with large-type print is another strategy for the client who maintains some vision. Evaluating the teaching should be done orally, with the client telling the nurse verbally what he or she has learned.

The Client With Hearing Impairment

For the hearing-impaired client, using visual aids such as charts, graphs, and written material is necessary. The nurse should instruct the client in a quiet room and limit words to facilitate the client's understanding. All teaching must also be written, preferably with specific steps that the client can follow. Teaching films or videos are also available from some agencies that are specifically geared to the learning needs of the hearing-impaired client. To evaluate the teaching, ask the client to verbally describe what he or she learned or to write down what was learned.

Cultural Issues

If English is not the client's primary language, the teaching plan should include having written teaching materials available in the client's primary language. Using an interpreter (who may be a family member) may be necessary to accomplish the teaching. Planning what you want to teach ahead of time can limit the possibility of misinterpretation by the client.

Because culture is an important influence in approaching client teaching, being knowledgeable about the client's culture is important. Although the nurse cannot become knowledgeable about all of the ethnocultural groups in the United States, becoming familiar with specific beliefs, practices, and traditions will help the teaching and learning process.

The Anxious Client

For the anxious client, several cues may be evident that will indicate to the nurse that the anxiety must be minimized before teaching can take place. Some of the cues to anxiety are that the client does not seem to be paying attention, or repeatedly asks the same questions over again. Anxiety may also be evident when the client tries to perform a repeat demonstration of a technique that the nurse has taught and the client is not able to accomplish the steps in the order that the nurse has taught. With insulin administration, for example, anxiety may manifest itself with an inability of the client to go from drawing up the insulin to the actual administration of the injection. Using written teaching materials with sequentially numbered steps for accomplishing the goal will reduce anxiety and reinforce the goal.

The Client in Denial

For the client in denial, the nurse may need to visit more often than originally planned. Acknowledging that the nurse's beliefs may not be the same as the client's beliefs is important. If the client needs to receive medication and is in denial, the nurse should administer the medication while working with the client and family to help them to acknowledge the health issue. Often negotiation is necessary to help a client move from denial to acceptance of his or her illness. The nurse cannot walk in to the client's home and expect to change behavior immediately. For example, the client with hypertension who needs to stop smoking should be approached with a realistic plan for decreasing smoking. The nurse may help the client who states that he or she wants to reduce his or her smoking by asking, "Instead of smoking 20 cigarettes today, do you think that you could reduce your smoking to 18 cigarettes?" It also would be helpful to ask the client to keep a diary for 1 week to write down the situations in which he or she smokes. Then the nurse can propose alternatives to smoking based on the particular circumstances.

SETTING GOALS IN TEACHING AND LEARNING

On completion of the first visit, the nurse, client, and family members should have agreed on a learning goal or goals with specific achievable and measurable steps for the next home visits. Frequently a learning contract is prepared by the nurse and client, which is a written contract with specific steps for achieving the goal. Although learning contracts are not required to be written, it is often helpful to have a written form that identifies the specific goal and the steps to achieve the goal. The specific timeframe for accomplishing the goal also can be written so that there is an awareness of when the goal should be completed. The learning contract may assist with required documentation for client teaching to be reimbursed as well. Further client teaching is frequently underdocumented, and the learning contract will provide a measurable tool to assist the nurse with documentation. The written learning contract will assist the nurse and client in staying within the planned number of visits for reimbursement eligibility.

THE LEARNING CONTRACT

Preparing a learning contract may make teaching in the home care setting easier for the nurse and client. It should be clearly identified as a contract between the nurse and client. The specific goal should be detailed first, and the steps or objectives for achieving the goal should be listed next. The nurse and client should agree on the target dates for achieving the objectives and the goal. Any specific interventions that the nurse and client must achieve should be outlined in the contract. The nurse and client should sign the learning contract to assure commitment to the goal and the timeframe for completion of the goal. The learning contract then provides a vehicle for the nurse and client to plan for each visit, to assess the steps to achieving each goal, and to reevaluate the progress in meeting the goal. Display 23-1 illustrates a learning contract that can be used for teaching in the home. The contract focuses each visit with measurable steps to achieve the ultimate goal. The final step is identifying a realistic timeframe for achieving the goal.

DISPLAY 23-1. **Example of a Learning Contract for the Home Care Setting**

Client Name: Nurse: Family:
Medical history:
Current medical/nursing status:
Medications:
Date:
Other health care providers involved in teaching/
   learning:
Goal: (Must include a measurable timeframe)

• Any educational needs or supports necessary for
  nurse and client to achieve the goal
• Specific steps or objectives to achieve the goal with
  measurable timeframes

A CLINICAL EXAMPLE OF TEACHING USING A LEARNING CONTRACT

The following clinical example will illustrate the application of teaching. The clinical example includes a case study with an individualized learning contract.

A Visually Impaired Client With Hypertension

A 46-year-old woman was diagnosed 2 years ago with a history of hypertension. She was found to have a blood pressure of 150/90 mm Hg at her

text continued on page 525

DISPLAY 23-2. **Learning Contract**

Client name: Nurse:
                                                Family member:

Medical history: Visual impairment due to cataracts

Current medical/nursing problems: Hypertension × 2 years, nonadherence with medicaion in the past, and a lack of knowledge about foods to snack on

Medications: Lasix 40 mg A.M. and 20 mg P.M.

Other health care providers involved in teaching/learning: Pharmacist

Goals:

1. Client will follow antihypertensive medication regimen by the second nursing visit.

2. Client will understand the dietary restrictions of a 2-g sodium, 150-mg cholesterol diet by the 3rd visit.

3. Client will understand potential complications of hypertension by the 4th visit.

continued

DISPLAY 23-2. Learning Contract Continued

Specific steps (behavioral objectives) to achieve goals:

- The nurse will instruct about need, action, and side effects of Lasix.
- The nurse will teach client to recognize medication by pill size or shape.
- The nurse will use pill box with mealtime slots with large type for visually impaired.
- The nurse will monitor client's adherence to medications by checking pill box at each visit.
- The nurse will instruct client on 2-g sodium, 150-mg cholesterol diet. (Begin with a diet history, as illustrated in Display 23-3.).
- The nurse will identify what client perceives as motivators and barriers to adhering to the diet.
- The nurse will instruct on the potential complications of hypertension, including cardiovascular effects, renal effects, and visual effects.

Signatures: Nurse: _____ Client: _____ Family: _____
Date by which goals will be achieved: _____

DISPLAY 23-3. **Diet History for the Home Care Client**

Client name:
Nurse:
Family/significant other:
Medical/nursing diagnoses:
Type of diet required:
Height:
Weight:
Frame (small, medium, large):
Ideal body weight:
Allergies (food or drug):
Medications:
When are medications taken (with meals or empty
  stomach):
Food preferences:
Food restrictions:
Describe your usual diet, including fluids:

---

last primary care visit 2 weeks ago. She reported not refilling her medications because she felt fine. Her Lasix was reordered, and she is to take 40 mg in the morning and 20 mg at 6:00 P.M. Client is visually impaired, and reads poorly. She uses a magnifying glass and corrective lenses to read magazines, but she is not able to easily read medication labels. She sees her greatest learning needs as: understanding why she must take medication and learning appropriate foods that she can snack on. Her visiting nurse agrees with the teaching needed, and together they formulate the goal with specific steps (behavioral objectives) to achieve the goal. Displays 23-2 and 23-3 were constructed for the client. The contract was both written and audiotaped to facilitate her ability to listen and reinforce the contract.

24

Quality Care in Home Health Nursing

Silvia M. Koerner, RN, MSN

Quality in health care. Everyone wants it. The government considers it a priority. Hospitals and home care agencies continually strive for it. The consumer says it is a right. Professionals say they provide it.

No wonder, with so many people and groups spouting the term, the task of defining, measuring, and providing quality has become enmeshed in a maze of confusing terms and approaches. In home care, as in hospitals, nurses hear of "CQI" and "TQM," "UR," and "client outcomes." They complete incident reports, track client complaints, and audit charts. They have to document, document, and document some more.

Nurses know what quality care is. So do clients. It is difficult to describe what quality is and demonstrate that we have achieved it. Perhaps one of the simplest definitions of quality is, "Doing the right thing and doing the thing right." Less simple is identifying what is "right," and then measuring and continuously improving on it.

Health care is so complex and involves so many variables that at best one can only measure small pieces of quality and put certain structures (rules) in place. For example, it can be required that all nurses attend a mandatory class or study whether prescribed processes, such as client teaching, were implemented. One can look at client outcomes such as, Was the client rehospitalized within 30 days of discharge? Each alone or taken together contributes to quality; none, standing alone, assures it.

Much of what we have in the past pointed to as quality has been a long list of measures, or indicators, that when viewed as a whole, were said to demonstrate quality care. Although this picture still exists, important changes have taken place in how quality is viewed. The role of the nurse providing quality care has also changed.

In the course of this century, concepts of quality have evolved in tandem with socioeconomic, organizational, industrial, and other far-reaching changes. Clients have become customers. Other departments within the organization have become customers. Referrers and payors are customers. Customer satisfaction has become a primary indicator of quality. Each employee in the organization is responsible and accountable for quality and quality improvement and for doing the right thing and doing it right. Understanding how we define, measure, and improve the quality of care provided in the home requires, first of all, an unscrambling of some of the terms that are most frequently used.

UNSCRAMBLING THE TERMS

Quality Control

Nurses conduct quality control when they follow the procedure for testing their blood glucose meters to ensure that the reading they get is correct. Quality control usually refers to written rules and regulations such as those found in policies and procedures. It is the intent of these rules to control practice in such a way that quality care occurs. Agencies need policies and procedures to set guidelines, cut risks, and provide a certain level or standard of care and service.

Quality control has its place and will remain a part of quality management programs. Standing alone, it does little to assure quality care.

Quality Assurance

Quality assurance (QA) is the process of checking that the right thing was done. In other words, QA is retrospective monitoring. By performing QA audits, it can be determined if standards were met, if mistakes were made, and if there are any trends or opportunities for improvement. QA has two major drawbacks. First, it measures what happened after the fact, when what was done cannot be changed. Second, it frequently leads to the unpopular blaming of individuals or shotgun corrective action plans aimed at the whole group. QA relies on defining multiple objective indicators of quality and simple statistical analysis. When problem areas or opportunities for improvement are identified, action plans are consequently developed and implemented.

Action plans are not always effective. QA does not give any direct evidence as to the cause of the problem or the best solution. With all of its limitations, many aspects of quality assurance too, will remain with the nurse. Alone, however, it is not an adequate approach to assuring quality in the environment of health care today.

Quality Management

Quality management (QM) is the program or plan in which the agency defines quality and its philosophy and approach to maintain and improve quality. Quality management programs include aspects of quality control, quality assurance as well as continuous quality improvement. It may even include total quality management. Aspects of risk management, utilization management, and contract management may also be incorporated.

Continuous Quality Improvement

Continuous quality improvement (CQI) is an approach to achieving quality that focuses on the study of processes and systems to improve customer service. The major shift that occurred with this approach was the focus on improving systems and processes to improve customer satisfaction. CQI seeks to find and correct the root problem by charging work groups to study and analyze systems and processes. CQI is a prevention-based strategy that uses specific tools such as graphs and charts to study processes.

Agencies vary in their adoption and adaptation of CQI techniques. Although accrediting agencies require that CQI takes place, they do not dictate how the agency achieves this.

A quality improvement project can be identified by anyone in the organization. Or a problem can be identified by QA activities. Typically a work group is assembled, including staff involved at all levels of the process under study. A group leader and facilitator help the group define and study each step of the process. If more information is needed, it is gathered and studied. Diagrams and graphs are widely used to ensure understanding by all participants. Finally, the process is refined, changed and improved, duplications are eliminated, and more customer-friendly approaches are integrated. Once the new process is implemented, improved quality should result. A CQI approach is widely used today. Multiple examples of successful work groups can be found in the literature. It is, however, a resource- and time-intensive approach, which presents a problem to many agencies.

Total Quality Management

Total quality management (TQM) is an approach to quality improvement that expands to include all processes, clinical and nonclinical, and seeks to improve service to all customers, internal as well as external. TQM goes further than CQI by permeating the organization both as a philosophy and as a way of doing business. In many ways, TQM is similar to CQI. It differs mainly in intensity and in the requirement that every role and function within the organization be geared to continuous improvement and customer satisfaction.

REGULATIONS GOVERNING HOME CARE

Home care agencies have a lot of people telling them what quality is and what they expect. Foremost among these are the governmental agencies, which seek to protect the public and ensure the quality of services they pay for. Both the federal and state governments have rules and regulations with which home health agencies must comply to operate.

Because deficiencies can lead to stiff penalties and can even lead to closing down an agency, these rules and regulations are given high priority in home health agencies. Many of these regulations can be found embedded in agency policies and procedures. Others are incorporated in what may seem to be excessive documentation requirements. Finally, the agency may actively monitor compliance to these regulations in its QM program. Although it is not necessary to know all of these regulations, it is helpful to understand why agencies place such an emphasis on compliance and why so many of the rules that may not seem to make sense to everyone are in fact nonnegotiable.

Medicare

Agencies that participate in the Medicare or Medicaid programs must comply with the federal Conditions of Participation (COP). Agencies found in compliance with these standards can bill Medicare and Medicaid directly and are called Certified Home Health Agencies (CHHAs). Licensed agencies that are contracted by certified agencies to serve their clients must also comply with Medicare regulations.

Medicare requires that an unannounced survey be conducted annually for all CHHAs. The survey may be conducted by the staff from the local Department of Health, or by an accrediting body, such as the Joint Commission on the Accreditation of Healthcare Organizations (JCAHO), or by the Community Health Accreditation Program (CHAP). These two groups have what is known as *deemed* status, meaning that they have met the Health Care Financing Administration (HCFA) requirements to conduct a Medicare survey.

Depending on the size of the agency, a Medicare survey will take 2 to 5 days. As in other surveys, policies and procedures are reviewed, client records are examined, and the surveyors make joint visits with the staff. The major distinction in this survey is that the focus is on the agency's compliance with the COPs.

The COPs spell out the basic structure and processes each CHHA must implement. These include regulations regarding administration, budget, service delivery, the governing body, home health aide training, and many other areas. Many of the documentation requirements in home care can be directly traced to the COPs. Many aspects of each agency's quality management program also originate in the COPs. The following are excerpts from the COPs:

- *The client has the right to be informed of his or her rights. These rights include the right to have property* treated with respect, the right to voice grievances and complaints, and the right to confidentiality of the clinical record. Under this standard, the agency must also advise clients of the State toll-free hotline.

Client rights may be the subject of a complaint or an incident. Agencies must have a process in place to document, track and resolve client complaints. An incident such as an allegation of theft or damage to property in the home places the agency at risk for liability.

- The CHHA must comply with all Federal, State and Local laws and regulations. Part of Medicare reviews include checking for compliance to federal regulations, such as those promulgated by Occupation Safety and Health Administration (OSHA), as well as compliance to state laws. Again, these are usually built into agency policies and procedures. Reviewers, however, also review records, observe practice and interview staff. Not only paper compliance, but also knowledge and implementation is required.

- The agency and its staff must comply with accepted professional standards and principles that apply to professionals supplying services. Reviewers expect a certain level of care to be provided, that is consistent with professional standards and state practice acts. Care provided but not documented can lead to deficiencies in this area. To ensure consistent practice, many agencies have spelled out expected standards of care or defined clinical pathways or guidelines.

- A group of professional personnel (frequently referred to as a Professional Advisory Committee) must establish and annually review the agency's policies and procedures, participate in the evaluation of the agency's program, and assist the agency maintain liaison with other health providers in the community.

This group, which usually reports directly to the Board of Directors, approves, monitors and evaluates the agency's quality management program.

• At least quarterly, appropriate health professionals representing at least the scope of the program review a sample of both active and closed clinical records. This is done to determine whether established policies are followed in furnishing services directly or under arrangement.

This group is usually called the Utilization Review Committee. All services have to be evaluated for consistency with professional practice standards for CHHAs, compliance with the plan of care, appropriateness, adequacy, and effectiveness of services offered, and evaluation of anticipated client outcomes. Nurses who have the opportunity to sit on this committee can learn much about home health care, documentation, and regulations.

• There is a continuing review of clinical records for each 62-day period that a client receives home health services. This is done to determine adequacy of the plan of care and appropriateness of continuation of care. This is usually referred to as a concurrent record review and can be defined as a quality assurance activity. Agencies define in their quality management plan the indicators used, how records are selected for this review, who reviews them, how problems and patterns are identified, and how plans of correction are developed and implemented.

State Departments of Health

State Departments of Health license, regulate, and survey Licensed Home Health Agencies (LHHAs). They also conduct Medicare surveys for CHHAs that are not accredited or opt not to be reviewed by CHAP or JCAHO. State regulations are less restrictive for LHHAs than for CHAAs. State regulations governing home care are in may ways very similar to the federal COPs.

In New York, for example, the section on clients' rights closely parallels the same section in the COPs. Very often, the states will add on or delineate additional requirements. For example, the federal COPs allow physical therapy to be the only service on a case. In Connecticut, the Department of Health requires that CHHA provide a minimum of one nursing visit per month. The New York regulations spell out detailed admission and discharge criteria. Such constraints vary among states. The state also makes unannounced visits to investigate client complaints. If deficiencies are found, the agency is required to correct them.

ACCREDITATION: A CLAIM TO EXCELLENCE

Accreditation is an acknowledgment made by an independent evaluating group that an agency meets high service standards. Hospitals have a much longer tradition of accreditation than the home health care industry. In fact, hospital survival today depends on obtaining a JCAHO mark of approval. Although this is not yet true in home care, competitiveness in the marketplace and survival needs are causing more and more agencies to seek accreditation. Two different groups accredit home health agencies: CHAP and JCAHO. Although similar in many ways, there are differences in the roots and approaches of these two accrediting bodies.

CHAP

CHAP, a subsidiary of the National League of Nursing, has been accrediting home and community care organizations since 1965. CHAP is an independent evaluating body founded on the principle that a voluntary commitment to excellence by home and community health care organizations is the only way to assure availability of quality community-based services and products. In 1992, the HCFA issued a regulation *deeming* agencies accredited by CHAP as meeting Medicare certification requirements.

CHAP accredits agencies for 3 years but makes site visits every 9 to 15 months. A full review is conducted at the start of each 3-year cycle. The interim reviews focus on recommendations and required actions from the previous visit. CHAP standards are outlined in their manual, *Standards of Excellence for Home Care.*

JCAHO

JCAHO has been accrediting hospitals since 1953 and home care agencies since 1988. Hospital-based home health agencies are usually JCAHO-accredited together with the hospital. JCAHO standards are outlined in the *JCAHO Accreditation Manual for Home Care.*

The standards are integrated, meaning that they apply to all services and departments of the agency. The major headings include:

Rights, responsibilities, and ethics
Assessment
Care, treatment, and services
Education
Continuum of care
Improving organizational performance
Management of the environment of care
Management of human resources
Management of information
Leadership
Surveillance, prevention, and control

Each standard is preceded by a preamble, which provides the goal and overall scope. After the statement of the standard, the intent is spelled out, together with examples illustrating how the standard is to be interpreted. Finally, how JCAHO will score the agency on the standard is outlined. CHAP and JCAHO are currently in the process of negotiating for reciprocity.

COMPONENTS OF A QUALITY MANAGEMENT PROGRAM

Each agency has a distinctive QM program, and each program is organized somewhat differently. There may be a director or manager of the program, or one person may have responsibility for several years, including the QM program. Still, there will be many commonalities as regulatory, accreditation, and professional standards cut across agencies. The following lists some of the most frequently seen components of QM programs:

Client Satisfaction Surveys

These are required by accrediting bodies and most managed care companies and are central to the CQI and TQM approaches. The trend today is to benchmark, that is, to compare the agency's client satisfaction rating with a previous rating, and with ratings achieved by other agencies. In many instances, client satisfaction ratings are published.

The major problems with these surveys is that agencies use different tools and methodologies. This makes it inappropriate to compare results. If a mail survey is used, the response rate is often too low to allow generalization to the entire population. Telephone surveys are intrusive and expensive. Several companies have recently developed client satisfaction surveys and are marketing these to home care agencies. These companies provide extensive analyses of responses as well as benchmark data.

Clients often mention the name of their nurse and other care givers and applaud (or complain about) them for excellent (or poor) care. The greatest value of client satisfaction surveys is that they give the agency an idea of how well they are doing and how they can improve their service. They are excellent sources for identifying new quality improvement initiatives.

In many agencies, referrer, physician, and intraorganizational satisfaction surveys are also conducted.

Client Complaints

As stated earlier, agencies, by Medicare and the State, are required to document, track, and resolve client complaints. Managed care companies are also increasingly requiring agencies to report complaints and their resolution as part of their contracts. Each agency has a policy and procedure as to how this is done.

Complaints provide an excellent resource for identifying ways to provide better care. Very often, for example, the complaint arises out of a misunderstanding or incomplete communication. Areas of most frequent misunderstanding can often be clarified with a pamphlet or clear directives to nurses on how to best explain certain agency procedures. The agency, too, can identify patterns of dissatisfaction and redesign processes to provide better customer-driven service.

Client Incidents

Incidents are broadly defined as unexpected occurrences that present a real or potential legal liability to the agency. Each agency defines reportable incidents more specifically in accordance with its risk management and QM objectives. Although incidents occurring in the home usually do not place agencies at risk to the same extent as client incidents in hospitals place hospitals at risk, the tracking and reporting process is very similar. Most agencies use incident reports that require documentation of what happened, how it happened, and what was done to prevent reoccurrence. These are forwarded to the QM or risk management staff, analyzed, and reported on in a manner similar to quality findings.

In home care, incidents may relate to a variety of occurrences, such as client injuries sustained while a worker was in the home, allegations of theft or property damage, allegations of abandonment or abuse by workers, and medication and treatment errors. Agency liability is dependent on the agency's role in the incident. If a client is competent and leaves the home against the nurse's and physician's advice and fractures his leg, the agency is probably not liable.

If there was an aide in the home assigned to provide continuous supervision to the client, and the client was left alone and fractured a leg, the agency may very well be liable. Similarly, if the nurse prepours or administers the wrong medication, that nurse is liable. In all cases, what determines an incident is a deviation from expected practice or behavior that leads to an adverse client response.

Utilization Review

Utilization review (UR) is a review process in which both active and discharged client records are reviewed for compliance with payor guidelines and efficient, effective use of services. Questions asked may include: Does this Medicare client meet Medicare criteria? Is the aide providing personal care services? Is the nursing visit frequency appropriate for this client's skilled needs? Are therapy visits being made frequently enough to achieve the goals of treatment? Was the client discharged prematurely? Both cost and effectiveness are important here.

In today's health care environment, utilization has become an important quality indicator. There has been a major increase of clients in commercial managed care plans, and both Medicare and Medicaid are increasing client enrollment in managed care programs. Furthermore, partial and full capitation programs as well as a prospective payment system (PPS) is on the horizon for home care. This means that only agencies who can provide quality care and achieve optimal client outcomes with fewer visits and services will survive and, maybe, prosper.

The nurse is in an ideal position to identify and provide those services that can move the client along more quickly toward self-sufficiency in the community. As coordinator of care, the nurse is a utilization manager.

Quality Care Review (Concurrent)

As part of their QM programs, agencies define those indicators of quality they consider most important to monitor or improve. Indicators can stem from regulations, accreditation standards, professional standards, or agency goals. Indicators may be classified as structure, process, or outcome indicators. Structures are rules and organizational procedures. For example, a structure indicator may be that all new staff participate in a planned orientation. Processes are procedures or things caregivers do. Most concurrently assessed review indicators are process indicators. For example, did the nurse assess the client's weight as part of the cardiovascular assessment? Outcome indicators describe the client's status at the end of the episode of care. An example of an outcome is that the client was not rehospitalized within 30 days of admission. If the client is hospitalized within 30 days, it may be an indication that the client was inappropriate for admission, or that signs of decompensation were not identified or treated on a timely basis. Indicators identify potential problems. Usually further analysis and professional judgment are needed to interpret indicators and assess quality.

Outcome-Based Quality Improvement

Outcome-based quality improvement (OBQI) is the new kid on the block. This is a model of quality improvement that is distinctive to home care and is very likely to be adopted nationally by the industry in the future. In fact, your agency may already be part of a national or state demonstration of OBQI in home care or may be developing an OBQI program on their own. Whatever the case in your agency, you will want to know the basics about this new approach to improving client care.

Why Outcomes?

The answer is very simple. Consumers and payors of health care want to know what they are getting for their dollar. They are asking questions such as "What difference does home care make?" and "In this era of cost conscientiousness, why put more money into home care?" Outcomes tell us what happened to the client as a result of the care we provided.

What Are Outcomes?

That is a little tougher to answer because the term *outcome* has been used and overused to the point where it is almost a cliché. In home care, however, a standard definition has been developed and is being used in OBQI. This definition is that a client-level **outcome** is a change in the client health status be-

tween two or more times. This is the definition proposed by Peter Shaughnessy, Director of the Center
for Health Policy Research at the University of Col-
orado.

How Are Outcomes Measured?

Outcomes can be measured with a valid reliable tool
called the Outcome Assessment Information Set
(OASIS). This tool was developed by Peter Shaughnessy and his group over years of research. The
OASIS consists of a series of client information items
that capture client demographics, living arrangements, supportive assistance, sensory status, integu-
mentary status, respiratory status, neuro/emotional/
behavioral status, activities of daily living (ADLs)/in-
strumental ADLs (IADLs), medications, and equipment management.

The major part of the tool is a checklist, which
can be completed (after practice) in approximately 15
minutes. The OASIS is administered on admission, at
60-day intervals, and on discharge. It provides standardized risk-adjusted client outcome measures in
terms of improvement, stabilization, or deterioration
of the client's physiologic, functional, cognitive, and
behavioral health.

How Do Outcomes Fit Into OBQI?

OBQI starts by examining outcomes achieved. In
areas in which outcomes are poorer than expected or
exemplary, a second process of care review is conducted. This is similar to the QA process. Here, what
was done or not done is examined in detail. Based on
the findings, a written plan of action to change or reinforce care behaviors relevant to the outcome is pre-

pared and implemented. The outcome then is monitored to assess the effectiveness of the plan.

Why Is OBQI Important Now?

Medicare is very interested in the outcomes of home care provided to their clients. HCFA has funded a 3 1/2-year demonstration of OBQI to be conducted in 50 CHHAs across the country. Some states, such as New York, are also conducting similar projects incorporating the OASIS in their assessment tools. The National Medicare Quality Assurance and Improvement Demonstration will be used to refine and develop OBQI for home care.

Medicare is considering requiring OBQIs of all CHHAs and using outcome data to supplant the current survey approach. The tool and approach were so well accepted by the industry that many agencies are adopting OBQI before completion of the demonstration.

25

Community Resources

Phyllis Cohen, MSW

A TEAM APPROACH TO ADDRESSING THE CLIENT'S PSYCHOSOCIAL NEEDS

The community health nurse and the social worker together offer a team approach to addressing the client's psychosocial needs. An understanding of each discipline's role is essential for the integration and functioning of the health care team. Although nursing is focused on the physical well-being of the client, nurses must be aware of psychosocial issues that may adversely impact on the client's recovery. The home care nurse is the coordinator of care for the client, and it is essential that the nurse and the home care social worker coordinate their services and engage in ongoing communication. The nurse is the first member of the health care team to visit and evaluate the client's illness, family structure, social support, environment, and finances. If the nurse has been oriented to the services provided by home care social work and has ongoing communication and collaboration with social work, the nurse will make an informed decision regarding when to refer the client to social work.

It is also important for clients and their families to recognize that this interdisciplinary team approach is designed to ensure that the client receives optimal care to achieve optimal recovery. The roles and responsibilities of the client, family, and health care team should be fully and clearly defined from the start of care. The importance of the team approach cannot be overemphasized. Ongoing communication and collaboration between the team members and the client and family ensures that the plan of care is consistent with client requirements and expectations.

There are times when the nursing role and the social work role overlap. For example, if a nurse is visiting a client and finds that the the client is at risk (without heat, hot water, or food, or there is obvious abuse occurring), the nurse will discuss with the client or the client's family the need for an emergency referral to the appropriate community resource. The nurse then calls the appropriate community resource and also informs the client that a social worker will be visiting to help resolve the problem. The nurse then makes the referral to social work.

In some cases, the issue of medical compliance may be addressed by the home care social worker. Financial, social, or emotional problems may be identified that must first be resolved for the patient to become medically compliant. For example, a new insulin-dependent diabetic may not have enough money for medication or proper food, or the client may be phobic about self-injecting.

THE ROLE OF THE SOCIAL WORKER IN THE HOME HEALTH SETTING

Because clients are being discharged from hospitals earlier and and not as fully recovered as in the past, the stress of being at home while in the early stages of recovery often is debilitating and frightening. The family also may be affected by the stress of caring for a sick or disabled loved one. This stress can upset family relationships. The client may be frightened, anxious, angry, or at a loss to comprehend the changes in his or her physical well-being. The family may be overwhelmed as they watch a loved one struggle to recover from a disabling illness or injury. In this crisis, familiar roles may be changed, lost, or reversed; finances and relationships may be strained. One spouse may be angry at the other for becoming ill, and the client may lose his or her identity.

Changes in family roles, employment status, physical loss, and the fear of death will add to the stress under which the client and family must live. Together, the nurse and the home care social worker can assist the client and family in coping with complex medical, emotional, and social problems arising from the client's illness.

Medicare has determined that the following skilled social work services are necessary to resolve social or emotional problems that are or are expected to be an impediment to the effective treatment of the client's medical condition or his or her rate of recovery:

Assessment of social and emotional factors: Skilled assessment of social and emotional factors related to the client's illness, need for care, response to treatment, and adjustment to care, followed by collaboration with the physician and nurse to develop a care plan

Counseling for long-range planning and decision making: Assessment of the client's needs for long-term care, including evaluation of home and family situation, enabling client/family to develop an in-home care system, exploring alternatives to in-home care, arranging for placement

Community resource planning: The promotion of community-centered service(s), education, advocacy, referral, and linkage

Short-term therapy: Goal-oriented intervention directed toward management of terminal illness, reaction/adjustment to illness, strengthening family/support system, conflict resolution related to chronicity of illness

Other: Includes other medical social services related to the client's illness and need for care. Problem resolution associated with high-risk indicators endangering clients's mental and physical health, including abuse/neglect, inadequate food/medical supplies; high suicide potential

The home care social worker is trained to assist clients and their families in working through crisis and stress to gain some measure of acceptance of the client's illness and to achieve an understanding of their feelings. The role of the home care social worker includes assessment of the client within the context of his or her illness and psychosocial environment. The home care social worker will assess the client's mental status, understanding of the illness and prognosis, current level of functioning, physical environment, and finances. The home care social worker also will assess the level of support that is available to the client from his or her family, community, or church, and any other source of emotional, spiritual, physical, or financial assistance.

The home care social work *Initial Psychosocial Assessment* is the basic tool for the development of the treatment plan. The Initial Psychosocial Assessment is completed by the home care social worker during the initial visit and includes the following information:

1. Name
2. Address and phone number
3. Date of birth, birthplace, and marital status
4. Language, education, occupation, and employer
5. Religion and ethnicity
6. Emergency contact person
7. Nurse coordinator and phone number
8. Reason for referral to the home care social worker
9. Current medical diagnoses
10. Past and present illnesses

11. Housing: apartment, private house, walk-up, elevator, condition of housing, etc.
12. Financial information: income, resources, including public benefits, assets, and expenses
13. Insurance information
14. Financial management (Who manages the client's finances; is there a power of attorney?)
15. Household composition (Who lives in the home; what relationship do they have to the client?)
16. Are there any pets?
17. Names and addresses of friends and relatives not in the client's household
18. Name and phone numbers of community agencies that currently provide services to the client or who have provided services in the past. The services provided should be identified.
19. Problem(s) from the client's or family members' perspective
20. History of pre-illness functioning, past or recent life changes or crises, abuse history (if any), and how the client and family have coped with prior problems
21. Current functioning of the client to include the client's mental status and orientation, the client's ability to perform instrumental activities of daily living (IADL) and activities of daily living (ADL) (for example, IADL is shopping, laundry, etc.; ADL is bathing, grooming, etc.)
22. Short-term client goals with timeframes (for example, client will identify problem(s) that interfere with medical compliance within two visits)
23. Long-term client goals with timeframes (for example, client will be medically compliant within four visits)

24. Treatment provided by the home care social worker during this visit
25. Total visits planned
26. Visit frequency
27. Duration of service
28. Date of next visit
29. The home care social worker's summary of the psychosocial assessment should include comments on observed coping skills and factors that may have a positive or adverse impact on the treatment plan and client's progress.

The home care social worker involves the client, family, and any significant others in the client's psychosocial assessment. The home care social worker also encourages the client, family, and significant others to assist in determining the client's needs and also encourages them to identify factors that could contribute to problems requiring social work intervention. For example, they may be asked how they or the client have coped with a prior life crises to anticipate how they will react to this crisis.

They will be asked how the home care social worker can best help them and what are their expectations. No plans, referrals, or decisions will be made concerning the provision of home care social work services without the client, family, and significant other being involved in the Initial Psychosocial Assessment and treatment planning process.

When the Initial Psychosocial Assessment is completed, the home care social worker conferences with the nurse to discuss the findings and agree on a treatment plan. The social worker and nurse should conference at least every 2 weeks thereafter to discuss progress, changes, or problems to ensure that the client has a well-coordinated interdisciplinary plan of care.

CRITERIA FOR REFERRAL FOR SOCIAL WORK SERVICES

Social work referrals are appropriate when a client is experiencing social, emotional, financial, or environmental problems that impede effective treatment. The following are indicators to identify clients who should be referred for social work services:

- The client is living alone and unable to care for self.
- The client is unable to care for self and is living with a significant other who is elderly or impaired who is unable to provide care for the client.
- The client is unable to care for self, yet has responsibility for caring for young children or physically or mentally impaired adults.
- The client is anxious, tearful, agitated, angry, and expresses suicidal thoughts.
- The client is exhibiting delusional, grandiose, paranoid, or hallucinatory behavior.
- The client is unable to provide a coherent personal history and exhibits rambling and repetitive speech.
- The client is living with family members who are unable or unwilling to provide care.
- The client has a history of psychiatric illness and is not on medication.
- The client is actively abusing alcohol or drugs.

- The client expresses hopelessness and helplessness, reports appetite loss and change of sleeping pattern, and is not motivated or interested in participating in his or her own care.
- The client is living alone and appears to be unable to participate in or make decisions concerning their care because of their confused mental status.
- The client is noncompliant with treatment.
- The client's family is noncompliant with treatment.
- The client has a terminal illness.
- The client is terminally ill and has responsibility for young children or elderly or impaired adults.
- The client has suffered a sudden illness or disability that will impact on his or her own or the family's functioning; for example, myocardial infarction, cerebral vascular accident, amputation, insulin-dependent diabetes mellitus, etc.
- The client has inadequate financial resources to meet basic needs or lives in substandard housing or has no food.
- The client is without heat and hot water.
- The client lives in an unsafe environment because of filth, lack of needed repairs, or insect or rodent infestation and is incapable of properly caring for pets.
- The client appears to be at risk of neglect, exploitation, or abuse or reports being neglected, abused, or exploited.
- The client requires referrals to community agencies for services while on the home care program or after discharge from the program; for example, home-delivered meals, nursing home placement, children's services, etc.

COMMUNITY RESOURCES: WHAT IS AVAILABLE AND HOW TO ASSESS A CLIENT'S ELIGIBILITY

There are various types of community resources. They are: (1) public benefits, which include benefits in kind; (2) services provided by federal, state, and local governments; and (3) other.

Public Benefits

Public benefits are generally called *entitlements.* These benefits may be *financial* or *benefits in kind.* For example:

Financial
  Public assistance such as welfare cash grants
  Supplemental Social Security such as cash grants
  HEAP (Home Energy Assistance Program): cash grants to assist with fuel and utility costs
Benefits in Kind
  Food stamps
  Medicaid payment to the provider for medical care, supplies, and services
  WIC (Women, Infants, and Children) vouchers for nutritional food supplements for pregnant women, infants, and children to age 5 years

Public benefits (entitlements) are always *means tested.* Means testing requires that the applicant is financially eligible to receive the benefits for which they are applying. Financial eligibility will vary between programs; financial eligibility also may vary in accordance with state and local government standards. Public benefits also usually require that the applicant be a legal resident in the United States.

The public benefits noted are federally sponsored and have basic standards and grants set and allocated by the federal government. State and local governments may impose impose additional eligibility requirements and establish the amount and extent of grants and services they will provide in addition to federally mandated minimums.

There are other public benefits programs that may be indigenous to individual states and local governments. For example:

EPIC (Elderly Pharmaceutical Insurance Coverage Program)

This program enables seniors to receive prescriptions at a discount (New York State program).

EISEP (Expanded In-Home Services for the Elderly Program)

EISEP provides personal care and housekeeping services for those who need services that are not Medicaid eligible or Medicare covered with sliding scale fees (New York State program).

ADAP PLUS (Aids Drug Assistance, Primary Care, and Home Care Program)

ADAP PLUS pays for health care services for human immunodeficiency virus (HIV)-positive persons who do not qualify for Medicaid, are awaiting Medicaid, or have limited health insurance (New York City and some counties in southern New York State).

Because public benefits are means tested, it is imperative that the Initial Psychosocial Assessment include a thorough financial and resource review.

Services Provided by Federal, State, and Local Governments

Federal, state, and local governments provide a wide variety of services that can be helpful in assisting clients and their families. Some of these services are:

Offices on Aging will help you locate:

Senior centers
Home-delivered meals
Senior transportation
Adult day care programs
Home care
Chore service
Public benefits for seniors
Home repair and weatherization for seniors
Training to assess eligibility for public benefits and completing public benefits applications
Services for Alzheimer's disease and other related dementias
Respite programs
Other services for seniors

Services for Developmentally Disabled will help you locate:

Residential placement
Day treatment programs
Sheltered workshops
Schools
Training programs
Transportation
Programs to evaluate the developmentally disabled client
Public benefits for the developmentally disabled client
Other services for the developmentally disabled client

Departments of Social Services or *Human Resources* will help you locate:

Public benefits offices, for example, public assistance, Medicaid, food stamps
Public housing
Training for those receiving public benefits
Children's day care programs
Training to assess eligibility for public benefits and application procedure
Other

Departments of Health will help you locate:

Well baby clinics
Immunization programs
Sexually transmitted disease clinics
Programs for children with special health needs
Tuberculosis treatment centers
Residential placement
Home care programs
Treatment programs for specific diseases
Programs for Alzheimer's disease and other related dementias
Other health-related services and programs

Services for the Visually and Hearing Impaired will help you locate:

Training programs
Schools
Support groups
Education
Camps
In-home training
Guide dog training
Home and medical appliances to ensure safety

Talking books
Magnification and amplification appliances
Other services for hearing and visually impaired

Services for the Mentally Ill/Departments of Mental Health will help you locate:

Services for evaluation
Day treatment programs
Residential placement
Clinics for treatment
Support groups
Psychiatric residences
Adult homes
Other services

Services for Drug and Alcohol Abusers will help you locate:

Treatment programs
Residential placement
Clinics
Support groups
Methadone maintenance treatment programs
Hospitalization
Detoxification programs
Day treatment
Other services

Services for the Mentally Ill Chemical Abuser (MICA) will help you locate:

Treatment programs
Residential placement
Clinics
Hospitalization
Support groups
Other services

Services for Crime Victims and Victims of Domestic Violence will help you locate:

Counseling
Support services
Legal services
Safe shelter
Advocacy
Information and referral
Medical care and services

Protective Services Agencies for Children will help you with children who are at risk of neglect and abuse by providing:

Parenting programs
Preventive programs
Foster homes for children
Family shelters
Legal services
Guardianship programs
Summer camps
Homemaking services
Other services to ensure the safety of children

Protective Services Agencies for Adults will help you with adults who are at risk for neglect and abuse by providing:

Psychiatric evaluations
Financial management
Guardianship
Placement in appropriate residences
Other services to protect adults at risk

Services for Vocational, Literacy, and General Equivalency Degree Training will help you locate:

Vocational testing services

Vocational training

High school general equivalency degree training programs

Literacy volunteer programs

English as second language programs

Other educational programs to meet your client's needs

Divisions of AIDS Services will help you locate:

Treatment programs

Housing

Information on public benefits

Residential health care facilities

Advocacy

Legal services

Support groups

Counseling

Children's services

Family services

Other services that may be required by your clients with acquired immune deficiency syndrome (AIDS)

Other Community Resources

In addition to these federal state and local agencies, there are voluntary organizations, such as charitable and religious organizations, self-help groups, disease-related associations (American Cancer Society, MS Society, Juvenile Diabetes Foundation) and community services for almost any health, social, emotional, financial, or environmental problem identified.

A thorough psychosocial and financial assessment is the critical first step in assisting the home care client in identifying his or her need and finding the right community resource to meet the need.

DEVELOPING A COMMUNITY RESOURCE DATABASE

It is important to gain a knowledge of the public benefits available to your clients, financial means testing, and the application process. This can be done by contacting your state or local office on aging or state or local department of social services or human resources.

Many government and community-based agencies provide training in evaluating your client's eligibility for public benefits as well as completing the required applications. Information concerning community resources can be obtained by contacting those resources listed previously.

In addition to those services, other means of finding community resources include:

Professional organizations
Workshops, conferences, seminars
Visiting community agencies
Working with community agencies
Networking
Local resource manuals

Neighborhood and community agencies frequently have developed directories of local health, welfare, and social services organizations within their service areas. Telephone directories also have listings of federal, state, and local government agencies as well as listings of social service, health care, religious, and community agencies. Information gathered from these sources can be the foundation on which you build your community resource database.

CHOOSING THE RIGHT COMMUNITY RESOURCE FOR YOUR CLIENT

To ensure you choose the right community resource for your client, you should:

Involve the client, family, and significant other in the identification of the problem and the development of the goals to cope with or resolve the problem.

Ensure that a thorough Initial Psychosocial Assessment *is completed.*

Use the appropriate community resources selected from your database.

Index

Numbers followed by f indicate a figure; t indicates tabular material; d indicates a display.

C